Endocrine Updates

Series Editor: *Shlomo Melmed, M.D.*

For further volumes:
http://www.springer.com/series/5917

Glenn D. Braunstein, MD

Editor

Thyroid Cancer

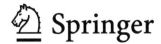 Springer

Editor
Glenn D. Braunstein, MD
Professor and Chairman, Department of Medicine
The James R. Klinenberg MD Chair in Medicine
Director of the Thyroid Cancer Center of Excellence
Cedars-Sinai Medical Center
Los Angeles, CA, USA
braunstein@cshs.org

ISSN 1566-0729
ISBN 978-1-4614-0874-1   e-ISBN 978-1-4614-0875-8
DOI 10.1007/978-1-4614-0875-8
Springer New York Dordrecht Heidelberg London

Library of Congress Control Number: 2011938203

Springer is part of Springer Science+Business Media (www.springer.com)

Preface

The American Cancer Society has estimated that in 2011, 48,020 new cases of thyroid cancer will be diagnosed in the United States, with three-quarters occurring in women. About two-thirds of the patients will be between the ages of 20 and 55. The disease will cause close to 1,740 deaths, of which 43% will be men. The overall 5-year survival rate is 97%, making it one of the least lethal cancers. The incidence of thyroid cancer has more than doubled over the last three decades, rising from 4.85 cases per hundred thousand people in 1975 to almost 12 cases per hundred thousand in 2007. This increase is seen exclusively in the well-differentiated thyroid cancers, which account for the vast majority of patients and carry the best prognosis. A good portion of this rise is due to increased detection of small tumors (microcarcinomas measuring less than 1 cm) because of the increased use of neck ultrasounds, CT scans, MRI, and PET scans, which detect these "incidentalomas." This may account for the rise in the incidence of microcarcinomas, but does not adequately explain the fact that the incidence of larger tumors also is increasing, and this increase is occurring around the world. The rise does not appear to be related to the two known causative factors for well-differentiated thyroid cancer: radiation exposure or genetic predisposition. Thus, it is likely that environmental factors such as the amount of iodine intake, industrial toxins (e.g., plasticizers, fire retardants, and pesticides), and other unknown exposures may contribute to the rising incidence of thyroid cancer.

Although numerically less frequent than the differentiated thyroid cancers, medullary cancer of the thyroid, anaplastic carcinoma, and thyroid lymphoma are important tumors to know about because their prognosis is less favorable and their treatment generally requires a more aggressive approach.

The management of thyroid cancer has changed greatly over the last several decades with the advent of new imaging techniques, the improved detection of biomarkers, a marked increase in our understanding of the genetic abnormalities that result in or accompany oncogenesis, and the development of targeted therapies that take advantage of the known molecular defects that result in thyroid cancer. One of the positive developments has been the emergence of multidisciplinary teams devoted to the management of the disease.

The Cedars-Sinai Thyroid Cancer Center residing in our Samuel Oschin Comprehensive Cancer Institute is composed of endocrinologists, surgeons, oncologists, radiation therapists, nuclear medicine physicians, pathologists, radiologists, nurses, speech therapists, and psychiatrists all of whom have a subspecialty interest in thyroid cancer. The team has developed protocols for the surgical management of patients and for determining who should or should not receive radioactive iodine or external beam radiotherapy, and have active clinical trials for patient management. Patients with complex or aggressive disease are presented at our monthly Thyroid Cancer tumor board, and continuing education is accomplished through a monthly Thyroid Cancer Grand Rounds. Since our Center is the only one for a wide geographic area, we see a large number of patients with thyroid nodules and cancer. Therefore, our medical students, residents, and fellows have extensive exposure to all aspects of thyroid disease. Both basic and clinical research is carried out under the Center's auspices.

When Shlomo Melmed, MD, Editor of the *Endocrine Updates Series*, and Springer Science+Business Media, LLC, invited me to edit a book on thyroid cancer, I readily agreed because I knew that I had a group of experts readily available within our Thyroid Cancer Center. Each was requested to write a chapter in their area of expertise, which together provides a broad overview and in-depth analysis of the current thinking in the diagnosis and management of differentiated, medullary, and anaplastic thyroid carcinoma, as well as thyroid lymphoma.

We appreciate the professionalism and excellence of the people who have been involved with this project from Springer, especially Ellen C. Green, Developmental Editor, and Richard Lansing, Executive Editor, Medicine. Also, we are grateful for the support of Boris Catz, MD, the Levy family and all of the staff of our Thyroid Cancer Center and, of course, to all of our patients who teach us many lessons daily about the complexity and natural history of thyroid cancer.

Los Angeles, CA, USA   Glenn D. Braunstein, M.D.

Contents

Contributors

Kenneth W. Adashek, MD, FACS Department of Surgery, Cedars-Sinai Medical Center, Los Angeles, CA, USA

Michel Babajanian, MD, FACS Department of Surgery, Cedars-Sinai Medical Center, Los Angeles, CA, USA

Shikha Bose, MD Department of Pathology and Lab Medicine, Cedars-Sinai Medical Center, Los Angeles, CA, USA

Glenn D. Braunstein, MD Divison of Endocrinology, Diabetes, and Metabolism, Department of Medicine, Cedars-Sinai Medical Center, Los Angeles, CA, USA

C. Michele Burnison, MD Department of Radiation Oncology, Cedars-Sinai Medical Center, Los Angeles, CA, USA

Wenwen Chien, PhD Division of Oncology/Hematology, Department of Medicine, Cedars-Sinai Medical Center, Los Angeles, CA, USA

C. Suzanne Cutter, MD Department of Surgery, Cedars-Sinai Medical Center, Los Angeles, CA, USA

David P. Frishberg, MD Department of Pathology and Lab Medicine, Cedars-Sinai Medical Center, Los Angeles, CA, USA

Gretchen E. Galliano, MD Department of Pathology and Lab Medicine, Cedars-Sinai Medical Center, Los Angeles, CA, USA

Jerome Hershman, MD, MS Divisions of Endocrinology, Diabetes and Metabolism, Greater Los Angeles VA and Cedars–Sinai Medical Center, Los Angeles, CA, USA

H. Phillip Koeffler, MD Division of Oncology/Hematology, Department of Medicine, Cedars-Sinai Medical Center, Los Angeles, CA, USA

Babak Larian, MD, FACS Department of Surgery, Cedars-Sinai Medical Center, Los Angeles, CA, USA

Stephen W. Lim, MD Department of Medicine and Samuel Oschin Comprehensive Cancer Center, Cedars-Sinai Medical Center, Los Angeles, CA, USA

Adam Lyko, MD Divisions of Endocrinology, Diabetes and Metabolism, Greater Los Angeles VA and Cedars–Sinai Medical Center, Los Angeles, CA, USA

Sandra M. McLachlan, PhD Division of Endocrinology, Diabetes, and Metabolism, Department of Medicine, Cedars-Sinai Medical Center, Los Angeles, CA, USA

Michelle Melany, MD Department of Imaging, Cedars-Sinai Medical Center, Los Angeles, CA, USA

Basil Rapoport, MB, ChB Division of Endocrinology, Diabetes, and Metabolism, Department of Medicine, Cedars-Sinai Medical Center, Los Angeles, CA, USA

Wendy Sacks, MD Divison of Endocrinology, Diabetes, and Metabolism, Department of Medicine, Cedars-Sinai Medical Center, Los Angeles, CA, USA

Nicole M. Tyer, MD Department of Medicine, Cedars-Sinai Medical Center, Los Angeles, CA, USA

Marina Vaysburd, MD Division of Hematology/Oncology, Department of Medicine, Cedars-Sinai Medical Center, Beverly Hills, CA, USA

Alan D. Waxman, MD Department of Imaging, Cedars-Sinai Medical Center, Los Angeles, CA, USA

Ronnie Meiyi Wong, MPH, MSW Divison of Endocrinology, Diabetes, and Metabolism, Department of Medicine, Cedars-Sinai Medical Center, Los Angeles, CA, USA

Run Yu, MD, PhD Divisions of Endocrinology, Diabetes, and Metabolism, Carcinoid and Neuroendocrine Tumor Center, Department of Medicine, Cedars-Sinai Medical Center, Los Angeles, CA, USA

Pathology and Classification of Thyroid Tumors

Gretchen E. Galliano and David P. Frishberg

Introduction

Nodules of the thyroid gland are common and frequently problematic specimens encountered by the diagnostic surgical pathologist. It is estimated that 4–7% of adults have a palpable thyroid nodule, and several times that many have nodules which are detectable at autopsy or by ultrasound [1]. Of the estimated 10–20 million clinically detectable thyroid lesions in the United States [2], approximately 5–30% will be malignant [3]. Thyroid nodules are more common in women, in people with a history of radiation exposure, and in those with goitrogenic-rich diets or iodine-deficient diets [1]. Carcinomas of follicular cell origin are the most common and greatly outnumber carcinomas of C-cell origin [4]. Secondary malignancies and lymphomas are far less common than follicular origin tumors, but they do occur and must be considered in the differential diagnosis of both benign and malignant thyroid abnormalities. The majority of carcinomas of follicular origin are indolent, with approximately 90% 10-year survival rates [4].

G.E. Galliano
Department of Pathology and Lab Medicine,
Cedars-Sinai Medical Center, 8700 Beverly Blvd,
Room 8725, Los Angeles, CA 90048, USA

D.P. Frishberg (✉)
Department of Pathology and Lab Medicine, Cedars-Sinai Medical Center, Los Angeles, CA, USA
e-mail: frishbergd@cshs.org

Intraoperative Diagnosis

General Considerations

Intraoperative consultation (IOC) for properly selected cases can be a useful tool for the surgical management of patients with thyroid nodules, but has significant limitations of which both the practicing pathologist and surgeon must be aware. In this regard, the application of clinical findings and fine-needle aspiration (FNA) results are of great help in selecting appropriate cases for IOC. These selection criteria depend on the two major limitations of sensitivity for intraoperative detection of cancer: the need to confirm (1) cytologic features of malignancy in papillary carcinoma and (2) vascular or capsular invasion in follicular carcinoma and its variants.

Technique

When a nodule, lobe, or gland is received for IOC, the surgical margins are inked, and the specimen is sectioned at 2–3-mm intervals, following which careful gross examination of the cut surfaces is performed, with notation of overall nodularity, the appearance of the cut surface, and encapsulation (if any) of identified lesion(s). A representative section of the nodule or tumor is sampled at the capsule or tumor interface with non-neoplastic thyroid [5]. This section is frozen in a semi-liquid medium and thin sections are

G.D. Braunstein (ed.), *Thyroid Cancer*, Endocrine Updates 30,
DOI 10.1007/978-1-4614-0875-8_1, © Springer Science+Business Media, LLC 2012

made and placed onto slides for staining. Our practice (and strong recommendation) is to make concurrent cytology preparations from the cut surface of the lesion. The histologic section(s) allow(s) for examination of the tumor and its capsule for interface irregularities with the adjacent non-neoplastic thyroid, morphology of the nodule, capsular or vascular invasion, and thyroid parenchymal invasion. Cytology preparations permit optimum evaluation of nuclear features. Representative sampling of the tumor or nodule of interest is performed; examination of the entire capsule is not routinely performed or recommended [5]. Increased colloid, lymphocytic thyroiditis, FNA biopsy site artifact, infarct, and freezing artifact can all hinder the diagnosis of papillary thyroid carcinoma (PTC), frequently making the cytology preparation essential for identification of diagnostic features.

Accuracy

The reported overall sensitivity of FS ranges from 68 to 77% [6], but this figure is misleadingly reassuring, as it reflects the high prevalence of benign lesions and thus a relatively high predictive value of a negative (benign) result. Sensitivity is, in fact, heavily dependent upon the type of lesion being evaluated, and can be abysmal for certain tumors of clinical importance. FS has a sensitivity as low as 21% for certain follicular lesions [2, 6]. The sensitivity drops even further, to 17%, for encapsulated and minimally invasive follicular carcinomas [6] because the entire capsule cannot be evaluated in routine frozen section (FS). FS has a higher sensitivity for papillary carcinomas (94% for classic PTC) than follicular carcinomas (44%), and a lower sensitivity for follicular variant of PTC (FVPTC) (27%) [6].

The specificity of FS is high (range 96–100%) [2, 7, 8], but the intraoperative management with respect to the FNA diagnosis of a thyroid lesion is rarely (3–5%) altered by FS diagnosis [2, 8–10], largely because FNA can preoperatively diagnose PTCs in >90% of cases [5], permitting definitive surgical management. In addition, FS diagnosis of well-circumscribed or

encapsulated follicular lesion must often be deferred pending complete permanent section examination of the lesion due to the low sensitivity of FS for follicular carcinoma and follicular variant of papillary carcinoma (17 and 27%, respectively) [6]. These limitations yield a 50–87% FS deferral rate in patients with a preoperative FNA diagnosis of follicular lesion/neoplasm [5, 9, 11]. Thus, the associated estimated cost per useful FS that ranges from $7,800 to $12,000 [9–12].

A further limitation of FS accuracy is in the diagnosis of malignancy associated with multinodular goiter. In one study of FS of 197 multinodular goiter patients with clinically suspicious nodules, FS was only 19% sensitive for malignancy and changed the operative management in 3% [13]. The greatest influence on the low sensitivity in this patient group was the size of tumor, with most false negatives seen in carcinomas <1 cm ($p=0.0012$) [13].

These data indicate that the best routine use of intraoperative diagnosis is in nodules with an indeterminate FNA diagnosis, FNA diagnosis suspicious for PTC, or in FLUS lesions in with nuclear abnormalities, suggesting the possibility of papillary carcinoma [6, 12]. In a study of 178 patients with indeterminate FNA, 36% had cancer on permanent sections, 47% of which were identified at FS. The author estimated a cost savings (based on reimbursement rates of 2002) of $1,298 per patient when FS is utilized after an indeterminate FNA diagnosis, attributed to saving a second operation for 30 patients [12].

Our Recommended Algorithm for Routine Cases

FNAs of patients undergoing surgery should be reviewed whenever possible by the pathology department of the institution where the operation is to be performed. In cases for which an unequivocal diagnosis of malignancy is rendered, proceeding to definitive surgery is reasonable, if appropriate for clinical parameters. Follicular lesions for which PTC is not entertained in the FNA diagnosis are probably most accurately and cost effectively handled by lobectomy, permanent section evaluation, and completion thyroidectomy if cancer is found on permanent sections. When FNA is suspicious but not definitive for malignancy, IOC, including FS and cytology preparations, is recommended as highly valuable and reasonably accurate to help guide the surgeon in further therapy, such as completion thyroidectomy or the need for lymph node exploration. Lastly, IOC can be helpful both for the diagnosis of unusual lesions and for guiding the collection of fresh tissue for research, molecular, or other studies.

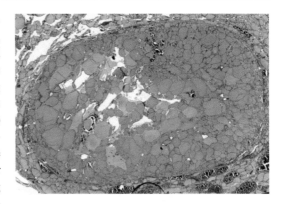

Fig. 1.1 Well-circumscribed hyperplastic nodule with large, colloid-filled follicles (H&E)

Follicular Neoplasms

Follicular lesions/neoplasms of the thyroid include adenomatoid (hyperplastic) nodules, follicular adenomas, and follicular carcinoma. All have follicular growth pattern or are follicle forming and lack the cytologic features of papillary carcinoma [14]. Follicular lesions often provoke controversy due to lack of specificity in their FNA diagnosis, morphologic overlap with one another, inter- and intraobserver variability, variable diagnostic criteria of malignancy, and controversies in treatment plans (thyroidectomy vs. lobectomy) of encapsulated and minimally invasive carcinomas [15–18].

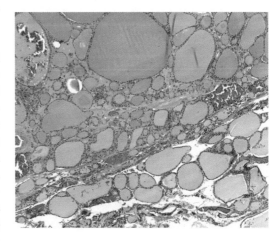

Fig. 1.2 Hyperplastic nodule. Note sharp circumscription of nodule from adjacent gland, despite lack of encapsulation (H&E)

Adenomatoid (Hyperplastic) Nodules

Dominant nodules can arise in a background of nodular goiter and may show partial or near-complete encapsulation [16, 17]. Microscopically, adenomatoid nodules can show partial or near-complete patterned growth with microfollicles [16] (Figs. 1.1 and 1.2) and can be difficult to distinguish from follicular adenomas, other than by incomplete encapsulation and the "definitional" solitary nature of the latter. Fortunately, this considerable overlap in diagnostic criteria has little prognostic significance since all behave in a benign fashion [16]. Degenerative changes such as cystic changes and hemorrhage can be found (Fig. 1.3) as well as pseudopapillary and

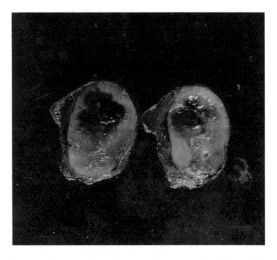

Fig. 1.3 Hemorrhage in a dominant hyperplastic nodule

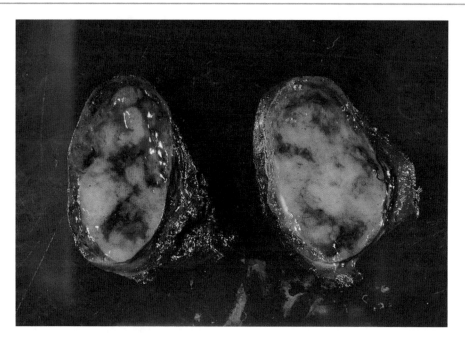

Fig. 1.4 Follicular adenoma. Note complete circumscription by thin fibrous capsule

hyperplastic areas. Multiple encapsulated nodules are termed adenomatoid hyperplasia [16]. Molecular studies indicate that up to 70% of nodules arising in goiter can be clonal [4, 16, 18].

Follicular Adenoma

Follicular adenoma (FA) is typically a solitary encapsulated follicular patterned lesion confined to a single lobe with a benign clinical course [4, 16]. Classically FAs are found in a background of normal thyroid, but may be diagnosed in thyroiditis and rarely goiter. Grossly, FAs are well circumscribed with a thick or variable fibrous capsule (Fig. 1.4). Cut surfaces are tan to red-brown and often bulging out of the capsule. Microscopically, follicular adenomas are classically composed of cytologically bland follicular cells forming small follicles (microfollicles; Figs. 1.5 and 1.6). There are a number of morphologic variants of follicular adenoma; although not clinically significant, awareness of such morphologic variability can help to avoid diagnostic pitfalls. These variants include microfollicular, macrofollicular, trabecular, and fetal/embryonal

patterns [4, 16]. Papillary/pseudopapillary formations can be seen and are typically oriented toward the center of the adenoma with edematous cores and small follicles within the cores [16]. Calcifications can be found, especially after FNA, and can even appear psammomatous [15]. Cystic and degenerative changes are generally absent, except after FNA [19, 20]. Commonly, follicular adenomas show a mixture of small follicles, microfollicles, and macrofollicles. Cytologic features of PTC are absent. Follicular adenomas lack capsular and vascular invasion; most (or if the size of the lesion is not prohibitive, preferably all) of the capsule should be histologically evaluated to exclude these [15, 16, 21]. Follicular adenomas may show the PPAR gamma rearrangements and RAS mutations seen in carcinomas. As of this writing, there is no reliable molecular test to distinguish among adenomatoid nodule, adenoma, and carcinoma [4, 17, 22] (Table 1.1).

Follicular Carcinoma

Follicular carcinoma (FC) accounts for 5–15% of thyroid carcinomas overall, but is more prevalent

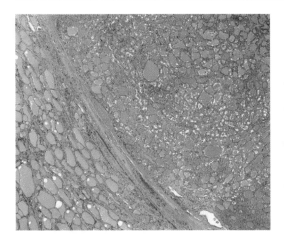

Fig. 1.5 Follicular adenoma. Capsule separates adenoma (*right*) from non-neoplastic thyroid. Follicles in adenoma are more densely packed (H&E)

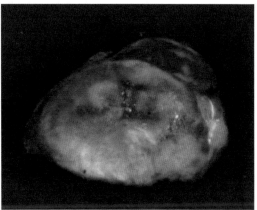

Fig. 1.7 Widely invasive follicular carcinoma. Note effacement of capsule in lower half of photo

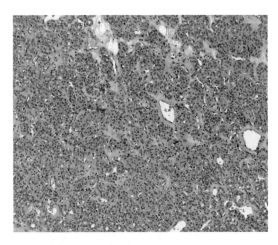

Fig. 1.6 Microfollicular pattern in follicular adenoma (H&E)

Table 1.1 Follicular adenoma

Definition
• Follicular patterned lesion with benign clinical course
Gross features
• Solitary encapsulated lesion confined to one lobe with red-brown or tan cut surface
Microscopic features
• Cytologically bland follicular cells
• Lack of vascular and capsular invasion
• Lack of cytologic features of papillary thyroid carcinoma
• Patterns: Macrofollicular, microfollicular, trabecular, and fetal
• Papillary structures can be seen

in iodine-deficient areas of the world where the incidence is higher (20–40%) [4, 15]. FTC is more common in women; its rare appearance in children is associated with congenital goiter in patients with thyroid gene mutations [4, 23, 24]. Peak age of presentation is in the 5th and 6th decades [4, 15]. FC spreads hematogenously with metastases to the brain, bone, liver, and lung [4, 15, 16].

FC is separated into two main groups with important prognostic significance: *widely invasive* and *minimally invasive*. Widely invasive FC is usually clinically and grossly detectable, with invasion into cervical veins and extension into extrathyroidal soft tissues [15, 16]. Prognosis is poor, with a mortality >50% [4, 15, 16]. As many as 20% are metastatic at presentation [25]. The tumors are usually > 1 cm, tan to brown with irregular borders, and extensive invasion into or complete effacement of the fibrous capsule [4, 25] (Fig. 1.7). Microscopically, widely invasive FCs are highly cellular and can show solid, microfollicular, or trabecular growth patterns and may have an associated poorly differentiated or insular component [26]. Capsular and/or vascular invasion is/are readily identified and may be extensive (Figs. 1.8 and 1.9). Other variants of follicular carcinoma include oncocytic variant (Hurthle cell carcinoma, discussed below) and clear cell variant, which is composed of clear cells and signet ring cells from glycogen, mucin, or lipid [4] (Table 1.2).

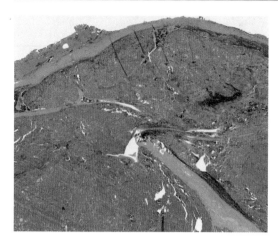

Fig. 1.8 Widely invasive follicular carcinoma with extensive growth beyond capsular breach (H&E)

Table 1.2 Follicular carcinoma – Widely invasive

Definition
• Follicular patterned lesion with grossly or clinically apparent vascular and/or capsular invasion
• More common in areas with endemic goiter and iodine deficiency
• Lack of cytologic features of papillary thyroid carcinoma[a]

Gross features
• Tan mass with irregular borders
• Clinically and grossly detectable invasion into cervical veins or extrathyroidal extension

Microscopic features
• Highly cellular with various growth patterns
• Solid, microfollicular, and trabecular growth
• May have poorly differentiated areas

Metastatic spread and outcome
• Metastasizes hematogenously to brain, bone, liver with low prevalence lymph node metastases (<5%)
• Poor prognosis (mortality >50%)

[a]See text. Features of papillary thyroid carcinoma can be multifocal and subtle

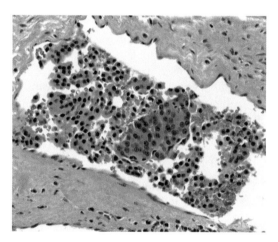

Fig. 1.9 Vascular invasion in widely invasive follicular carcinoma (H&E)

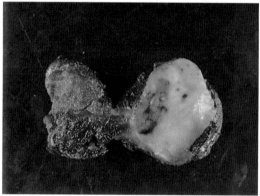

Fig. 1.10 Minimally invasive follicular carcinoma. Tumor largely replaces lobe, but gross encapsulation appears maintained

Most minimally invasive FCs have a good prognosis. This tumor grossly resembles a follicular adenoma and is typically a solitary well-defined tan nodule with a thick or variably thick fibrous capsule [4, 15, 16] (Fig. 1.10). Extensive histologic evaluation of the tumor–capsule–thyroid interface reveals foci of capsular (Fig. 1.11) invasion with at least focal complete capsular penetration or vascular invasion (Fig. 1.12) into the fibrous capsule vessels or larger vessels outside of the main nodule [15, 16, 18, 21]. The tumor/capsule–normal surrounding thyroid interface reveals tongues or invasive "hooks" of tumor infiltrating the capsule with connection to the main tumor [15, 16, 18, 21, 27]. Vascular invasion is defined as the presence of tumor embolus in capsular vessels or vessels outside the capsule [15, 21]. Archtypically, tumor emboli are intermixed with fibrin and blood and show attachment to the endothelial wall. If the tumor thrombus is not attached to the vessel wall in the examined section, to qualify as defining vascular invasion it should be covered by endothelium on at least three sides [15, 21] (Table 1.3).

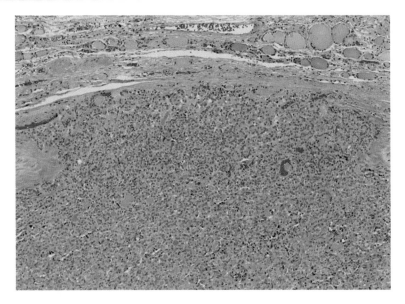

Fig. 1.11 Early transcapsular invasion in minimally invasive follicular carcinoma (H&E)

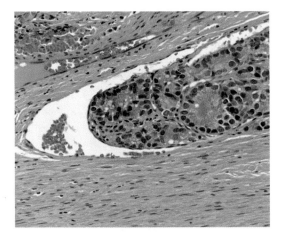

Fig. 1.12 Vascular invasion in minimally invasive follicular carcinoma (same case as seen in Fig. 1.11; H&E)

Capsular irregularities are frequently found in encapsulated thyroid tumors. These irregularities, and changes at FNA biopsy sites, often make interpretation of capsular and vascular invasion challenging for even experienced surgical pathologists [15, 16, 19, 20]. Tumor impingement on blood vessels and/or the presence of nonendothelialized tumor in blood vessels are not considered vascular invasion [15, 16, 21].

There has been significant debate on accepted criteria for minimally invasive FC. Several stud-

Table 1.3 Follicular carcinoma – Minimally invasive

Definition
- Follicular patterned lesion with multifocal and minimal capsular and vascular invasion
- Extensive capsular sampling may be required for diagnosis
- Lack of cytologic features of papillary thyroid carcinoma[a]

Gross features
- Solitary, encapsulated tan or red-brown mass
- Resembles follicular adenoma grossly

Microscopic features
- Foci of capsular invasion seen at tumor thyroid interface and/or vascular invasion[b]
- Patterns can be microfollicular or normofollicular or a mix of patterns

Metastatic spread and outcome
- Metastases can present 10 years or more after presentation
- Risk of metastatic spread is associated with increased number of foci of invasion (especially ≥4)
- Overall prognosis is good (mortality of 3–5% with survival curves approaching normal population)

[a]See text. Features of papillary thyroid carcinoma can be multifocal and subtle
[b]see text for definitions and controversies in vascular and capsular invasion

ies have shown high interobserver variability in the diagnosis of follicular carcinoma and encapsulated follicular lesions [14, 28]. Most minimally invasive FCs show several foci of capsular or vascular invasion [15, 16, 29], but detection of these multiple foci may require exhaustive examination of the complete tumor capsule with multiple histologic sections on several paraffin blocks. Rarely, an encapsulated follicular lesion may present with a single focus of capsular invasion, causing great difficulty in classification. Such lesions are controversial, with differing opinions on how to classify them. Some authorities state that encapsulated follicular tumors with partial capsular invasion only have little to no chance of causing metastatic disease and in order to avoid overtreatment may use the term "thyroid tumor of uncertain malignant potential" [15, 16, 29, 30]. Conversely, several studies have shown evidence for the metastatic potential of such tumors, and equally prominent authorities assert that encapsulated follicular tumors with any capsular invasion (partial or complete) or vascular invasion should be classified as minimally invasive follicular carcinoma [4, 15, 16, 21, 27, 29].

Metastases can present long after resection (>10 years are more) [4, 21]. The risk of metastatic disease is associated with the number of foci of vascular invasion and capsular invasion (especially >4 foci) [4, 27].

Hurthle Cells

A Hurthle cell is a follicular cell with distinctive cytomorphology. The cell size is larger (2–3×) than that of an ordinary follicular cell, the cytoplasm is brightly eosinophillic and granular, the nucleus is larger, and the nucleolus is prominent (Fig. 1.13). Ultrastructurally, the cytoplasm is swollen with numerous mitochondria, possibly the result of abnormalities in mitochondrial DNA [31, 32].

Commonly in histologic and cytologic samplings, follicular cells are observed which have overlap features between Hurthle cells and non-Hurthle follicular cells. Pathologists may call such cells as "Hurthle-like," "Hurthleoid," "oncocytic," "oxyphilic," and "Hurthle cell transition" forms. Hurthle cells are common in many conditions including thyroiditis, Grave's dis-

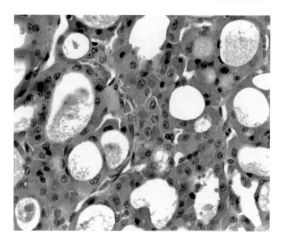

Fig. 1.13 Hurthle cells. Note abundant granular eosinophilic cytoplasm, coarse chromatin, and prominent nucleoli (H&E)

ease, goiter, aging, adenomatoid nodules, and neoplasms [31, 33]. Hurthle cell neoplasms were historically considered all malignant [4, 31, 33], but the current WHO [4] classification categorizes Hurthle cell adenomas and carcinomas as variants of follicular adenomas and carcinomas, respectively, with the same criteria for malignancy as non-Hurthle neoplasms [4, 33]. Hurthle cell lesions display the same immunophenotype as non-Hurthle follicular cells (TTF-1 positive, CK7 positive, thyroglobulin positive, and CK20 negative) [4].

Hurthle Cell Adenomas (Follicular Adenoma, Oncocytic Variant)

Hurthle cell adenomas are solitary, well circumscribed, encapsulated, and composed of >75% Hurthle cells [4, 31, 33]. Other terms for such lesions are follicular adenoma, oncocytic variant, and oncocytic adenoma. Oncocytic adenomatoid nodules, especially in Hashimoto's thyroiditis, can be difficult to distinguish from adenomas [4, 31]. Grossly, cut surfaces are mahogany brown to yellow-tan and can have a central area of scarring [4]. Microscopically, Hurthle cell adenomas can show the variety of growth patterns of follicular adenomas with microfollicular, macrofollicular, trabecular, and solid growth patterns. Occasional

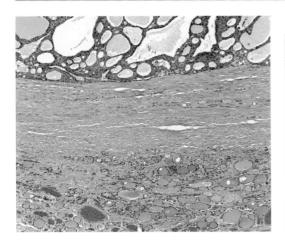

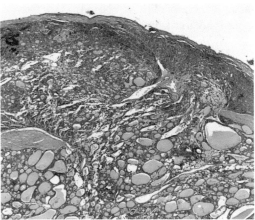

Fig. 1.14 Thickly encapsulated Hurthle cell adenoma (H&E)

Fig. 1.15 Widely invasive Hurthle cell carcinoma (H&E)

papillary structures can be seen [4, 31, 33]. There is a lack of capsular and vascular invasion (Fig. 1.14). Some nuclear features of PTC (such as chromatin clearing and nuclear grooves) may be seen focally in rare cases, but are neither extensive nor diagnostic of PTC. Occasionally, Hurthle cell adenomas can undergo infarction, spontaneously or following FNA [31, 33]. Extensive necrosis is not a criterion of malignancy and other features such as capsular and vascular invasion remain the defining features [4, 27, 31, 33, 34].

Hurthle cell adenomas with cytologic atypia, increased mitotic activity, spontaneous infarction and necrosis, and trapping of tumor cells within the capsule may be considered "atypical Hurthle cell adenomas"; however, since these behave in a benign fashion with long-term follow-up [31], the value of this term as a taxonomic category is dubious.

Hurthle Cell Carcinoma

Hurthle cell carcinomas are malignant tumors composed of >75% oncocytic cells and which lack the cytologic features of papillary carcinoma. Hurthle cell carcinomas account for up to 3–4% of thyroid cancers [4]. The age at diagnosis is about 60, with a female predominance (female to male 6.5:3.5) [4]. Patients most commonly present with a solitary thyroid mass but can present with

increasing pressure after long-standing goiter [35]. Aggressive carcinomas can present with hoarseness, stridor, and dyspnea [35]. In up to 23–39% of patients there is a history of radiation [36, 37].

Criteria for malignancy are the same for both Hurthle and non-Hurthle neoplasms, but the rate of malignancy may be higher in Hurthle cell tumors than in follicular tumors (30–45% compared to 2–3% of classic follicular neoplasms) [31, 33]. Hurthle cell carcinomas metastasize to cervical lymph nodes as well as bone and lung and metastases can be present in up to 9–17% of patients at initial diagnosis [35, 36].

Hurthle cell carcinomas are divided into minimally invasive and widely invasive (Fig. 1.15), similar to non-Hurthle cell FCs and are considered variants of FC under the WHO [4]. However, oncocytic tumor type may be associated with a worse prognosis compared to classical follicular carcinomas [31, 38]. Stage for stage, Hurthle cell carcinomas behave more aggressively than non-Hurthle follicular carcinomas [31].

Grossly, widely invasive Hurthle cell carcinomas are large dominant masses with irregular borders. Cut surfaces show a mahogany brown to tan tumor with scarring and hemorrhages and a capsule remnant may or may not be present. Microscopically, oncocytic carcinomas show the same variety of growth patterns seen in other FCs [4, 31]. Widely invasive tumors have extensive transcapsular and vascular invasion [4, 31] (Fig. 1.15). Oncocytic carcinomas may undergo infarction, especially after FNA [4, 33]. Infarction alone is not a criterion for malignancy or biologically aggressive behavior, but can render specimens difficult to interpret with regard to potential biologic behavior. The prognosis for widely invasive Hurthle cell carcinoma is poor with a mortality of 50–60% at 5 years [31]. Stage, age, and size (>4 cm) are predictors of prognosis [36].

Minimally invasive oncocytic carcinomas are grossly indistinguishable from oncocytic adenomas, present as a dominant encapsulated mahogany brown to tan mass composed of >75% oncocytes, and lack the cytologic features of papillary carcinoma [4, 31]. The microscopic patterns of growth are similar to those found in widely invasive oncocytic carcinoma and non-Hurthle follicular carcinomas. Increased cellularity, nuclear atypia, tumor necrosis, and increased mitoses are not determinant criteria for malignancy nor predict biologically aggressive behavior. Minimally invasive oncocytic carcinoma exhibits capsular or vascular invasion with the same criteria applied as for FC [15, 34]. In general, minimally invasive Hurthle cell carcinoma is associated with a good prognosis, with survival curves similar to non-Hurthle minimally invasive follicular carcinomas [4, 31, 34]. However, minimally invasive Hurthle cell carcinomas have a propensity to present with more extensive vascular invasion than their non-Hurthle counterparts [34]. As with conventional FC, vascular invasion, especially if greater than 4 foci are present, is associated with a poorer prognosis [27, 34].

Medullary Carcinoma

Medullary thyroid carcinoma (MTC) is a malignant tumor of C-cell derivation. C cells (also called parafollicular cells) are neuroendocrine cells that produce calcitonin in response to hypercalcemia. C-cells can undergo hyperplasia (unifocal and multifocal) or form large neoplastic nodules as microcarcinomas (<1 cm) or macrocarcinomas (>1 cm). MTCs account for 3–10% of thyroid cancers and are either sporadic or familial, with inherited forms accounting for about 30% [4, 39, 40]. These are associated with

gain-of-function mutations in the RET oncogene in the multiple endocrine neoplasia syndromes MEN 2a and MEN 2b [4].

Clinical

Most patients present with a solitary nodule and increased serum calcitonin and CEA levels [4, 41]. Mean patient age ranges from 45 to 51 years [4, 40, 42]. Lymph node metastases are present in up to 50% of patients, and extensive local growth is associated with vocal cord paralysis, dysphagia, or other signs of upper airway obstruction [4]. Familial forms are often detected at an earlier stage due to screening by serum calcitonin levels [40, 41] and thus present as microcarcinomas. MTC is not associated with neck radiation [4], and it has been suggested that chronic hypercalcemia may be a contributing factor for some patients [4, 41, 43].

Gross Pathology

The tumor is more often located in the upper two-thirds of the gland [43] where a higher concentration of C cells is found. Most medullary carcinomas are circumscribed but nonencapsulated firm tan to yellow or grayish tumors (Fig. 1.16). Some tumors infiltrate the surrounding thyroid parenchyma. Occasionally, necrosis or hemorrhage may be seen [43].

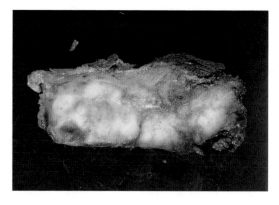

Fig. 1.16 Medullary carcinoma. Note circumscription but lack of encapsulation

Microscopic

MTCs vary both in their architectural growth patterns and in cytomorphology. The tumors may grow in tongues, nests, cords, in a pseudopapillary fashion, in trabecular, or as solid bands (Fig. 1.17). There are thin intervening fibrous bands and a fine capillary network throughout the tumor [43]. Often, there is dense amorphous eosinophillic material with the staining characteristics of amyloid, e.g., Congo Red positivity [4, 43] (Fig. 1.18). In a Swedish study with long-term follow-up, Bergholm et al. showed that an association of a paucity or absence of amyloid is associated with a poorer prognosis [40]. MTCs can also produce

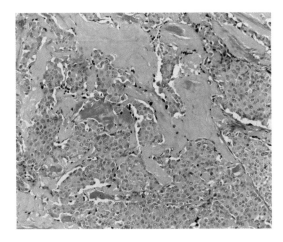

Fig. 1.17 Medullary carcinoma. Nested growth of polygonal cells in amyloid stroma (H&E)

mucin, melanin, and an array of polypeptides (such as VIP and somatostatin) [4, 43].

Cells of MTC may be round, polygonal, plasmacytoid, or spindled. Nuclei are round to oval with coarse chromatin. Nucleoli are not prominent, but can be seen. The cytoplasm has both eosinophilic and basophilic staining properties and irregular margins so that distinction between adjacent cells may not be possible [4]. Tumor cells can also show "small cell" change, causing confusion with other small-cell tumors such as lymphomas or insular carcinoma. MTC cells may show large nuclei, hyperchromasia, and irregular nuclear membranes, but these features do not portend more aggressive behavior. Mitotic figures are typically rare.

Variants of MTC include pseudopapillary, glandular, giant cell, spindle cell, paraganglioma-like, oncocytic cell, clear cell, angiosarcoma-like, melanin producing, and squamous cell. MTCs stain with TTF-1, but do not express thyroglobulin. They are immunopositive for calcitonin (Fig. 1.19), carcinoembryonic antigen, cytokeratin, and neuroendocrine markers such as synaptophysin and chromogranin.

C-cell hyperplasia may be present in the background, more frequently, but not exclusively in familial cases [41]. Chronic lymphocytic thyroiditis can be found but its association with MTC is unclear [4].

The histologic differential diagnosis includes hyalinizing trabecular adenoma, oncocytic tumors,

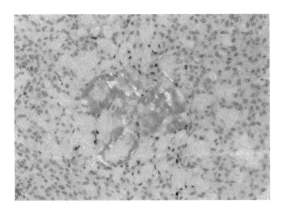

Fig. 1.18 Amyloid in medullary carcinoma (Congo Red, polarized)

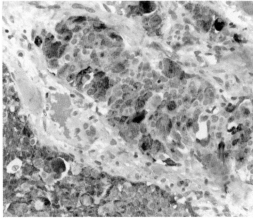

Fig. 1.19 Medullary carcinoma (Calcitonin immunoperoxidase)

Table 1.4 Medullary carcinoma

Definition
- Malignant tumor of thyroid C-cell derivation
- Can be inherited, most are sporadic
- Can present with elevated serum CEA and/or calcitonin

Gross features
- Nonencapsulated firm tan to grayish tumor

Microscopic features
- Variable growth patterns
- Round, polygonal, plasmacytoid or spindled cells
- Dense amyloid deposits
- Round to oval nuclei with coarse chromatin, can have nuclear pseudoinclusions

Metastatic spread and outcome
- Can spread to regional lymph nodes
- Older age, higher stage, extrathyroidal extension, male sex associated with lower survival

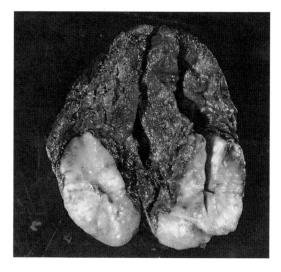

Fig. 1.20 Hyalinizing trabecular tumor. Well-circumscribed firm mass

paraganglioma, follicular carcinoma with trabecular growth pattern, parathyroid tumors, papillary carcinoma, and lymphoma (if small-cell pattern MTC) [4, 43].

The 10-year survival for MTC ranges from 61 to 75% and overall 15-year survival is about 65% [39, 40, 42, 44]. Patients with familial MTC may have a better prognosis due to early detection by serum calcitonin levels [40, 41]. When familial cases of MTC were excluded from a study of 247 Swedish patients, the 10-year and 15-year survival rates dropped to 60.8% and 53.7%, respectively. Older age, higher stage (> stage I), extrathyroidal extension, and male sex are associated with lower survival rates and higher recurrence rates [4, 42, 44] (Table 1.4). Incomplete removal of the tumor, tumor necrosis, and decreased amyloid are factors associated with poorer prognosis [40, 42, 44]. N1 (regional lymph node metastases) patients have a risk of disease progression higher than N0 patients (2–6 fold higher) [44], in contrast to patients with PTC. The staging scheme for medullary carcinoma is different from papillary and follicular carcinoma [45].

Hyalinizing Trabecular Tumor

Hyalinizing trabecular tumor (HTT) is a tumor of follicular cell origin which shows overlapping morphologic features with PTC and MTC. Most HTTs behave in a benign fashion, but because rare cases with lymph node metastases have been reported the term hyalinizing trabecular *tumor* is preferred over hyalinizing trabecular *adenoma* [4].

Clinical Features

HTT typically presents as a palpable solitary mass lesion in the 4th decade [4, 46]. A few patients have goiter or a history of radiation [4, 46].

Gross Pathology

HTTs are solitary well-circumscribed and/or encapsulated tumors ranging in size from less than 1 cm to 4 cm. Cut surfaces are firm, tan to yellow, and show bulging of their capsules [46] (Fig. 1.20).

Microscopic Pathology

HTTs are solid with thin fibrous capsules. Growth is trabecular (Fig. 1.21) or lobular; when present, trabeculae are two to four cells thick. There is a fibrovascular network coursing throughout the tumor with associated pink hyaline material [4, 46]. The hyaline material resembles amyloid but is PAS positive and Congo Red negative [4].

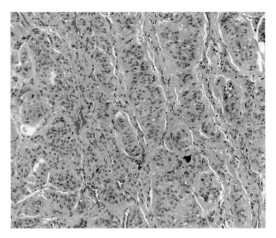

Fig. 1.21 Trabecular growth pattern in hyalinizing trabecular tumor (H&E)

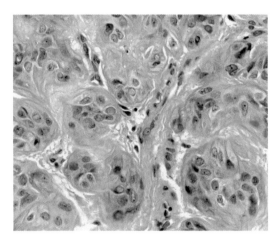

Fig. 1.22 Hyalinizing trabecular tumor. Nuclear features show striking overlap with papillary carcinoma, including nuclear enlargement and envelope irregularities, dispersed chromatin, and many intranuclear inclusions (H&E)

The cells are medium sized with clear, amphophillic, or pink granular cytoplasm with variable epithelioid and spindled morphology [4, 46] (Fig. 1.22). The nuclear to cytoplasmic ratio is typically low and chromatin is dispersed [46, 47]. Nuclei are round to oval and there are abundant intranuclear cytoplasmic inclusions, nuclear grooves, and nuclear overlapping. Intranuclear cytoplasmic inclusions are more abundant than in papillary carcinoma [47]. Mitotic figures are sparse to absent [46]. Psammomatous calcifications may be identified, and multinucleated giant cells are typically absent [4, 47]. It is important for clinicians to be aware that HTTs may be pre-

Table 1.5 Hyalinizing trabecular tumor

Definition
• Tumor of follicular cell origin with overlapping morphologic features between papillary thyroid carcinoma and medullary carcinoma
• Most behave in a benign fashion
Gross features
• Well-circumscribed and/or encapsulated tumor with tan or light yellow cut surface
Microscopic features
• Trabecular or lobular growth
• Associated with pink hyaline stromal material
• Intranuclear cytoplasmic inclusions, which may be more abundant than papillary thyroid carcinoma
Metastatic spread and outcome
• Rare cases of lymph node spread
• Can have RET/PTC rearrangements (up to 28%)

operatively diagnosed as papillary carcinoma on FNA, as the distinction between these tumors can be impossible on cytologic grounds.

Prognosis

There are isolated reports of HTT with capsular and vascular invasion [48–50], but the classification of such cases is controversial [4]. Eleven were reported by Carney et al., with no recurrence or evidence of metastatic disease over a mean follow-up period of 10 years [46]. HTTs have been shown to have rearrangements of the *RET/PTC* oncogene and these rearrangements occur in a comparable proportion to PTC [51]. The morphologic and molecular similarities with PTC further support "hyalinizing trabecular *tumor*" as the preferred term for this entity.

The differential diagnosis of this tumor includes PTC due to overlapping nuclear features, MTC due to the pink matrix, and variable spindled and epithelioid appearance of the cells. Immunohistochemical stains can help to exclude MTC, but are not helpful in distinguishing HTT from papillary carcinoma. HTT is immunopositive for thyroglobulin and TTF-1 and negative for calcitonin, and the hyaline matrix is negative for Congo Red. MTC is positive for CEA, synaptophysin, and calcitonin and negative for thyroglobulin and its pink matrix (amyloid) is positive for Congo Red (Table 1.5).

Papillary Carcinoma

General

PTC is a primary thyroid cancer of follicular epithelial cell origin with distinctive nuclear features, and is the most common cancer of the endocrine system with approximately 22,000 new cases a year in the US [4, 22]. There is an increasing incidence of PTC, particularly of cancers 1 cm and smaller due in part to increasingly sensitive detection methods [52].

Clinical Features

Most PTCs occur in adults from 20 to 50 years of age, but can be encountered in children and in the elderly [53]. There is a female predominance with a female to male ratio of 4:1 [4, 22]. Prior radiation exposure to the thyroid is an important risk factor, but many PTCs occur in patients with no radiation history [4]. There is also an association with environmental factors (iodine deficiency) and genetics [4, 22]. Patients with chronic thyroiditis (especially chronic lymphocytic thyroidts) are at a higher risk. PTC can occur in any part of the thyroid or in ectopic thyroid tissue (mediastinum and ovary).

Gross Pathology

PTC typically presents as an irregular tan to gray firm mass (Fig. 1.23), but the gross features may vary considerably. The tumor can be encapsulated (follicular variant), cystic, nodular, and/or sclerotic with abundant calcifications. Microscopic foci of PTC may not be visible on the gross level, especially in the presence of concomitant lymphocytic thyroiditis, goiter, or prior biopsy. Calcifications can occasionally be identified grossly.

Microscopic Pathology

The diagnosis of PTC depends on its nuclear characteristics, irrespective of whether features overlapping with other thyroid malignancies are

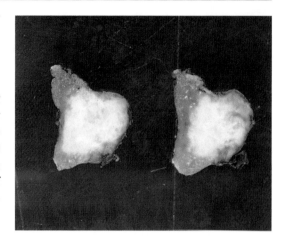

Fig. 1.23 Papillary carcinoma, classical variant. Pale, sclerotic cut surface with infiltrative borders

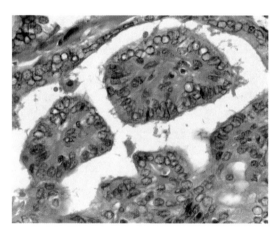

Fig. 1.24 Papillary carcinoma, classical variant. Nuclear irregularities including elongation, crowding with overlap, and chromatin clearing ("Orphan Annie" nuclei; H&E)

seen. The classic features that define papillary carcinoma include nuclear crowding with overlap, nuclear enlargement, chromatin clearing or ground glass appearance ("Orphan Annie eyes"), nuclear elongation, nuclear grooves, irregular nuclear membranes, intranuclear cytoplasmic inclusions, and eccentric inconspicuous nucleoli [4, 19, 54] (Figs. 1.24 and 1.25). Other minor features that can be seen, but which are insufficient for a diagnosis of papillary carcinoma if seen without the nuclear features, include papillary architecture (classical variant; Figs. 1.26 and 1.27) with complexity, psammomatous calcifications (Fig. 1.28), squamous metaplasia, dense

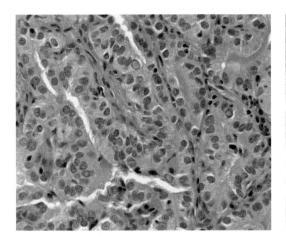

Fig. 1.25 Papillary carcinoma. Nuclear elongation, crowding with overlap, grooves, and prominent intranuclear inclusions. This focus was present in a lymph node metastasis (H&E)

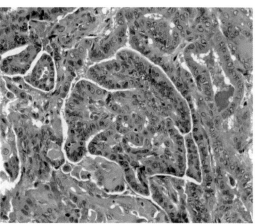

Fig. 1.27 Papillary carcinoma, classical variant, showing papillary architecture. Nuclei are crowded and overlapping, elongated, and many show grooves (H&E)

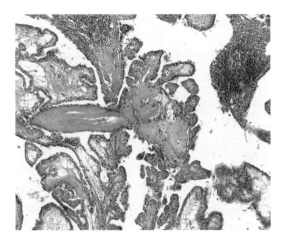

Fig. 1.26 Papillary architecture in classical variant of papillary carcinoma. Note small focus of lymphocytic thyroiditis on the upper right (H&E)

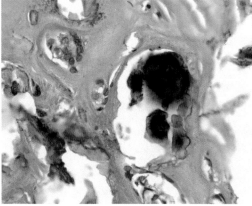

Fig. 1.28 Psammoma body in papillary carcinoma (H&E)

cytoplasm, brightly eosinophilic ("bubble gum") colloid , and multinucleated giant cells [4]. Other than classical PTC, many variants have been described, of which a few are considered clinically important.

Follicular Variant of PTC

FVPTC represents 9–22% of PTCs [27]. Grossly, these tumors are well circumscribed and often encapsulated (Fig. 1.29). FVPTC is composed nearly entirely of small to medium-sized follicles lined by cells with the nuclear features of PTC [4, 27] (Figs. 1.30 and 1.31). Colloid is brightly eosinophllic ("bubble gum"), with the follicles often showing circumferential scalloping [4].

Many cases of FVPTC show diffuse nuclear features of PTC and the diagnosis is straightforward. However, there is a subset of tumors that are entirely encapsulated and show follicular patterned growth with multiple discrete foci having nuclear features of PTC, but other areas lacking these features. There is high interobserver and intraobserver variability in the diagnosis of such lesions, even among expert thyroid pathologists,

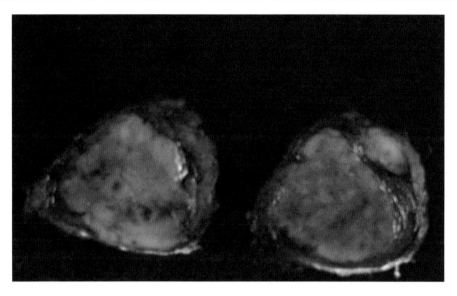

Fig. 1.29 Follicular variant, papillary thyroid carcinoma. Note circumscription and fleshy appearance with greater similarity to follicular tumors than to classical papillary carcinomas

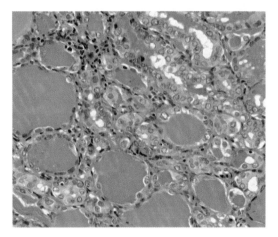

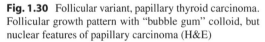

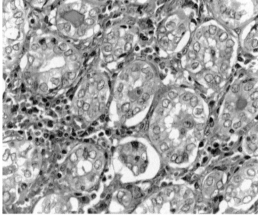

Fig. 1.30 Follicular variant, papillary thyroid carcinoma. Follicular growth pattern with "bubble gum" colloid, but nuclear features of papillary carcinoma (H&E)

Fig. 1.31 Optically clear ("Orphan Annie") nuclei in follicular variant, papillary carcinoma (H&E)

with differing thresholds for diagnosis in different centers and different countries [28, 55, 56]. On one side of the controversy are those experts who assert that these lesions are overdiagnosed as PTC, leading to overtreatment with total thyroidectomy in a tumor that has excellent long-term prognosis [57]. Anchoring the counterargument is Baloch and Livolsi's series of five cases of encapsulated tumors with microscopic features that simulated follicular adenomas with only focal nuclear fea-

tures of papillary carcinoma that metastasized to bone [58]. In the absence of evidence pointing otherwise, it is a common practice (and our own) to diagnose lesions with unequivocal multifocal nuclear features of papillary carcinoma as encapsulated FVPTC and to measure the whole nodule for staging purposes; [15] however, clinicians should be aware that this diagnostic assignment is subjective and that there is no industry-wide "gold standard" for the diagnosis.

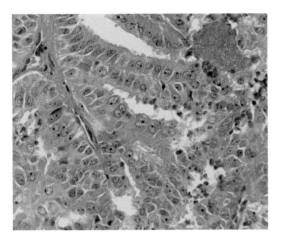

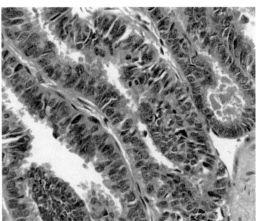

Fig. 1.32 Tall cell variant, papillary thyroid carcinoma. Cell height is at least twice the cell width; such cells must comprise at least 50% of tumor (H&E)

Fig. 1.33 Columnar cell variant, papillary thyroid carcinoma. Elongated columnar cells with nuclear stratification. Nuclear overlapping and envelope irregularities are prominent, but chromatin is coarser than in other papillary carcinoma variants (H&E)

Tall Cell Variant

Tall cell variant of PTC is uncommon, but important for its association with a more aggressive clinical course [4, 59, 60]. By convention, tall cells have a height that is at least twice the width of the cell, eosinophillic cytoplasm, and characteristic nuclear features of papillary carcinoma [59] (Fig. 1.32). The tumor typically grows as cords, but solid, papillary, cribriform, and rare follicular growth patterns may all be seen. The proportion of cells with tall cell features deemed needed to make the diagnosis of tall cell variant has ranged from 30 to70% in the literature [59, 60], but a cutoff of>=50% is proposed [59]. Regardless of the definitional threshold for tall cell composition, there is a higher frequency of extrathyroidal extension, presentation at higher stage, larger size, and older age at diagnosis (mean 57 years), and death due to tumor compared to other variants [59, 60].

Columnar Cell Variant

Columnar cell variant is a rare variant of PTC that is also associated with a more aggressive clinical course [61, 62]. Growth patterns may be papillary, follicular, solid, cribriform, or fascicular [62]. The cells are elongated columnar cells with prominent nuclear stratification (comprising >50% of the tumor) and elongated nuclei. Chromatin ranges from finely granular to coarse, and optically clear nuclei may not be found. Similarly and importantly, intranuclear cytoplasmic inclusions may not be found and nuclear grooves may be rare. Cytoplasm ranges from clear to amphophillic. Subnuclear cytoplasmic vacuoles may be identified [4, 62] (Fig. 1.33). Columnar cell variant is more often associated with extrathyroidal extension, recurrence, and aggressive local growth [4, 62], but tumors that present at a low stage and are entirely encapsulated appear to have low metastatic potential [4].

Macrofollicular Variant

Macrofollicular PTC, the rarest variant, is composed of greater than 50% macrofollicles lined by cells with nuclear features of PTC [4, 63, 64]. The importance of this variant is not prognostic, but rather for pathologists its easy diagnostic confusion with adenoma or adenomatous hyperplasia [4]. Mean age at presentation is 35 years (range 15–69 years) [64]. Extrathyroidal extension, metastases, and dedifferentiation have been reported [63, 64]. Metastases can retain the macrofollicular architecture [4].

Oncocytic Variant

Oncocytic variant of PTC is a rare variant with grossly mahogany brown to tan appearance, papillary or follicular growth pattern, oncocytic cytoplasm, and nuclear features of PTC [4]. It is important to recognize for its distinction from oncocytic variants of follicular adenoma and follicular carcinoma [33]. Making the distinction between oncocytic variant of PTC and a Hurthle cell neoplasm may be difficult in some cases, as "true" Hurthle cell neoplasms can show cleared nuclei and papillary and pseudopapillary structures [33]. Mean age at presentation is 57 years (range 34–86 years) [65]. There is a "Warthin-like" variant with prominent papillary structures and lymphoid follicles and aggregates present within the papillae in a thyroid with background lymphocytic thyroiditis [4, 65, 66], simulating Warthin's tumor of the salivary gland. This variant can be mistaken for a lymphoepithelial lesion of the thyroid commonly seen in lymphocytic thyroiditis [66]. The prognosis is similar to usual PTC and is dependent upon stage [4].

Diffuse Sclerosing Variant of Papillary Thyroid Carcinoma

Diffuse sclerosing variant of PTC is an uncommon variant of papillary carcinoma which presents in younger patients (mean age 18 years; range 6–49 years) and which is biologically more aggressive [4, 67]. Tumors can present with a dominant mass, but are more often bilateral [4, 67]. All cases show conventional papillary, solid, or follicular growth pattern with increased stromal fibrosis and sclerosis, squamous metaplasia, lymphocytic infiltrate, and psammoma bodies [4, 67] (Figs. 1.34 and 1.35). Extensive lymphovascular invasion with small papillae within lymphatic spaces, extrathyroidal extension, and increased incidence of cervical lymph node metastases are also characteristic [4, 67, 68]. There is an increased incidence of lung metastases as well [68]. Despite the high metastatic rate, 5-year survival can be 95% and higher

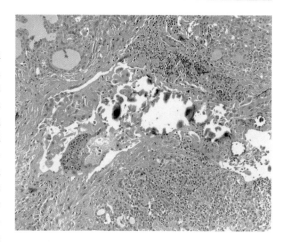

Fig. 1.34 Diffuse sclerosing variant, papillary thyroid carcinoma. Note inflammatory background, prominent intralymphatic tumor, and psammoma bodies (H&E)

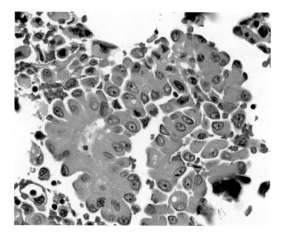

Fig. 1.35 Diffuse sclerosing variant, papillary thyroid carcinoma. Note abundant eosinophilic cytoplasm of tumor cells (H&E)

with appropriate treatment [67, 69]. Chronic lymphocytic thyroiditis is often found in the background [4, 69].

Cribriform-Morular Variant of Papillary Thyroid Carcinoma

Cribriform-morular variant of PTC is a rare one, but clinically important for its association with familial adenomatous polyposis syndrome; [4] however, sporadic cases do occur. Typically, the growth pattern is solid, trabecular, or follicular with cribriform areas (glands within glands) and epithelial morules – whorled cellular balls of tumor cells with dense squamoid cytoplasm [70]. Nuclear features of papillary carcinoma are present throughout the tumor.

Papillary Microcarcinomas

The term *microcarcinoma* is applied to PTCs less than 1 cm in greatest dimension. These tumors are discovered incidentally, and in up to 24% of thyroids removed for other reasons such as chronic lymphocytic thyroiditis, goiter, and Graves' disease [71]. They can also be found in otherwise normal thyroids at autopsy in up to one-third of patients who have died of nonendocrine causes [4]. Histologic mimics include ultimobrachial body rests or reactive nuclear changes in chronic lymphocytic thyroiditis [71]. Up to 11% can exhibit local recurrence or regional metastases [4, 71]. Multifocality can be seen in up to 20–46% of cases; the chance of recurrence or metastasis increases with multifocality [71]. However, a majority of these tumors have an indolent behavior [4, 71].

Prognosis

Overall, the prognosis for PTC is excellent, with a 10-year survival of over 90% [4, 53]. While the most important prognostic indicator is stage, age (>45 years), larger size (>1 cm), extrathyroidal extension, large vessel invasion, and insular component are all poor prognostic indicators [4, 53]. (Table 1.6)

Poorly Differentiated Thyroid Carcinoma

Poorly differentiated thyroid carcinoma is a follicular cell-derived tumor with solid/trabecular/insular growth pattern and one that lacks the nuclear features of PTC. The prognosis is intermediate

Table 1.6 Papillary thyroid carcinoma

Definition
- Primary epithelial carcinoma of the thyroid with distinctive nuclear features
- Most common cancer of the thyroid gland

Gross features
- Irregular tan scirrhous mass
- May also have variable gross appearance – cystic, encapsulated, nodular

Microscopic features
- Nuclear overlapping
- Chromatin clearing or ground glass appearance
- Nuclear grooves
- Intracytoplasmic nuclear inclusions
- Psammomatous calcifications, squamous metaplasia, and papillary architecture
- Tall cell variant, diffuse sclerosing variant, columnar cell variant associated with aggressive clinical course

Metastatic spread and outcome
- Spreads via lymphatic channels
- RAS mutation in 10%, BRAF mutation in up to 70%,
- 10-year survival of over 90% with treatment

between differentiated thyroid carcinoma (FC and PTC) and anaplastic thyroid carcinoma. The concept of this tumor as a distinct entity began to evolve in the early 1980s and has a controversial history, including varying criteria for diagnosis by experts and high intraobserver variability [26, 72, 73]. The prevalence is variable (up to 4–6% of thyroid carcinomas in some countries) and possibly related to the variable thresholds for diagnosis [4, 74]. Poorly differentiated thyroid carcinoma often arises in association with a smaller component of conventional PTC or FC, and it is postulated that the poorly differentiated component represents dedifferentiation of these entities [4, 26]. However, it can arise de novo (or at least without morphologic evidence of PTC or FC) [4]. A synonym for this entity is *insular carcinoma*, which characterizes a common growth pattern seen in these tumors.

This neoplasm presents as a dominant thyroid mass or as a rapidly growing area in a long-standing mass [4]. The mean age at presentation is comparable to conventional PTC (55 years old, SD 18 years) [74].

Fig. 1.36 Poorly
differentiated carcinoma.
Tumor largely replaces
lobe

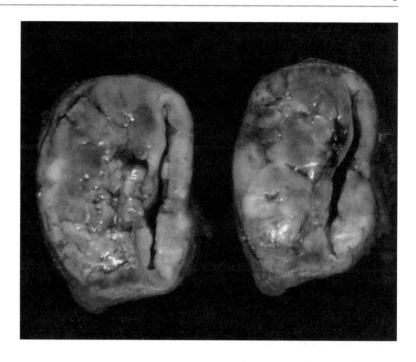

Gross Features

Most tumors are singular and large (3–5 cm),
with pushing borders [4, 74]. An entire lobe may
be replaced. Partial encapsulation or pseudoen-
capsulation can be seen [4, 73]. Cut surfaces are
gray to tan and firm and satellite nodules are
common [4] (Fig. 1.36).

Microscopic Features

Solid, insular, trabecular, and alveolar patterns
may all be seen [72]. For insular growth pattern,
tumor cells are arranged in cellular solid nests
with occasional microfollicles surrounded by a
thick hyalinized stroma [75] (Fig. 1.37). Cells
are small to intermediate in size with decep-
tively bland nuclei [4]. On closer inspection, the
nuclei are hyperchromatic with finely granular
chromatin and convoluted with raisin-like, cup-
shaped, or trifold forms [72]. The mitotic rate is
typically elevated (>3 per 10 high power field,
range 1–10 per high power field) [72, 74].
Tumor necrosis is frequently present [72]
(Fig. 1.38). Occasional groves and pseudoinclusions can be seen, especially when a PTC is
dedifferentiated [72].

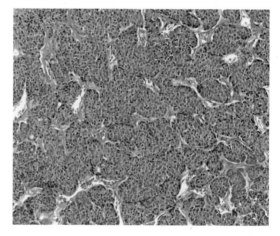

Fig. 1.37 Insular growth pattern in poorly differentiated
carcinoma (H&E)

Differential Diagnosis

The differential diagnoses are MTC, solid variant
PTC, and follicular carcinoma with solid growth
[4, 72]. Distinction from MTC can be aided with
immunohistochemistry. MTC is immunopositive
for synaptophysin, calcitonin, and CEA, and negative for thyroglobulin. Distinction from solid
variant PTC can be difficult and subject to great
intraobserver variability [72]. A panel of experts
in thyroid pathology has proposed "Turin criteria"

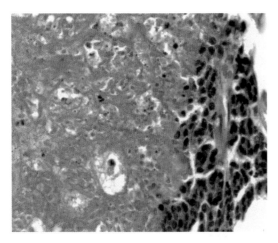

Fig. 1.38 Cellular necrosis in poorly differentiated carcinoma (H&E)

Table 1.7 Poorly differentiated thyroid carcinoma

Definition
- Follicular cell-derived tumor with solid, trabecular, insular growth pattern
- Lacks nuclear features of papillary thyroid carcinoma
- Can arise in association with well-differentiated thyroid carcinomas (follicular and papillary thyroid carcinomas)

Gross features
- Dominant thyroid mass or rapidly growing area in a long-standing mass
- Replacement of the entire lobe is often seen

Microscopic features
- Small to intermediate-sized cells
- Hyperchromatic nuclei with finely granular chromatin, convoluted raisin-like or cup-shaped nuclei
- Elevated mitotic rate and tumor necrosis

Metastatic spread and outcome
- Poorer prognosis than papillary thyroid carcinoma but better prognosis than undifferentiated carcinoma
- Lung metastases and bone metastases more frequent than papillary thyroid carcinoma

for poorly differentiated carcinoma. If typical nuclei of PTC are present throughout a thyroid tumor with solid, trabecular, or insular growth, then it is more aptly classified as solid variant PTC. If nuclear features of PTC are absent, and there is also a lack of the convoluted nuclei, mitoses, and necrosis in a thyroid carcinoma with solid, trabecular, or insular growth that characterize poorly differentiated thyroid carcinoma, then a diagnosis of solid variant FC is likely [72].

Prognosis

Poorly differentiated thyroid carcinoma has a worse prognosis than PTC, with a 5-year survival rate from 20 to 60% [4, 73–75]. Patients with poorly differentiated thyroid carcinoma have a higher rate of metastatic spread to regional lymph nodes (84.6% vs. 73% for PTC) [75]. Lung metastases and bone metastases are also more frequent than in papillary and follicular carcinomas [75]. There may also be a higher frequency of extrathyroidal extension [73]. The proportion of the poorly differentiated component also has a negative impact on survival. Patients with a predominantly poorly differentiated component (>50% of tumor is poorly differentiated) have a poorer outcome and significantly higher rate of metastatic disease than patients with a focal poorly differentiated component (<50% of tumor is poorly differentiated) [74] (Table 1.7).

Anaplastic (Undifferentiated) Thyroid Carcinoma

In stark contrast to other thyroid carcinomas, undifferentiated thyroid carcinoma is one of the most aggressive malignancies known [4, 76]. It accounts for <5–14% of thyroid malignancies, but is responsible for over half of all deaths attributable to thyroid cancer in the US [4, 76]. The incidence is about one to two cases/million, but varies by geographic region and is higher in regions with endemic goiter [4]. Undifferentiated (anaplastic) carcinoma is a tumor composed of undifferentiated tumor cells with immunohistochemical or ultrastructural evidence of epithelial derivation and/or arises in association with a more differentiated carcinoma [4]. Most cases of undifferentiated carcinoma arise in association with a differentiated carcinoma, predominantly PTC and poorly differentiated carcinoma [4, 76], but other carcinomas such as Hurthle cell carcinoma and follicular carcinoma can undergo anaplastic transformation [76].

Clinical Features

Undifferentiated carcinoma is a tumor primarily of the elderly with only 25% of patients younger than 60 years at diagnosis [4, 76]. The female:male ratio of 1.5:1 is less female-predominant than other thyroid malignancies [4]. Most patients present with a rapidly enlarging neck mass; dysphagia and/or dyspnea are present in up to 35% of cases [76]. Vocal cord paralysis and invasion into surrounding muscles into the neck may be evident [4]. Subsets of patients can present years after treatment for a differentiated thyroid carcinoma [76]. Others experience rapid growth of a previously stable goiter [76]. From 10 to 40% of patients present with metastatic disease involving the lung, bones, or brain [4, 76].

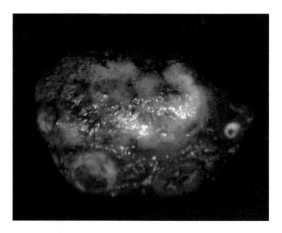

Fig. 1.39 Variegated cut surface of undifferentiated (anaplastic) carcinoma

Gross Features

Tumors are large and irregular with white to tan fleshy cut surfaces (Fig. 1.39). Hemorrhage and necrosis are common [4]. Borders are infiltrative and tumor may invade into surrounding soft tissues such as the trachea, pharynx, esophagus, and regional lymph nodes [4, 76]. Bilateral involvement of the gland (25%) and multiple nodules (40%) are common [4].

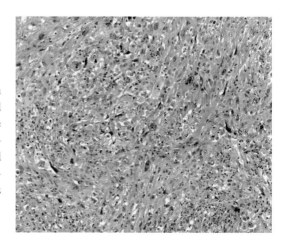

Fig. 1.40 Unpatterned growth of wildly pleomorphic cells in anaplastic carcinoma (H&E)

Microscopic Features

Tumors consist of spindled cells, pleomorphic giant cells, and epithelioid cells in variable proportions [4, 76, 77] (Fig. 1.40). Squamous differentiation can be seen in up to 20% of cases [76] (Fig. 1.41). Giant cells may be pleomorphic and sarcomatoid or multinucleated and osteoclast-like [4, 76]. The cells may be arranged in syncytial sheets with enlarged nuclei and prominent nucleoli [78]. Extensive vascular invasion with obliteration of vessels is common [4]. Some tumors exhibit sarcomatoid features with a storiform appearance reminiscent of malignant fibrous histiocytoma or resemble differentiated sarcomas such as fibrosarcoma, angiosarcoma, or leiomyosarcoma. Other sarcomatous areas may show rhabdoid features [76]. Undifferentiated carcino-

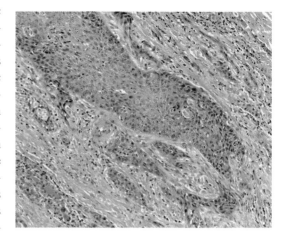

Fig. 1.41 Squamoid differentiation in anaplastic carcinoma (H&E)

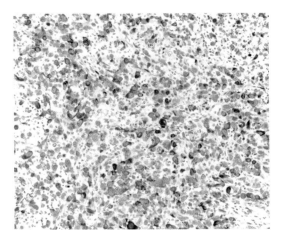

Fig. 1.42 Keratin staining in anaplastic carcinoma tumor cells (AE1/AE3 immunoperoxidase)

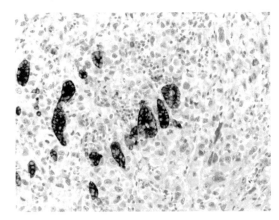

Fig. 1.43 Negative thyroglobulin staining in anaplastic carcinoma; positive cells are background non-neoplastic follicles (Thyroglobulin immunoperoxidase)

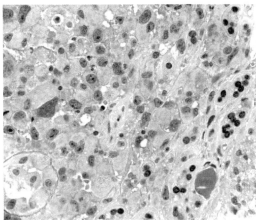

Fig. 1.44 Weak TTF-1 staining in anaplastic carcinoma. Note benign follicular cells on right with stronger staining and small round nuclei for comparison (Thyroid Transcription Factor-1 immunoperoxidase)

Table 1.8 Anaplastic (undifferentiated) thyroid carcinoma

Definition
• One of the most aggressive malignancies known
• Primary thyroid carcinoma lacking specific (follicular or C-cell) differentiation
• Can arise in association with poorly differentiated thyroid carcinoma, papillary thyroid carcinoma, and follicular carcinoma
Gross features
• Large irregular white to tan fleshy masses with hemorrhage and necrosis
• Soft-tissue invasion into trachea, pharynx, esophagus, and regional lymph node spread
Microscopic features
• Spindled cells, pleomorphic giant cells, and epithelioid cells
• Squamous differentiation in up to 20% of cases
• Extensive vascular invasion with vessel obliteration is common
• Some tumors can exhibit sarcoma-like areas, but rarely some are paucicellular
Metastatic spread and outcome
• Prognosis is extremely poor with median survival of 2–7 months

mas are usually highly cellular, but there are rare paucicellular examples that show divergent differentiation (spindled morphology, squamoid morphology, etc.) [78].

Up to 80% of tumors will be at least focally immunopositive for keratin [76, 77] (Fig. 1.42). Thyroglobulin staining is markedly decreased (1–5% of cells) and is present in few cases [76, 77] (Fig. 1.43). TTF-1 is rarely expressed [4] (Fig. 1.44). Most tumors (93%) stain for the nonspecific marker vimentin (93%) [76]. Pertinent negative immunostains are stains for lymphoma, differentiated sarcomas, and melanoma. Proliferation markers (Ki67) are high due to high cell turnover.

Prognosis

Prognosis of anaplastic carcinoma is extremely poor, with a 5-year survival from 0 to 14% [4, 76] and a median survival from 2 to 7 months [4, 76]. Rare cases have a slightly better prognosis if discovered at a smaller size [4, 76] (Table 1.8).

Lymphoma

Lymphomas of the thyroid gland are uncommon, but may be encountered in a busy surgical pathology practice and represent about 5% of all thyroid malignancies and 2–7% of extranodal lymphomas [4, 79]. Most arise in patients with a history of chronic lymphocytic thyroiditis and are extranodal marginal zone B-cell lymphomas (mucosa-associated lymphoid tissue lymphoma or MALT lymphoma) or diffuse large B-cell lymphomas [4, 79]. Diffuse large B-cell lymphoma can occur alone or as large-cell transformation in a patient with marginal zone B-cell lymphoma. Rarely, follicular lymphomas, plasmacytomas, anaplastic large-cell lymphomas, and T-cell lymphomas can be seen [4, 80]. Patients with Hashimoto's thyroiditis have a much higher risk than the general population (40–80 times) [79].

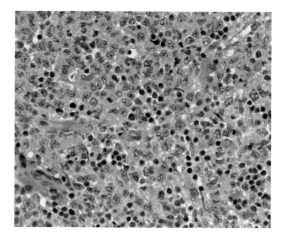

Fig. 1.45 Diffuse large cell lymphoma (H&E)

Clinical Features

Patients' age ranges from 28 to 95 years, with a mean of 64 years and they can present with pain, dyspnea, hoarseness, a noticeably enlarging mass in the gland, or hypothyroidism in the setting of Hashimoto's thyroiditis [4, 79]. As the proportion of the large-cell component increases, there is an association with an increase in symptoms related to compression and infiltration of neck structures [79]. Female to male ratio is 2.7:1 [79].

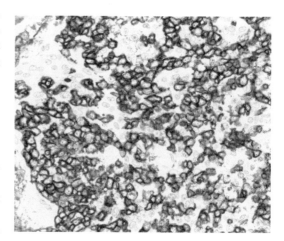

Fig. 1.46 B-cell immunophenotype in diffuse large-cell lymphoma (CD20 immunoperoxidase)

Microscopic Features

Tumors are composed of atypical lymphocytes that form noncohesive sheets, nodules, or infiltrate singly throughout the gland (Figs. 1.45 and 1.46). Lymphoma cytology is dependent upon the type. Marginal zone lymphomas are classically composed of small atypical lymphocytes and monocytoid lymphocytes with condensed chromatin, and may subtly colonize germinal centers. Large-cell lymphomas are composed of large cells with variable chromatin and prominent nucleoli. Mitotic activity can be brisk in large-cell lymphomas and when very high should raise the possibility of Burkitt-like diffuse large

Gross Features

Tumor size ranges from microscopic to massive (up to 20 cm) and can be a single mass, multinodular, or show diffuse effacement of the thyroid parenchyma [4]. Cut surface appearances are variable depending on the type of lymphoma but range from tan to gray to pink with a characteristic "fish-flesh" appearance [4]. Hemorrhage and necrosis can be seen in the setting of diffuse large B-cell lymphomas.

Table 1.9 Lymphoma

Definition
- Uncommon
- Most arise in patients with a history of chronic lymphocytic thyroiditis

Gross features
- Microscopic to very large in size
- Often with diffuse effacement of the thyroid gland parenchyma; "fish-flesh" appearance

Microscopic features
- Atypical lymphocytes in sheets, nodules, or infiltrating singly throughout the gland
- Marginal zone lymphomas are composed of small atypical monocytoid cells
- Large-cell lymphomas are composed of large cells in sheets with prominent nuclei and brisk mitotic activity
- Proper classification required additional studies

Metastatic spread and outcome
- MALT lymphomas have a good prognosis
- Large-cell lymphomas have a poorer prognosis

B-cell lymphoma. Proper classification of lymphomas generally requires additional studies including immunohistochemistry and/or flow cytometry. If lymphoma is suspected, it is highly advisable to collect unfixed tissue intraprocedurally for flow studies.

Prognosis

Prognosis is dependent upon stage and type [4, 79, 80]. Small MALT-type lymphomas have a good prognosis. Large tumors, diffuse large B-cell lymphoma or a large-cell component, vascular invasion, and high mitotic rate are associated with a poor prognosis [4, 79, 80] (Table 1.9).

Unusual Tumors of the Thyroid

The thyroid gland can be involved by unusual tumors specific to the thyroid or can be involved by tumors more common in other body sites.

Squamous Cell Carcinoma

Squamous cell carcinoma accounts for about 1% of thyroid malignancies and occurs primarily in older women (mean peak incidence in the 6th decade) [4] and is a malignant epithelial tumor with squamous differentiation [78]. Squamous epithelium can be found in the thyroid in persistent thyroglossal ducts, ectopic thymic elements, and as a metaplastic and reactive phenomenon of follicular cells in association with thyroiditis [78]. Grossly, the tumor is typically large and firm and white to gray with areas of necrosis or cheesy material representing keratinization [4, 78]. Tumor spreads by local extension and airway obstruction with nodal metastases common and distant metastases in 20% [4, 78]. Microscopically, the tumor is composed of entirely of malignant squamous cells in islands with invasion into thyroid parenchyma without evidence of other types of thyroid carcinoma [4]. Prominent vascular and perineural invasion is common [4]. Mitotic activity is high [78]. Squamous cell carcinoma of the thyroid is typically positive for CK19 [4]. Prognosis is poor and similar to undifferentiated thyroid carcinoma; the staging scheme used is the same as undifferentiated carcinoma [4, 78].

Primary Mucoepidermoid Carcinoma

Mucoepidermoid carcinoma is the most common malignant tumor of the salivary glands and is composed of various proportions of squamous cells, mucinous cells, intermediate cells, and clear cells. Primary mucoepidermoid carcinoma of the thyroid gland is rare (0.5% of thyroid malignancies) and occurs more frequently in women than in men (2:1) with a mean age at incidence of 46 years (range 29–57 years) [4, 81]. The histogenesis of this tumor has been debated [81–83]. Theories include origin from follicular cells which have undergone metaplasia [81] and origin from solid cell nests (remnants of ultimobranchial body) [83, 84]. It presents as a painless solitary well-circumscribed but nonencapsulated mass measuring up to 10 cm [4, 84]. Tumors are rubbery and firm with tan to yellowish cut surfaces [4]. Microscopically, there is focal infiltration into thyroid parenchyma [81]. The tumor is composed of predominantly nests of squamoid cells with keratin pearls and cysts which are admixed with mucinous glandular cells and intermediate cells (cells with features of mucinous cells and squamous cells) surrounded by a fibrous stroma [4, 81]. There is typically mild nuclear pleomorphism, mild increase in nuclear to cytoplasmic ratio, and scattered mitotic figures [81]. There are both intracellular and extracellular mucin and hyaline (colloid-like) intracellular droplets [4, 81]. Psammomatous calcifications can be seen [84]. Tumor cells are positive for TTF-1, thyroglobulin, and cytokeratin and are negative for calcitonin [84]. Mucoepidermoid carcinomas are considered indolent low-grade tumors despite relatively common cervical lymph node metastases [4, 81, 84]. Nevertheless, up 20% of patients with mucoepidermoid carcinoma have died of disease [4].

Primary Sclerosing Mucoepidermoid Carcinoma with Eosinophilia

Sclerosing mucoepidermoid carcinoma with eosinophilia has a similar clinical presentation and behavior as other mucoepidermoid carcinomas of the thyroid [84], but this rare tumor occurs almost exclusively in women [4] and is characterized by features of mucoepidermoid carcinoma with prominent stromal sclerosis and eosinophillic and lymphocytic infiltration [4, 84]. There is a strong association with Hashimoto's thyroiditis [82, 84, 85]. In about half the cases there is involvement with perithyroidal soft tissues [4, 85]. The squamous and glandular components characteristic of mucoepidermoid carcinoma are seen microscopically, along with prominent hyaline stroma and eosinophilia [84, 85]. Follow-up and prognosis information are limited. About half of the patients have an aggressive course with local or distant spread [4, 85]. Despite the clinical and morphologic similarities with primary mucoepidermoid carcinoma, sclerosing mucoepidermoid carcinoma with eosinophilia is usually negative for thyroglobulin immunostaining, suggesting that

these two tumors may have a different histogenesis [4, 82].

Tumors of Possible Thymic or Ultimobranchial Origin

Spindle Epithelial Tumors with Thymus-Like Differentiation

Spindle epithelial tumor with thymus-like differentiation (SETTLE) is a rare malignant tumor of the thyroid with lobulated growth and spindle shaped and epithelioid cells that merge into glandular cells in a biphasic pattern [4]. Morphologic and immunophenotyic studies show similarities with thymic or branchial pouch differentiation [78]. However, the histogenesis of these tumors has been debated [84]. SETTLE occurs mostly in children and adolescents with a rare reported case in adults [4, 78, 86]. There is a slight male predominance, in contrast to most other thyroid malignancies [4, 78]. Patients most commonly present with a painless thyroid mass, which can be rapidly enlarging [4, 78]. Grossly, the tumor is encapsulated, nodular, or partially circumscribed [78]. Microscopically, SETTLE is very cellular and shows spindled growth blending imperceptibly into areas with epithelial differentiation with glomeruloid, papillary, tubular, and glandular structures lined by cuboidal to columnar cells [78, 87]. Hassall's corpuscles can be seen [78]. Tumors express high-molecular-weight keratin, CK7, Bcl2 (88%), CD99 (75%), and CD117 (75%), among other markers [87]. Tumor cells are negative for thyroglobulin, calcitonin, S100, and CD5 [4].

In the differential diagnosis, undifferentiated thyroid carcinoma must be excluded as well as synovial sarcoma which can show epithelial and spindled elements [4]. Ectopic thymoma is also in the differential diagnosis and can be distinguished by the rich lymphocytic infiltrate typically present in thymomas [4].

SETTLEs are slow growing but may metastasize (up to 60% with late presentation of metastases) [4, 78, 84].

Carcinoma Showing Thymus-Like Differentiation

Carcinoma showing thymus-like differentiation (CASTLE) is a carcinoma of the thyroid gland which shows morphologic similarities to thymoma [4]. Some studies show phenotypic similarities to solid cell nests/ultimobrachial remnants of the thyroid, suggesting these may be the origin of these tumors [88]. CASTLE is very rare and affects middle-age adults [4]. There is a slight female predominance (1.3:1) [78]. Patients present with a painless mass thyroid mass or symptoms related to upper-airway compression or hoarseness [4]. Grossly, the tumor is lobulated and tan to gray with well-defined borders [4, 78, 88]. Microscopically, tumor cells are squamoid, spindled, or syncytial with smooth contoured tumor islands [4, 78, 88]. Cytoplasm is pale to eosinophilic and nuclei are oval with pale or vesicular chromatin, small nucleoli, and mild to moderate nuclear atypia [4, 78, 88]. Tumor islands infiltrate through a fibrous stroma [4]. Keratin pearls and Hassel's corpuscles can be seen [78]. Tumor cells are positive for CD5 and cytokeratin and negative for thyroglobulin [78, 88]. CASTLE can have an indolent course or be rapidly progressive [4, 89]. The 10-year survival according to a study of 25 patients was 82% [89]. Early regional lymph node metastases are common (up to 32%) [89]. Distant metastases to lung, liver, bone, mediastinum, and pleura have been reported [89].

Teratoma

Primary teratomas of the thyroid are extremely rare and comprise <0.1% of all tumors of the thyroid gland. These germ cell-derived tumors show mature or immature components of ectoderm, endoderm, and mesoderm [4, 90]. Because of the rarity of these tumors and paucity of large case series, established classification schemes typically applied to teratomas in other locations are employed [90]. They can be separated into three categories: benign, immature, and malignant [90]. Benign teratomas are composed entirely of mature components [90]. Immature teratomas have tissue resembling fetal tissues (most often neuroectodermal elements) [90]. Malignant teratomas have a prominent immature component (>4 low power fields) along with mitoses and cellular atypia [90]. Teratomas can occur at any age (newborn to 56 years, with a mean of 12.4 years). Greater than 90% of tumors in the neonatal group are benign and >50% in adults are malignant [4, 91, 92]. Patients present with a mass in the neck and may experience dyspnea or stridor [4, 90]. Other congenital anomalies may be present in newborns [4]. Grossly, tumors can range from 2 to 13 cm with a smooth or bosselated surface and gray to yellow cut surfaces with solid and cystic areas with white creamy material within cysts in mature teratomas (sebaceous material/cyst contents) [4, 90]. Microscopically, there are a variety of growth patterns within one lesion [90]. Cystic epithelial elements can include respiratory, squamous, columnar, or transitional epithelium [4]. Cartilage, bone, smooth muscle, and skeletal muscle can be seen [4]. Immature neural elements have hyperchromatic, medium-sized nuclei with associated mitotic figures arranged in sheets or rosettes [4, 90]. Immunohistochemical stains used to identify neural tissue or skeletal muscle (S100 and myoD1) may be helpful in characterizing immature elements [4]. Malignant teratomas can recur and metastasize in 30% of cases [4, 90].

Mesenchymal Tumors

Vascular tumors. Reactive endothelial hyperplasias (Masson pseudotumor), benign hemangiomas, and malignant angiosarcomas can occur in the thyroid [4, 84].

Benign reactive endothelial hyperplasias can occur in long-standing goiter or in association with post-FNA reactive changes and can result from hemorrhage and granulation tissue formation [93]. They can appear as florid vascular proliferations and the differential diagnosis can include angiosarcoma [93]. There should be a lack of cytologic atypia and mitotic activity [93].

Angiosarcoma of the thyroid, also known as "hemangiosarcoma" or "malignant hemangioendothelioma," has been described in the Alpine regions of Switzerland, Austria, and Northern Italy where the incidence was much higher than the rest of the world (2–10% of thyroid malignancies in that region), and was linked to dietary iodine deficiency [4, 94]. This tumor does occur in non-Alpine, nonmountainous regions, but is much rarer [4, 94]. Tumors present as a "cold" nodule in elderly patients in their 6th and 7th decade with a female to male ratio of 4.5:1 [4, 94].

Grossly, tumors range from 3 to 10 cm and are circumscribed with infiltrative borders [4, 94]. Cut surfaces show a variegated tumor with cystic spaces and hemorrhage within the cysts [4, 94]. Microscopically, tumors are polymorphous with atypical spindled cells arranged in fascicles and anastomosing channels with papillary formations and extensive necrosis and hemorrhage. The channels and papillae are lined by plump pleomorphic epithelioid and polygonal cells with abundant eosinophillic cytoplasm, round vesicular nuclei, and prominent eosinophillic nucleoli [4, 94]. Cells may contain intracytoplasmic lumens with fragments of erythrocytes within the lumens [93, 94]. Mitotic activity is high and there is abundant brown hemosiderin present in the background [94]. Tumor cells are positive for immunostains which stain vessels (CD31 and CD34) and keratins in epithelioid areas [94].

The differential diagnosis is undifferentiated/anaplastic thyroid carcinoma and the distinction between the two can be quite difficult [4, 93, 94]. Prognosis is very poor with most patients dying within 6 months [4, 94, 95]. If the tumor is limited to the thyroid without extrathyroidal extension, survival may be longer than expected [4, 94].

Smooth muscle tumors. Smooth muscle tumors including benign leiomyomas and malignant leiomyosarcomas are very rare in the thyroid and usually attributed to vessels at the periphery of the gland [4]. Leiomyomas occur in women and present as a small isolated well-circumscribed mass with identical histologic and immunophenotypic features as leiomyomas in other locations [4, 84]. Leiomyosarcomas can be large and occur in the elderly with equal male and female incidence [4, 84]. Leiomyosarcomas are malignant smooth muscle sarcomas with nuclear pleomorphism, vascular invasion, necrosis, and hemorrhage [4].

Neural tumors. Neural tumors are rare and can be benign schwannomas or malignant peripheral nerve sheath tumors with the morphologic and immunohistochemical features of schwannomas and malignant peripheral nerve sheath tumors seen in other body sites [4]. There is no gender or age predilection [4].

Solitary fibrous tumor. Solitary fibrous tumor (SFT) is a rare spindle-cell mesenchymal tumor which is classically associated with the pleura but has been reported in most other body sites. SFTs occur predominantly in middle-age adults with a slight female predilection [4, 84] and present as well-circumscribed masses with gray to brown firm cut surfaces [4]. Tumor growth is storiform or hemangiopericytoma-like and composed of spindled cells with scant or indistinct cytoplasm and oval vesicular nuclei with fine and dispersed chromatin [4]. SFT should be distinguished from leiomyoma. SFTs have the potential to recur and spread and aggressive features include nuclear atypia, large size, and necrosis; however, no cases of recurrent or metastatic SFT of the thyroid have been reported to date [4]. Spindle cells are positive for CD34, CD99, and BCL2.

Secondary Tumors of the Thyroid Gland

Metastatic involvement of the thyroid gland by tumors can occur by direct extension or by hematogenous spread [4]. Tumors from the larynx, pharynx, lymph nodes, parathyroid, mediastinum, and soft tissue can directly infiltrate the thyroid. Metastases to the thyroid can be found in up to 25% of patients with disseminated cancer [4]. Tumors that most commonly metastasize to the

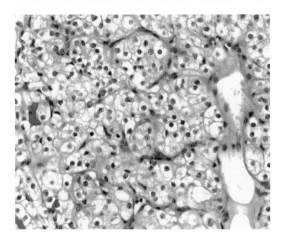

Fig. 1.47 Metastatic renal cell carcinoma (H&E)

thyroid include renal cell carcinoma, lung, uterus, melanoma, breast and stomach [4] (Fig. 1.47).

Molecular Pathology

RET/PTC Rearrangements

Rearrangement of RET (rearranged during transfection)-proto-oncogene is a major event in papillary thyroid carcinogenesis [96]. RET is located on chromosome 10 and encodes a tyrosine kinase receptor for neurotropic factors and when activated by constitutively expressed genes produces a fusion oncogene PET/PTC [97]. RET/PTC rearrangement can be found in 3–60% of PTCs and about 10% of poorly differentiated carcinomas [22, 96]. RET/PTC rearrangements vary significantly by geographic location, and in the adult non-radiation-exposed population in the United States its frequency is estimated at about 35% [22, 97]. The prevalence of RET/PTC is higher in the radiation-exposed population (60–70%) [97]. There are several RET rearrangements (up to 10) of which RET/PTC1 is the most common rearrangement (60–70%) followed by RET/PTC3 (20–30%) and RET/PTC 2 (<10%) [97]. RET/PTC may be responsible for the nuclear features seen in PTC, and classical papillary thyroid tends to have a higher frequency of RET/PTC [97]. Follicular variant of PTCs have lower frequency of RET/PTC, and solid variant is more often associated with RET/PTC3 [22]. RET/PTC rearrangements also occur in HTTs and have been found in patients with Hashimoto's thyroiditis [97]. Point mutations of RET can be seen in MTCs (sporadic and familial) [4].

BRAF Mutations

The RAS-RAF-MEK-ERK-MAP kinase pathway is a signal transduction pathway that regulates cell proliferation [98]. RAF proteins are serine/threonine kinases that are involved in activation of the MAPK pathway and involved in proliferation, apoptosis, and differentiation [4, 22]. BRAF mutations have been found in 29–70% of PTCs and are associated with classical, tall cell, and oncocytic variants of papillary carcinoma [4, 22]. The most common mutation is V600E and is a valine to glutamine substitution at amino acid residue 600 [22]. BRAF mutations can occur along with RET–PTC mutations [22]. BRAF mutations have been shown to be associated with a poorer outcome [99]. In a study of 219 patients with PTC, Xing et al. found a significant association between BRAF mutations and extrathyroidal extension, lymph node metastasis, and advanced tumor stage [99].

RAS Mutations

RAS genes are GTPases involved in signal transduction for cell proliferation in the RAS-RAF-MEK-ERK-MAP kinase pathway. RAS activating point mutations are found in less than 10% of PTCs [4, 100]. RAS has been found in greater proportion of follicular variant of papillary carcinomas [4]. RAS mutations have recently been found in strictly classified poorly differentiated thyroid carcinomas as the almost exclusive genetic event [100].

PAX8/PPARγ

PAX8/PPARγ(gamma) is an oncogene created by a balanced translocation between chromosome 2 and 3 [101]. PPAR is the peroxisome proliferator-activated receptor gamma, which is a part of a family of nuclear receptors which act as transcription factors for gene regulation [101]. PAX8 is involved in the terminal differentiation step in follicular cell development [101]. The fusion protein has been identified in about 36% follicular thyroid carcinomas, 11% of follicular adenomas, and 13% of follicular variant of PTCs [101].

Summary

Among primary thyroid malignancies, papillary thyroid carcinoma is the most common tumor of the thyroid, far outnumbering others. The increase in the reported incidence of papillary thyroid carcinoma is likely related to the increased detection of tumors by ultrasound imaging. Variants of papillary carcinoma associated with a more aggressive course include tall cell variant, columnar cell variant, and diffuse sclerosing variant. The diagnosis of follicular variant of papillary thyroid carcinoma remains particularly challenging for cytopathologists and surgical pathologists because the nuclear features of papillary carcinoma can be focal and/or subtle. Moreover, the behavior and molecular pathology of encapsulated follicular variant of papillary carcinoma suggest that this may represent an "intermediate" category of tumor between classical follicular adenoma/carcinoma and papillary carcinoma, and in clinical behavior. Molecular alterations in thyroid carcinoma are currently a subject of great research. RET/PTC rearrangements, BRAF mutations, RAS mutations, or PAX8/PPARγ are important genetic alterations in the majority of thyroid cancers. Most of these tests are currently available for tumors from formalin-fixed surgical specimens. Current efforts are to make these tests available on cytologic specimens to assist in management decisions for indeterminate thyroid nodules.

References

1. Faquin WC. Recurring problems in histologic and cytologic evaluation. Arch Pathol Lab Med. 2008; 132:622–32.
2. Peng Y, Wang HH. A meta-analysis of comparing fine-needle aspiration and frozen section for evaluating thyroid nodules. Diagn Cytopathol. 2008;36:916–20.
3. Kingston GW, Bugis SP, Davis N. Role of frozen section and clinical parameters in distinguishing benign from malignant follicular neoplasms of the thyroid. Am J Surg. 1992;164:603–5.
4. DeLellis RA, Lloyd RV, Heitz PU, Eng C. Pathology and genetics: tumors of endocrine organs. Lyon: IARC Press; 2004.
5. Livolsi VA, Baloch ZW. Use and abuse of frozen section in the diagnosis of follicular thyroid lesions. Endocr Pathol. 2005;16:285–93.
6. Leteurtre E, Leroy X, Pattou F, Wacrenier A, Carnaille B, Proye C, et al. Why do frozen sections have limited value in encapsulated or minimally invasive follicular carcinoma of the thyroid? Am J Clin Pathol. 2001; 115:370–4.
7. Rosen Y, Rosenblatt P, Saltzman E. Intraoperative pathologic diagnosis of thyroid neoplasms: report on experience with 504 specimens. Cancer. 1990;66: 2001–6.
8. Brooks AD, Shaha AR, DuMornay W, Huvos AG, Zakowski M, Brennan MF, et al. Role of fine needle aspiration biopsy and frozen section analysis in the surgical management of thyroid tumors. Ann Surg Oncol. 2001;8:92–100.
9. McHenry CR, Raeburn C, Strickland T, Marty JJ. The utility of routine frozen section examination for intraoperative diagnosis of thyroid cancer. Am J Surg. 1996;172:658–61.
10. Udelsman R, Westra WH, Donovan PI, Sohn TA, Cameron JL. Randomized prospective evaluation of frozen section analysis for follicular neoplasms of the thyroid. Ann Surg Oncol. 2001;233:716–22.
11. Callcut RA, Selvaggi SM, Mack E, Ozgul O, Warner T, Chen H. The utility of frozen section evaluation for follicular thyroid lesions. Ann Surg Oncol. 2003; 11:94–8.
12. Roach JC, Heller KS, Dubner S, Sznyter LA. The value of frozen section examinations in determining the extent of thyroid surgery in patients with indeterminate fine needle aspiration cytology. Arch Otolaryngol Head Neck Surg. 2002;128:263–7.
13. Zambudio AR, Gonzales JMR, Perez JS, Cogollos TS, Fernandez PJG, Paricio PP. Utility of frozen section examination for diagnosis of malignancy associated with multinodular goiter. Thyroid. 2004;14: 600–4.
14. Franc B, De La Salmoniere P, Lange F, Hoang C, Louvel A, De Roquancourt A, et al. Interobserver and intraobserver reproducibility in the histopathology of follicular thyroid carcinoma. Hum Pathol. 2003;34: 1092–100.

15. Baloch ZW, LiVolsi VA. Our approach to follicular patterned lesions of the thyroid. J Clin Pathol. 2007;60:244–50.
16. Baloch ZW, LiVolsi VA. Follicular patterned lesions of the thyroid: the bane of the pathologist. Am J Clin Pathol. 2002;117:143–50.
17. Livolsi VA, Baloch ZW. Follicular neoplasms of the thyroid: views, biases, and experiences. Adv Anat Pathol. 2004;11:279–87.
18. Serra S, Asa SL. Controversies in thyroid pathology: the diagnosis of follicular neoplasms. Endocr Pathol. 2008;19:156–65.
19. Baloch ZW, Livolsi VA. Cytologic and architectural mimics of papillary thyroid carcinoma. Am J Clin Pathol. 2006;125 Suppl 1:S135–44.
20. Pandit AA, Phulpagar MD. Worrisome histologic alterations following fine needle aspiration of the thyroid. Acta Cytol. 2001;45:173–9.
21. Thompson LDR, Wieneke JA, Paal E, Frommelt RA, Adair CF, Heffess CS. A clinicopathologic study of minimally invasive follicular carcinoma of the thyroid gland with a review of the English literature. Cancer. 2001;91:505–24.
22. DeLillis RA. Pathology and genetics of thyroid carcinoma. J Surg Oncol. 2006;94:662–9.
23. Medeiros-Neto G, Gil-Da-Costa MJ, Santos CLS, Medina M, Silva JCE, Tsou RM, et al. Metastatic thyroid carcinoma arising from congenital goiter due to mutation in the thyroid peroxidase gene. J Clin Endocrinol Metab. 1998;83:4162–6.
24. Alzahrani AS, Baitei EY, Zou M, Shi Y. Metastatic follicular thyroid carcinoma arising from congenital goiter as a result of a novel splice donor site mutation in the thyroglobulin gene. J Clin Endocrinol Metab. 2006;91:740–6.
25. Lin JD, Chao TC, Hsueh C. Follicular carcinomas with lung metastases: a 23 year retrospective study. Endocr J. 2004;51:519–225.
26. Ashfaq R, Vuitch F, Delgado R, Albores-Saavedra J. Papillary and follicular thyroid carcinomas with insular component. Cancer. 1994;73:416–23.
27. Ghossein R. Problems and controversies in the histopathology of thyroid carcinomas of follicular cell origin. Arch Pathol Lab Med. 2009;133:683–91.
28. Hirokawa M, Carney JA, Goellner JR, DeLellis RA, Heffess CS, Katoh R, et al. Observer variation of encapsulated follicular lesions of the thyroid gland. Am J Surg Pathol. 2002;26:1508–14.
29. Goldstein NS, Czako P, Neill JS. Metastatic minimally invasive (Encapsulated) follicular and Hurthle cell carcinoma: a study of 34 patients. Mod Pathol. 2000;13:123–30.
30. Hofman V, Lasalle S, Bonnetaud C, Butori C, Laoubatier C, Ilie M, et al. Thyroid tumors of uncertain malignant potential: frequency and diagnostic reproducibility. Virchows Arch. 2009;455:21–33.
31. Montone KT, Baloch ZW, LiVolsi VA. The thyroid Hurthle (Oncocytic) Cell and its associated pathologic conditions: a surgical pathology and cytopathology review. Arch Pathol Lab Med. 2008;132:1241–50.
32. Maximo V, Soares P, Lima J, Cameselle-Teijeiro J, Sobrinho-Simoes M. Mitochondrial DNA somatic mutations (point mutations and large deletions) and mitochondrial DNA variants in human thyroid pathology: a study with emphasis on Hurthle cell tumors. Am J Pathol. 2002;160:1857–65.
33. Asa SL. My approach to oncocytic tumors of the thyroid. J Clin Pathol. 2004;57:225–32.
34. Ghossen RA, Hiltzik DH, Carlson DL, Patel S, Shaha A, Shah JP, et al. Prognostic factors of recurrence in encapsulated Hurthle cell carcinoma of the thyroid gland. Cancer. 2006;106:1669–76.
35. Har-el G, Hadar T, Segal K, Levy R, Sidi J. Hurthle cell carcinoma of the thyroid gland: a tumor of moderate malignancy. Cancer. 1986;57:1613–7.
36. Lopez-Penabad L, Chiu AC, Hoff AO, Schultz P, Gaztambide S, Ordonez NG, et al. Prognostic factors in patients with Hurthle cell neoplasms of the thyroid. Cancer. 2003;97:1186–94.
37. Arganini M, Behar R, Wu TC, Straus F, McCormick M, DeGroot LJ, et al. Hurthle cell tumors: a twenty-five year experience. Surgery. 1986;100:1108–15.
38. Shaha AR, Loree TR, Shah JP. Prognostic factors and risk group analysis in follicular carcinoma of the thyroid. Surgery. 1995;118:1131–8.
39. Kaserer K, Scheuba C, Neuhold N, Weinhausel A, Haas OA, Vierhapper H, et al. Sporadic versus familial medullary thyroid microcarcinoma: a histopathologic study of 50 consecutive patients. Am J Surg Pathol. 2001;25:1245–51.
40. Etite D, Faquin WC, Gaz R, Randolph G, DeLellis RA, Pilch BZ. Histopathologic and clinical features of medullary microcarcinoma and C-cell hyperplasia in prophylactic thyroidectomies for medullary carcinoma: at study of 42 cases. Arch Pathol Lab Med. 2008;132:1767–73.
41. Livolsi VA, Feind CR. Incidental medullary thyroid carcinoma in sporadic hyperparathyroidism. An expansion of the concept of C-cell hyperplasia. Am J Clin Pathol. 1979;71:595–9.
42. Bergholm U, Bergstrom R, Ekbom A. Long term follow up of patients with medullary carcinoma of the thyroid. Cancer. 1997;79:132–8.
43. Scopsi L, Sampietro G, Boracchi P, Del Bo R, Gullo M, Placucci M, et al. Multivariate analysis of prognostic factors in sporadic medullary carcinoma of the thyroid: a retrospective review of 109 consecutive patients. Cancer. 1996;78:2173–83.
44. Franc B, Rosenberg-Bourgin M, Caillou B, Dutrieux-Berger N, Floquet J, Houcke-LeComte M, et al. Medullary thyroid carcinoma: Search for histological predictors of survival (109 Proband cases analysis). Hum Pathol. 1998;29:1078–84.
45. Edge SB, Byrd DR, Compton CC, Fritz AG, Fl G, Trotto A, editors. AJCC Cancer staging manual. 7th ed. New York, NY: Springer; 2010.
46. Carney JA, Ryan J, Goellner JR. Hyalinizing trabecular adenoma of the thyroid gland. Am J Surg Pathol. 1987;11:583–91.

47. Casey MB, Sebo TJ, Carney JA. Hyalinizing trabecular adenoma of the thyroid gland: cytologic features in 29 cases. Am J Surg Pathol. 2004;28:859–67.
48. McCluggage WG, Sloan JM. Hyalinizing trabecular carcinoma of thyroid gland. Histopathology. 1996;28: 357–62.
49. Gonzalez-Campora R, Fuentes-Vaamonde E, Hevia-Vazquez A, Otal-Salaverri C, Villar-Rodriguez JL, Galera-Davidson H. Hyalinizing trabecular carcinoma of the thyroid gland: report of two cases of follicular cell thyroid carcinoma with hyalinizing trabecular pattern. Ultrastruct Pathol. 1998;22:39–46.
50. Molberg K, Albores-Saavedra J. Hyalinizing trabecular carcinoma of the thyroid gland. Hum Pathol. 1994;25:192–7.
51. Papotti M, Volante M, Giuliano A, Fassina A, Fusco A, Bussolati G, et al. RET/PTC activation in hyalinizing trabecular tumors of the thyroid. Am J Surg Pathol. 2000;24:1615–21.
52. Davies L, Welch HG. Increasing incidence of thyroid cancer in the United States, 1973–2002. JAMA. 2006;295:2164–7.
53. Gilliland FD, Hunt WC, Morris DM, Key CR. Prognostic factors for thyroid carcinoma: a population based study of 15, 698 cases from the surveillance, epidemiology, and end results (SEER) program 1973–1991. Cancer. 1997;79:564–73.
54. Baloch ZW, LiVolsi VA. Etiology and significance of the "optically clear nucleus". Endocr Pathol. 2002; 13:289–99.
55. Llyod RV, Erickson LA, Casey MB, Lam KY, Lohse CM, Asa SL, et al. Observer variation in the diagnosis of follicular variant of papillary thyroid carcinoma. Am J Surg Pathol. 2004;28:1336–40.
56. Elsheikh TM, Asa SL, Chan JKC, DeLellis RA, Heffess CS, LiVolsi VA, et al. Interobserver and intraobserver variation among experts in the diagnosis of thyroid follicular lesions with borderline nuclear features of papillary carcinoma. Am J Clin Pathol. 2008;130:736–44.
57. Chan JKC. Strict criteria should be applied in the diagnosis of encapsulated follicular variant of papillary thyroid carcinoma. Am J Clin Pathol. 2002;117:16–8.
58. Baloch ZW, LiVolsi VA. Encapsulated follicular variant of papillary thyroid carcinoma with bone metastases. Mod Pathol. 2000;13:861–5.
59. Ghossein R, LiVolsi VA. Papillary thyroid carcinoma tall cell variant. Thyroid. 2008;18:1179–81.
60. Johnson TL, Lloyd RV, Thompson NW, Beierwaltes WH, Sisson JC. Prognostic implications of the tall cell variant of papillary thyroid carcinoma. Am J Surg Pathol. 1988;12:22–7.
61. Gaertner EM, Davidson M, Wenig BM. The columnar cell variant of thyroid papillary carcinoma: case report and discussion of an unusually aggressive thyroid papillary carcinoma. Am J Surg Pathol. 1995;19:940–7.
62. Wenig BM, Thompson LDR, Adair CF, Shmookler B, Heffess CS. Thyroid papillary carcinoma of columnar cell type: a clinicopathologic study of 16 cases. Cancer. 1998;82:740–53.
63. Lugli A, Terracciano LM, Oberholzer M, Bubendorf L, Tornillo L. Macrofollicular variant of papillary carcinoma of the thyroid: a histologic, cytologic, and Immunohistochemical study of 3 cases and review of the literature. Arch Pathol Lab Med. 2004;128:54–8.
64. Albores-Saavedra J, Gould E, Vardaman C, Vuitch F. The macrofollicular variant of papillary thyroid carcinoma: a study of 17 cases. Hum Pathol. 1991;22:1195–205.
65. Berho M, Suster S. The oncocytic variant of papillary carcinoma of the thyroid: a clinicopathologic study of 15 cases. Hum Pathol. 1997;28:47–53.
66. Baloch ZW, LiVolsi VA. Warthin-like papillary carcinoma of the thyroid. Arch Pathol Lab Med. 2000;124:1192–5.
67. Thompson LDR, Wieneke JA, Heffess CS. Diffuse sclerosing variant of papillary thyroid carcinoma: a clinicopathologic and immunophenotypic analysis of 22 cases. Endocr Pathol. 2005;16:331–48.
68. Carcangiu ML, Bianchi S. Diffuse sclerosing variant of papillary thyroid carcinoma: clinicopathologic study of 15 cases. Am J Surg Pathol. 1989;13:1040–9.
69. Fujimoto Y, Obara T, Ito Y, Kodama T, Aiba M, Yamaguchi K. Diffuse sclerosing variant of papillary carcinoma of the thyroid: clinical importance, surgical treatment, and follow up study. Cancer. 1990;66: 2306–12.
70. Hirokawa M, Kuma S, Miyauchi A, Qian ZR, Nakasono M, Sano T, et al. Morules in cribriform-morular variant of papillary thyroid carcinoma: immunohistochemical characteristics and distinction from squamous metaplasia. APMIS. 2004;112:275–82.
71. Baloch ZW, LiVolsi VA. Microcarcinoma of the thyroid. Adv Anat Pathol. 2006;13:69–75.
72. Volante M, Collini P, Nikiforov YE, Sakamoto A, Kakudo K, Katoh R, et al. Poorly differentiated thyroid carcinoma: the Turin proposal for the use of uniform diagnostic criteria and an algorithmic diagnostic approach. Am J Surg Pathol. 2007;31:1256–64.
73. Sanders EM, LiVolsi VA, Brierley J, Shin J, Randolph GW. An evidence based review of poorly differentiated thyroid cancer. World J Surg. 2007;31:934–45.
74. Rufini V, Salvatori M, Fadda G, Pinnarelli L, Castaldi P, Maussier ML, et al. Thyroid carcinomas with variable insular component: prognostic significance of histopathologic patterns. Cancer. 2007;110:1209–17.
75. Pellegriti G, Giuffrida D, Scollo C, Vigneri R, Regalbuto C, Squatrito S, et al. Long term outcome of patients with insular carcinoma of the thyroid: the insular histotype is an independent predictor of poor prognosis. Cancer. 2002;95:2076–85.
76. Venkatesh YSS, Ordonez NG, Shultz PN, Huckey RC, Goepfert H, Sammaan NA. Anaplastic carcinoma of the thyroid: a clinicopathologic study of 121 cases. Cancer. 1990;66:321–30.
77. Hurlimann J, Gardiol D, Scazziga B. Immunohistology of anaplastic thyroid carcinoma. A study of 43 cases. Histopathology. 1987;11:567–80.
78. Papi G, Corrado S, LiVolsi VA. Primary spindle cell lesions of the thyroid gland. Am J Clin Pathol. 2005;124 Suppl 1:S95–S123.

79. Derringer GA, Thompson LDR, Frommelt RA, Bijwaard KE, Heffess CS, Abbondanzo SL. Malignant lymphoma of the thyroid gland: a clinicopathologic study of 108 cases. Am J Surg Pathol. 2000;24:623–39.

80. Skacel M, Ross CW, His ED. A reassessment of primary thyroid lymphoma: high-grade MALT-type lymphoma as a distinct subtype of diffuse large B cell lymphoma. Histopathology. 2000;37:10–8.

81. Wenig BM, Adair CF, Heffess CS. Primary mucoepidermoid carcinoma of the thyroid gland: a report of six cases and a review of the literature of a follicular epithelial derived tumor. Hum Pathol. 1995;26:1099–108.

82. Baloch ZW, Solomon AC, LiVolsi VA. Primary mucoepidermoid carcinoma and sclerosing mucoepidermoid carcinoma with eosinophilia of the thyroid gland: a report of nine cases. Mod Pathol. 2000;13:802–7.

83. Ando M, Nakanishi Y, Asai M, Maeshima A, Matsuno Y. Mucoepidermoid carcinoma of the thyroid gland showing marked ciliation suggestive of its pathogenesis. Pathol Int. 2008;58:741–4.

84. Baloch ZW, LiVolsi VA. Unusual tumors of the thyroid gland. Endocrinol Metab Clin North Am. 2008; 37:297–310.

85. Sim SJ, Ro JY, Ordonez NG, Cleary KR, Ayala AG. Sclerosing mucoepidermoid carcinoma with eosinophilia of the thyroid: report of two patients, one with distant metastasis, and review of the literature. Hum Pathol. 1997;28:1091–6.

86. Cheuk W, Jacobson AA, Chan JKC. Spindle epithelial tumor with thymus-like differentiation (SETTLE): a distinctive malignant thyroid neoplasm with significant metastatic potential. Mod Pathol. 2000;13:1150–5.

87. Folpe AL, Lloyd RV, Bacchi CE, Rosai J. Spindle epithelial tumor with thymus-like differentiation: a morphologic, immunohistochemical, and molecular genetic study of 11 cases. Am J Surg Pathol. 2009;33:1179–86.

88. Reimann JDR, Dorfman DM, Nose V. Carcinoma showing thymus-like differentiation of the thyroid (CASTLE): a comparative study. Evidence of thymic differentiation and solid cell nest origin. Am J Surg Pathol. 2006;30:994–1001.

89. Ito Y, Miyauchi A, Nakamura Y, Miya A, Kobayashi K, Kakudo K. Clinicopathologic significance of intrathyroidal epithelial thymoma/carcinoma showing thymus-like differentiation. A collaborative study with member institutes of the Japanese Society of Thyroid Surgery. Am J Clin Pathol. 2007;127: 230–6.

90. Thompson LDR, Rosai J, Heffess CS. Primary thyroid teratomas: a clinicopathologic study of 30 cases. Cancer. 2000;88:1149–58.

91. Martins T, Carrillo M, Gomes L, Mesquita C, Martins M, Carvalheiro M. Malignant teratoma of the thyroid: case report. Thyroid. 2006;16:1311–3.

92. Nishihara E, Miyauchi A, Hirokawa M, Kudo T, Ohye H, Ito M, et al. Benign thyroid teratomas manifest painful cystic and solid composite nodules. Endocr J. 2006;30:231–6.

93. Papotti M, Arrondini M, Tavaglione V, Veltri A, Volante M. Diagnostic controversies in vascular proliferation of the thyroid gland. Endocr Pathol. 2008;19:175–83.

94. Ryska A, Ludvikova M, Szepe P, Boor A. Epithelioid haemangiosarcoma of the thyroid gland. Report of six cases from a non-Alpine region. Histopathology. 2004;44:40–6.

95. Maiorana A, Collina G, Cesinaro AM, Fano RA, Eusebi V. Epithelioid angiosarcoma of the thyroid. Clinicopathological analysis of seven cases from non-Alpine areas. Virchows Arch. 1996;429: 131–7.

96. Soares P, Trovisco V, Rocha AS, Lima J, Castro P, Preto A, et al. BRAF mutations and RET/PTC rearrangements are alternative events in etiopathogenesis of PTC. Oncogene. 2003;22:4578–80.

97. Nikiforov YE. RET/PTC Rearrangement in thyroid tumors. Endocr Pathol. 2002;13:13.

98. Xiulong X, Quiros RM, Gattuso P, Ain KB, Prinz RA. High prevalence of BRAF gene mutation in papillary thyroid carcinomas and thyroid tumor cell lines. Cancer Res. 2003;63:4561–7.

99. Xing M, Westra WH, Tufano RP, Cohen Y, Rosenbaum E, Rhoden KJ, et al. BRAF mutation predicts a poorer clinical prognosis for papillary thyroid cancer. J Clin Endocrinol Metab. 2005;90: 6373–9.

100. Volante M, Rapa I, Gandhi M, Bussolati G, Giachino D, Papotti M, et al. RAS mutations are the predominant molecular alteration in poorly differentiated thyroid carcinomas and bear prognostic impact. J Clin Endocrinol Metab. 2009;94:4735–41.

101. Eberhardt NL, Grebe SKG, McIver B, Reddi HV. The role of PAX8/PPARγ fusion oncogene in the pathogenesis of follicular thyroid cancer. Mol Cell Endocrinol. 2010;321:50–6.

Molecular Biology of Thyroid Cancer

Wenwen Chien and H. Phillip Koeffler

Introduction

Our medical discoveries often follow advancement in biologic techniques. The use of karyotypic analysis, fluorescent in situ hybridization, candidate gene sequencing, microarray expression analysis, and whole-genome associations has helped determine the molecular defects causing thyroid cancer. These and future discovered defects will allow clear classifications, precise prognosis, and targeted therapy. Genetic events involved in the development of well-differentiated papillary thyroid carcinoma (PTC) include rearrangement of the tyrosine receptor kinase RET and TRK and activating mutations of the intracellular signaling effectors BRAF (B-type Raf kinase) and RAS (see Fig. 2.1) [1]. Rearrangement of PAX8/PPARγ (peroxisome proliferator–activated receptor) and RAS mutations are frequent in well-differentiated follicular thyroid carcinoma (FTC). These mutations occasionally have been identified in benign follicular adenoma (FA). Also, loss of phosphate and tensin homolog (PTEN) and activation of PI3K/AKT are involved in FTC pathogenesis.

Progression of PTC and FTC to anaplastic thyroid carcinoma (ATC) is associated with mutation of p53, β catenin, as well as members of PI3K/AKT pathway. Recent reports suggest that additional molecular mechanisms such as epigenetic modification and microRNA deregulation are involved in the development of thyroid tumorigenesis. This review summarizes the molecular characterization of thyroid cancer and the molecular mechanisms involved in thyroid carcinogenesis. Table 2.1 lists the nomenclature for the various abbreviations used throughout the text.

Gene Rearrangement

Translocation of chromosomes can fuse two genes together to produce a novel protein with oncogenic properties. About 36% of FTC, 11% of FA, and 13% PTCfv (follicular variant of PTC) have a chromosomal translocation t(2;3)(q13;p25) which fuses a thyroid-specific transcription factor PAX8 to PPARγ, a nuclear hormone receptor normally involved in the differentiation of cells of different tissues especially adipocytes (see Fig. 2.2) [2–4]. This gene rearrangement has

W. Chien • H.P. Koeffler (✉)
Division of Oncology/Hematology, Department
of Medicine, Cedars-Sinai Medical Center,
8700 Beverly Blvd., NT Lower Level, AC1060,
Los Angeles, CA 90048, USA
e-mail: koeffler@cshs.org

G.D. Braunstein (ed.), *Thyroid Cancer*, Endocrine Updates 30,
DOI 10.1007/978-1-4614-0875-8_2, © Springer Science+Business Media, LLC 2012

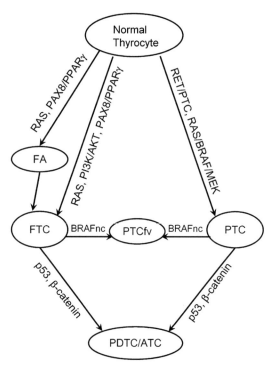

Fig. 2.1 Genetic events involved in thyroid tumorigenesis. *FA* follicular adenoma; *FTC* follicular thyroid carcinoma; *PTC* papillary thyroid carcinoma; *PTCfv* follicular variant of PTC; *PDTC* poorly differentiated thyroid carcinoma; *ATC* anaplastic thyroid cancer; *BRAFnc* nonconventional BRAF mutations (non-BRAF V600E). Adapted from Eberhardt et al. [1]

Table 2.1 Abbreviations used in this chapter

AKAP9	A-kinase anchor protein 9
AKT	Serine/thyreonine-specific protein kinase
APC	Adenomatosis polyposis coli
ATC	Anaplastic thyroid carcinoma
BRAF	V-raf murine sarcoma viral oncogene homolog B1
CK19	Cytokeratin 19
CS	Cowden syndrome
DAPK	Death-associated protein kinase
EGFR	Epidermal growth factor receptor
FA	Follicular adenoma
FAP	Familial adenomatous polyposis
FTC	Follicular thyroid carcinoma
GSK3	Glycogen synthase kinase-3 beta

Table 2.1 (continued)

HBME-1	Monoclonal antibody against a mesothelial cell antigen
HDAC	Histone deacetylase
Histone H4	Histone protein in nucleosome
HMGA2	High mobility group AT-hook 2
IRAK1	IL-receptor-associated kinase 1
LEF	lymphoid enhancing binding factor
MAPK	Mitogen-activated protein kinase
MEK	Mitogen-activated protein kinase 1
miRs	MicroRNAs
Myc	Transcription factor a portion of whose gene is similar to myelocytomatosis viral oncogene
NCOA4	Nuclear receptor coactivator 4
NFkB	Nuclear factor kappa B
NIS	Sodium iodide symporter
NTRK1	Neutropic thyrosine kinase receptor type 1
p53	Protein 53; a tumor suppressor protein
PAX8	Paired box gene 8
PDGFR	Platelet-derived growth factor receptor
PI3K	Phosphoinositide-3-kinase
PPARγ	Peroxisome proliferator-activated receptor (gamma)
PTC	Papillary thyroid carcinoma
PTCfv	Follicular variant of papillary thyroid carcinoma
PTEN	Phosphate and tensin homolog
RAS	Rat sarcoma oncogene; a transforming oncogene
RET	Rearranged during transfection; a proto-oncogene encoding a receptor tyrosine kinase
TCF	T-cell-specific transcription factor
TIMP3	Tissue inhibitor of metalloproteinase-3
TLR	Toll-like receptor
TMP3	Non-muscle tropomyosin
TRAF6	Tumor necrosis factor receptor-associated factor 6
TRK	Tyrosine receptor kinase
TSHR	Thyroid stimulation hormone receptor
TTF-1 -2	Transcription termination factor 1 and 2
3′ UTR	3′ untranslated region of mRNA
VEGF	Vascular endothelial growth factor
VEGFR	Vascular endothelial growth factor receptor
XRCC1	X-ray repair complementing defective repair in Chinese hamster cells 1

PAX8: Chromosome 2q13

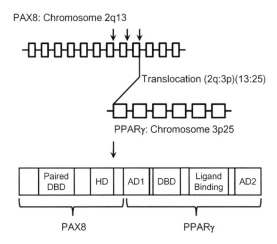

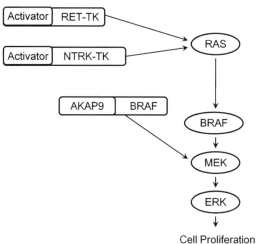

Cell Proliferation

Fig. 2.2 Schematic diagram of translocation between PAX8 on chromosome 2q13 and PPARγ on chromosome 3p25. *DBD* DNA-binding domains; *HD* homeodomain; *AD* transactivation domain; the different spliced isoforms of PAX8 which can fuse with PPARγ [4]

Fig. 2.3 Gene rearrangements in PTC. *TK* tyrosine kinase domain; *MEK* mitogen-activated protein kinase; *ERK* extracellular signal-regulated kinase

been identified as an early event in the development of FA and FTC. Opinions differ as to how the fusion product PAX8/PPARγ is oncogenic. Initial studies showed that the fusion protein can function as a dominant-negative suppressor of PPARγ-induced gene transcription [2] which confers anti-apoptotic properties [5]. Other studies showed that the fusion product can disrupt PAX8 transcriptional activity resulting in deregulation of expression of its target thyroid-specific genes such as thyroglobulin (Tg), thyroperoxidase (TPO), and sodium-iodide symporter (NIS) [6].

PTC is frequently (40–70%) associated with an RET gene rearrangement, in which the tyrosine kinase domain of the normally silent RET is fused with various constitutively expressed genes (see Fig. 2.3) [7]. The most common gene rearrangement products are RET/PTC1 (inv(10)(q11.2;q21)) and RET/PTC3 (inv(10)(q11.2;q10)). Both involve inversion of the long arm of chromosome 10, generating a fusion between RET and either histone H4 (histone protein in nucleosome) or nuclear receptor coactivator 4 (NCOA4) gene, respectively, for RET/PTC1 and RET/PTC3. Another gene rearrangement in PTC is an inversion of chromosome 7q generating fusion between BRAF and AKAP9 (A-kinase anchor protein 9 gene)

containing BRAF kinase domain without the N-terminal auto-inhibitory domain. This fusion protein has elevated kinase activity. BRAF mutation is common in sporadic PTC, while this novel AKAP9/BRAF (inv(7)(q21–22q34)) rearrangement occurs in radiation-induced thyroid carcinomas [8]. The other less common (<12%) gene rearrangement in PTC involves the fusion between the 3′ terminal sequences encoding the kinase domain of NTRK1 (neutropic tyrosine kinase receptor type 1) on chromosome 1 and 5′ terminal sequences of various genes resulting in activated TRK oncogenes [9]. The most frequent fusion product is between NTRK1 and TMP3 (nonmuscle tropomyosin). In PTC, fusion proteins with constitutively activated kinase produced by gene rearrangements stimulate downstream mitogen-activated protein kinase (MAPK) signaling and finally promote thyroid carcinogenesis.

Somatic Mutation

PTC frequently (30–69%) has a missense somatic mutation of BRAF at nucleotide 1799 substituting an A for a T, which changes valine to glutamic acid at amino acid 600 [10]. It is the most frequently known genetic event in PTC; and this mutation is associated with a block in differentiation of PTC. The change activates BRAF kinase leading to stimulation of the MAPK pathway, which blocks the normal differentiation of thyroid cells. The BRAF mutation occurs in about 40% of papillary and 25% of anaplastic thyroid tumors. Although this V600E BRAF mutation is highly prevalent in adult PTC, it is infrequent in childhood thyroid cancer as well as in radiation-induced thyroid tumors [11, 12]. RAS is a kinase that is upstream of BRAF. Three RAS (H-, N-, and K-) forms exist. RAS mutation occurs in 10–20% of PTC, 40–50% of FTC, and in more than 50% ATC. These mutations always localize to either codon 12, 13, or 61 [13, 14]. Mutations of either H-RAS or N-RAS at codon 61 are the most frequent RAS changes in thyroid cancer. This

mutation inactivates the intrinsic GTPase activity, and, in turn, mutant RAS constitutively activates the MAPK and PI3K/AKT signaling pathways.

Signaling Pathways

Many of the genetic changes including RET/PTC gene rearrangements and RAS and BRAF mutations cause activation of the MAPK and PI3K/AKT signaling pathways (see Fig. 2.4) [15]. PTEN is a phosphatase that acts as a suppressor of PI3K/AKT pathway. Both allelic imbalance, including deletion of the PTEN locus at 10q23 (20–60% of thyroid malignancies), and silencing of PTEN by aberrant promoter methylation (>50% of FTC) enhance PI3K signaling

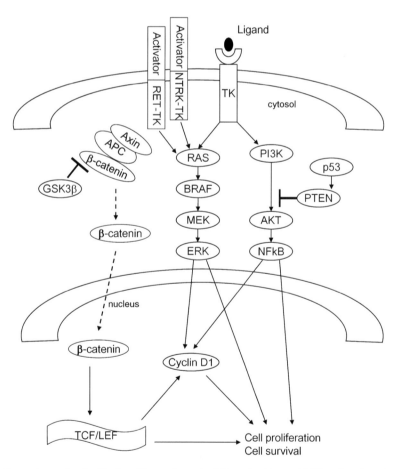

Fig. 2.4 Signaling pathways involved in thyroid tumorigenesis. *TK* tyrosine kianse; *NFkB* nuclear factor kappa B; *GSK3β* glycogen synthase kinase 3 beta; *TCF/LEF* T-cell specific transcription factor/lymphoid enhancer binding factor

and is associated with progression of thyroid tumors [16–18]. Beta-catenin signaling has emerged as another pathway of significance in thyroid cancer since proteins that regulate β-catenin (beta) activity are frequently activated, including AKT [19]. Beta-catenin is a part of a cytoplasmic complex also containing APC (adenomatosis polyposis coli) and axin, which is regulated by glycogen synthase kinase-3 (GSK3β). When the complex is phosphorylated by GSK3β, it undergoes ubiquitination and degradation. AKT phosphorylates and inactivates GSK3β releasing β-catenin from the complex, allowing it to be translocated to nucleus. In the nucleus, β-catenin activates T-cell-specific transcription factor/lymphoid enhancer binding factor (TCF/LEF) target genes such as cyclin D1 and myc, which promote cell proliferation. In some poorly differentiated PTC and undifferentiated ATC, β-catenin harbors a mutation in exon 3 where phosphorylation sites are involved in β-catenin degradation. Therefore, the mutation is associated with aberrant nuclear localization of the protein and stimulation of cell proliferation. These mutations of β-catenin are associated with a poor prognosis [20]. In PTC cell lines transfected with RET/PTC, β-catenin nuclear localization was dependent on RET/PTC kinase activity; and silencing of β-catenin by siRNA suppressed cell proliferation [21].

Epigenetic Regulation Of Genes

Two mechanisms are commonly involved in epigenetic regulation of genes: DNA methylation and histone modifications. Many thyroid-specific genes such as those for the sodium iodide symporter (NIS) and thyroid-stimulating hormone receptor (TSHR) are methylated in their promoter and their expression in thyroid cancer is frequently lost. Exposure of these cells to a histone deacetylase (HDAC) inhibitor in vitro can induce NIS expression in thyroid cancer cell lines, suggesting a role of deacetylation of histones in thyroid tumorigenesis [22]. Studies have shown that thyroid cancer cells with a BRAF mutation can be associated with methylation of iodide-metabolizing

genes [23, 24]. Treatment of a human PTC-derived cell line that has a BRAF V600E mutation with a mitogen-activated protein kinase 1 (MEK) inhibitor restored the expression of TSHR and NIS [25]. Aberrant promoter methylation of the tumor suppressor gene PTEN occurs in more than 50% of FTC, which leads to gene silencing of PTEN resulting in activation of the PI3K/AKT signaling pathway [26]. In PTC, aberrant methylation of tumor suppressor genes such as TIMP3 (tissue inhibitor of metalloproteinase-3) and DAPK (death-associated protein kinase) has been associated with tumor aggressiveness [27].

Micro RNA

MicroRNAs (miRs) are short noncoding RNAs involved in gene silencing by binding to complementary sequences in the 3′UTR (untranslated region) of target mRNAs. A multitude of genes are regulated by miRs, including those involved in cell proliferation, apoptosis, and differentiation. Aberrant expression of miRs occurs in human cancers. miR expression profile analysis by microarrays containing precursor and mature miR oligonucleotide probes have been examined in thyroid cancer and have identified a distinct set of miR transcripts including upregulation of miR-221, -222, -181b, and -146 in PTC compared to normal thyroid tissue [28–30].

Laboratory studies using human PTC-derived cell lines have shown that overexpression of miR-221 in these cells lead to their enhanced proliferation; in contrast, inhibition of miR-221 expression by an antisense oligonucleotide inhibited their cell growth [30]. One of the predicted target genes of miR-221 is Cyr61 which was shown to be downregulated in a study that examined both RNA levels and protein expression by tissue microarrays on 107 PTC samples compared to normal thyroid tissue [31]. Further studies are required to elucidate the role of Cyr61 in thyroid pathogenesis. Another miR of interest is miR-146a. A common (6%) polymorphism in the precursor of this miR causes decreased expression of the mature miR-146a, which reduces the inhibition of its target genes [32]. Two of these are IL-1 receptor-associated kinase 1 (IRAK1) and TNF receptor-associated factor 6 (TRAF6), two key molecules in the toll-like receptor (TLR) signaling pathway. Activation of TLR signaling activates the NFκB pathway and promotes thyroid tumorigenesis [33, 34]. This suggests that patients carrying this common polymorphism in their germ line have a predisposition to PTC.

Genetic Signatures of Malignancy

Microarray technology has provided molecular characterization of thyroid pathologies. Up to 20% of thyroid nodules cannot be diagnosed by fine-needle aspiration biopsy. Microarrays and multigene assays can be used as adjuncts to morphology after obtaining a biopsy. Gene expression analysis demonstrated that cyclin D1 is overexpressed in PTC, which is not detectable in normal thyroid tissue [35]. This suggests that the levels of cyclin D1 can be used as a diagnostic marker. Changes in gene expression profiles provide insights into stages of tumor progression. For example, a study of 100 benign and 105 malignant thyroid tumors using a panel of 57 molecular markers found an association of tumor pathology with the expression of a subset of markers including cytokeratin 19 (CK19), galectin-3, HBME-1, vascular endothelial growth factor (VEGF), androgen receptor, p16, and aurora-A kinase [36]. They showed that this subset of markers can discriminate benign versus differentiated thyroid carcinoma. Among the markers, CK19, galectin-3, HBME-1, and VEGF have been successfully used as preoperative diagnostic markers from tissue obtained by fine-needle aspiration and biopsy [37–40]. In another microarray analysis of 54 benign and 44 malignant tumors, 12 genes were identified as differentially expressed. Nine genes were overexpressed [high mobility group AT-hook 2 (HMGA2), leucine-rich repeat kinase 2, pleiomorphic adenoma gene 1, dipeptidyl-peptidase 4, P-cadherin, CD66c, serine protease 3, testican-1, and phosphodiesterase 5 A] and three were underexpressed (recombination activating gene 2, angiotensin II receptor type 1, and thyroid peroxidase transcript variant 5) in malignant thyroid tumor compared with benign thyroid masses [41]. Expression of HMGA2 correlates with malignant phenotype of thyroid tumors and can be used as a tool to differentiate malignant from benign lesions [42, 43].

Genetic Susceptibility

Genome-wide association studies enable identification of genetic susceptibility loci for the development of tumors (Table 2.2) [15, 44–48]. In one study of a European population, common variants on 9q22.33 and 14q13.3 were associated with thyroid cancer [44]. Individuals who were homozygous for both variants were at a 5.7-fold greater risk of developing either PTC or FTC. Two transcription factors, TTF-1 and -2 (transcription termination factor 1 and 2), are located at these regions. Both transcription factors are involved in the regulation of thyroglobulin and TPO which are crucial for thyroid organogenesis and differentiation. Also, a putative noncoding RNA gene AK023948 on chromosome 8q24 has

Table 2.2 Genetic susceptibility loci for thyroid cancer

Chromosome	Gene	Function	Specific type of thyroid cancer
1q41–42	ADPRT	ADP-ribosyltransferase	PTC and FTC [47]
2q12–14	VDR	Vitamin D receptor	FTC [46]
5q33	Pre-MiR-146a	Gene regulation	PTC [32]
8q24	AK023948	Noncoding RNA	PTC [45]
9q22.33	FOXE1	Thyroid differentiation	PTC and FTC [44]
12q24	P2X7R	Purinergic receptor	PTCfv [48]
14q13.3	TTF-1	Thyroid differentiation	PTC and FTC [44]
19q13.2–13.3	XRCC1	DNA repair	PTC and FTC [47]

Adapted from Kouniavsky and Zeiger [15]

been identified as a susceptibility gene for PTC [45]. Expression analysis showed that AK023948 is downregulated in PTC. In another study, a vitamin D receptor polymorphism was associated with an increased risk of FTC [46]. In addition, polymorphism of a DNA repair gene XRCC1 (X-ray repair complementing defective repair in Chinese hamster cells 1) is associated with either radiation-induced or sporadic PTC [47]. Approximately 5% of thyroid cancers are associated with hereditary germline genetic changes (see Fig. 2.5) [49]. Identification of the susceptibility genes for these familial cancer syndromes can aid in early diagnosis (see Table 2.3) [49]. Inactivating mutation of APC tumor suppressor gene results in familial adenomatous polyposis (FAP) and some of these patients will develop PTC which is associated with acquiring an additional RET/PTC somatic mutation. Cowden syndrome (CS) is an autosomal-dominant disorder resulting from a PTEN germline mutation. Approximately two-thirds of

Table 2.3 Familial thyroid cancer syndromes

Name	Gene mutation	Histological features
FAP	APC	Cribriform variant of PTC
Gardner's syndrome	APC	Cribriform variant of PTC
Cowden's disease	PTEN	FTC
Werner's syndrome	WRN	PTC,FTC,ATC
Carney's complex	PRKAR1alpha	PTC,FTC

FAP familial adenomatous polyposis. Adapted from Vriens et al. [49]

the CS patients will develop benign thyroid lesions and 10% have an increased risk for developing thyroid cancer [50].

Conclusions

Advancement of molecular biology technique provides insights into cause, classification, and prognosis of thyroid cancer. The early genetic events such as mutation of BRAF and rearrangement of PAX8/PPARγ leading to PTC and FTC are mutually exclusive events, suggesting their downstream pathways may intersect. These, as well as RAS mutations, can provide accurate diagnostic markers for initial fine-needle aspiration. Gene expression analysis has begun to elucidate a diagnostic signature of thyroid cancer versus non-neoplastic masses. Further enhancement of accurate diagnosis will be attained when more biological markers have been identified and validated.

During the progression of thyroid tumors, overexpression of EGFR (epidermal growth factor receptor), PDGFR (platelet-derived growth factor receptor), and VEGFR (vascular endothelial growth factor receptor) often occurs. Clinical studies with inhibitors of several tyrosine kinase receptors have shown that these activated growth factor receptors can be suppressed resulting in stabilization or partial remissions of the thyroid cancer [51–54]. Identification of additional molecular targets will enhance the identification of more effective approaches to advanced thyroid cancer.

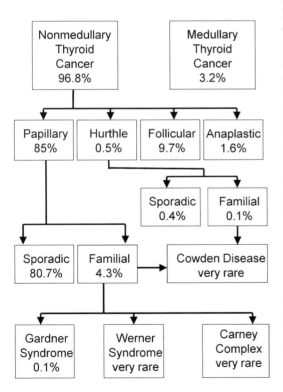

Fig. 2.5 Relative frequency of different types of familial/thyroid cancer

References

1. Eberhardt NL, Grebe SKG, McIver B, Reddi HV. The role of the PAX8/PPAR gamma fusion oncogene in the pathogenesis of follicular thyroid cancer. Mol Cell Endocrinol. 2010;321:50–6.
2. Kroll TG, Sarraf P, Pecciarini L, et al. PAX8-PPAR gamma 1 fusion in oncogene human thyroid carcinoma. Science. 2000;289:1357–60.
3. Castro P, Rebocho AP, Soares RJ, et al. PAX8-PPAR gamma rearrangement is frequently detected in the follicular variant of papillary thyroid carcinoma. J Clin Endocrinol Metab. 2006;91:213–20.
4. Reddi HV, McIver B, Grebe SKG, Eberhardt NL. The paired box-8/peroxisome proliferator-activated receptor-gamma oncogene in thyroid tumorigenesis. Endocrinology. 2007;148:932–5.
5. Martelli ML, Iuliano R, Le Pera I, et al. Inhibitory effects of peroxisome proliferator-activated receptor gamma on thyroid carcinoma cell growth. J Clin Endocrinol Metab. 2002;87:4728–35.
6. Au AYM, McBride C, Wilhelm Jr KG, et al. PAX8-peroxisome proliferator-activated receptor gamma (PPAR gamma) disrupts normal PAX8 or PPAR gamma transcriptional function and stimulates follicular thyroid cell growth. Endocrinology. 2006;147:367–76.
7. Zitzelsberger H, Bauer V, Thomas G, Unger K. Molecular rearrangements in papillary thyroid carcinomas. Clin Chim Acta. 2010;411:301–8.
8. Ciampi R, Knauf JA, Kerler R, et al. Oncogenic AKAP9-BRAF fusion is a novel mechanism of MAPK pathway activation in thyroid cancer. J Clin Invest. 2005;115:94–101.
9. Greco A, Miranda C, Pierotti MA. Rearrangements of NTRK1 gene in papillary thyroid carcinoma. Mol Cell Endocrinol. 2010;321:44–9.
10. Kimura ET, Nikiforova MN, Zhu Z, et al. High prevalence of BRAF mutations in thyroid cancer: Genetic evidence for constitutive activation of the RET/PTC-RAS-BRAF signaling pathway in papillary thyroid carcinoma. Cancer Res. 2003;63:1454–7.
11. Kumagai A, Namba H, Saenko VA, et al. Low frequency of BRAFT1796A mutations in childhood thyroid carcinomas. J Clin Endocrinol Metab. 2004;89:4280–4.
12. Lima J, Trovisco V, Soares P, et al. BRAF mutations are not a major event in post-Chernobyl childhood thyroid carcinomas. J Clin Endocrinol Metab. 2004;89:4267–71.
13. Vasko V, Ferrand M, Di Cristofaro J, et al. Specific pattern of RAS oncogene mutations in follicular thyroid tumors. J Clin Endocrinol Metab. 2003;88:2745–52.
14. Nikiforova MN, Lynch RA, Biddinger PW, et al. RAS point mutations and PAX8-PPAR gamma rearrangement in thyroid tumors: Evidence for distinct molecular pathways in thyroid follicular carcinoma. J Clin Endocrinol Metab. 2003;88:2318–26.
15. Kouniavsky G, Zeiger AM. Thyroid tumorigenesis and molecular markers in thyroid cancer. Curr Opin Oncol. 2010;22:23–9.
16. Yeh JJ, Marsh DJ, Zedenius J, et al. Fine-structure deletion mapping of 10q22-24 identifies regions of loss of heterozygosity and suggests that sporadic follicular thyroid adenomas and follicular thyroid carcinomas develop along distinct neoplastic pathways. Genes Chromosomes Cancer. 1999;26:322–8.
17. Frisk T, Foukakis T, Dwight T, et al. Silencing of the PTEN tumor-suppressor gene in anaplastic thyroid cancer. Genes Chromosomes Cancer. 2002;35:74–80.
18. Alvarez-Nunez F, Bussaglia E, Mauricio D, et al. PTEN promoter methylation in sporadic thyroid carcinomas. Thyroid. 2006;16:17–23.
19. Abbosh PH, Nephew KP. Multiple signaling pathways converge on beta-catenin in thyroid cancer. Thyroid. 2005;15:551–61.
20. Garcia-Rostan G, Camp RL, Herrero A, et al. Beta-catenin dysregulation in thyroid neoplasms. Am J Pathol. 2001;158:987–96.
21. Castellone MD, De Falco V, Rao DM, et al. The beta-catenin axis integrates multiple signals downstream from RET/Papillary Thyroid Carcinoma leading to cell proliferation. Cancer Res. 2009;69:1867–76.
22. Akagi T, Luong QT, Gui D, et al. Induction of sodium iodide symporter gene and molecular characterisation of HNF3β/FoxA2, TTF-1 and C/EBPβ in thyroid carcinoma cells. Br J Cancer. 2008;99:781–8.
23. Hoque MO, Rosenbaum E, Westra WH, et al. Quantitative assessment of promoter methylation profiles in thyroid neoplasms. J Clin Endocrinol Metab. 2005;90:4011–8.
24. Liu D, Liu Z, Jiang D, Dackiw AP, Xing M. Inhibitory effects of the mitogen-activated protein kinase inhibitor CI-1040 on the proliferation and tumor growth of thyroid cancer cells with BRAF or RAS mutations. Clin Cancer Res. 2007;92:4686–95.
25. Liu D, Hu S, Hou P, Jiang D, Condouris S, Xing M. Suppression of BRAF/MEK/MAP kinase pathway restores expression of iodide-metabolizing genes in thyroid cells expressing the V600E BRAF mutant. J Clin Endocrinol Metab. 2007;13:1341–9.
26. Hou P, Ji M, Xing M. Association of PTEN gene methylation with genetic alterations in the phosphatidylinositol 3-kinase/AKT signaling pathway in thyroid tumors. Cancer. 2008;113:2440–7.
27. Hu SH, Liu D, Tufalno RP, et al. Association of aberrant methylation of tumor suppressor genes with tumor aggressiveness and BRAF mutation in papillary thyroid cancer. Int J Cancer. 2006;119:2322–9.
28. Nikiforova MN, Nikiforov YE. Molecular diagnostics and predictors in thyroid cancer. Thyroid. 2009;19:1351–61.
29. He HH, Jazdzewski K, Li W, et al. The role of microRNA genes in papillary thyroid carcinoma. Proc Natl Acad Sci USA. 2005;102:19075–80.
30. Pallante P, Visone R, Ferracin M, et al. MicroRNA deregulation in human thyroid papillary carcinomas. Endocr Relat Cancer. 2006;13:497–508.

31. Wasenius V-M, Hemmer S, Kettunen E, Knuutila S, Franssila K, Joensuu H. Hepatocyte growth factor receptor, matrix metalloproteinase-11, tissue inhibitor of metalloproteinase-1, and fibronectin are up-regulated in papillary thyroid carcinoma. Clin Cancer Res. 2003;9:68–75.

32. Jazdzewski K, Murray EL, Franssila K, Jarzab B, Schoenberg DR, de la Chapelle A. Common SNP in pre-miR-146a decreases mature miR expression and predisposes to papillary thyroid carcinoma. Proc Natl Acad Sci USA. 2008;105:7269–74.

33. McCall KD, Harii N, Lewis CJ, et al. High basal levels of functional toll-like receptor 3 (TLR3) and noncanonical Wnt5a are expressed in papillary thyroid cancer and are coordinately decreased by phenylmethimazole together with cell proliferation and migration. Endocrinology. 2007;148:4226–37.

34. Pacifico F, Mauro C, Barone C, et al. Oncogenic and anti-apoptotic activity of NF-κB in human thyroid carcinomas. J Biol Chem. 2004;279:54610–9.

35. Basolo FC, Pinchera MA, Fedeli M, et al. Cyclin D1 overexpression in thyroid carcinomas: relation with clinico-pathological parameters, retinoblastoma gene product, and Ki67 labeling index. Thyroid. 2000;10:741–6.

36. Wiseman SM, Melck A, Masoudi H, et al. Molecular phenotyping of thyroid tumors identifies a marker panel for differentiated thyroid cancer diagnosis. Ann Surg Oncol. 2008;15:2811–26.

37. Nasser SM, Pitman MB, Pilch BZ, Faquin WC. Fine-needle aspiration biopsy of papillary thyroid carcinoma. Cancer. 2000;90:307–11.

38. Sanabria A, Carvalho AL, Piana de Andrade V, Pablo Rodrigo J, et al. Is galectin-3 a good method for the detection of malignancy in patients with thyroid nodules and a cytologic diagnosis of follicular neoplasm? A critical appraisal of the evidence. Head Neck. 2007;29:1046–54.

39. de Micco C, Savchenko V, Giorgi R, Sebag F, Henry JF. Utility of malignancy markers in fine-needle aspiration cytology of thyroid nodules: comparison of Hector Battifora mesothelial antigen-1, thyroid peroxidase and dipeptidyl aminopeptidase IV. Br J Cancer. 2008;98:818–23.

40. Hedayati M, Kołomecki K, Pasieka Z, Korzeniowska M, Kuzdak K. Assessment of VEGF and VEGF receptor concentrations in patients with benign and malignant thyroid tumors. Endokrynol Pol. 2005;56:252–8.

41. Prasad NB, Somervell H, Tufano RP, et al. Identification of genes differentially expressed in benign versus malignant thyroid tumors. Clin Cancer Res. 2008;14:3327–37.

42. Belge G, Meyer A, Klemke M, et al. Upregulation of HMGA2 in thyroid carcinomas: a novel molecular marker to distinguish between benign and malignant follicular neoplasias. Genes Chromosomes Cancer. 2008;47:56–63.

43. Chiappetta G, Botti G, Monaco M, et al. HMGA1 protein overexpression in human breast carcinomas. Clin Cancer Res. 2004;10:7637–44.

44. Gudmundsson J, Sulem P, Gudbjartsson DF, et al. Common variants on 9q22.33 and 14q13.3 predispose to thyroid cancer in European populations. Nat Genet. 2009;41:460–4.

45. He H, Nagy R, Liyanarachchi S, et al. A susceptibility locus for papillary thyroid carcinoma on chromosome 8q24. Cancer Res. 2009;69:625–31.

46. Penna-Martinez M, Ramos-Lopez E, Stern J, et al. Vitamin D receptor polymorphisms in differentiated thyroid carcinoma. Thyroid. 2009;19:623–8.

47. Chiang FY, Wu CW, Hsiao PJ, et al. Association between polymorphisms in DNA base excision repair genes XRCC1, APE1, and ADPRT and differentiated thyroid carcinoma. Clin Cancer Res. 2008;14:5919–24.

48. Dardano A, Falzoni S, Caraccio N, et al. 1513A>C Polymorphism in the P2X7 receptor gene in patients with papillary thyroid cancer: correlation with histological variants and clinical parameters. J Clin Endocrinol Metab. 2009;94:695–8.

49. Vriens MR, Suh I, Moses W, Kebebew E. Clinical features and genetic predisposition to hereditary nonmedullary thyroid cancer. Thyroid. 2009;19:1343–9.

50. Blumenthal GM, Dennis PA. PTEN hamartoma tumor syndromes. Eur J Hum Genet. 2008;16:1289–300.

51. Sherman SI, Wirth LJ, Droz JP, et al. Motesanib diphosphate in progressive differentiated thyroid cancer. N Engl J Med. 2008;359:31–42.

52. Eder JP, Shapiro GI, Appleman LJ, et al. A phase I study of foretinib, a multi-targeted inhibitor of c-Met and vascular endothelial growth factor receptor 2. Clin Cancer Res. 2010;16:3507–16.

53. Cohen EE, Rosen LS, Vokes EE, et al. Axitinib is an active treatment for all histologic subtypes of advanced thyroid cancer: results from a phase II study. J Clin Oncol. 2008;26:4708–13.

54. Britten CD, Kabbinavar F, Hecht JR, et al. A phase I and pharmacokinetic study of sunitinib administered daily for 2 weeks, followed by a 1-week off period. Cancer Chemother Pharmacol. 2008;61:515–24.

Thyroid Nodules

Glenn D. Braunstein and Wendy Sacks

Introduction

Thyroid nodules are quite common, and are often discovered as an incidental finding on a physical examination, through imaging modalities or at autopsy. The vast majority of these nodules are benign and do not require any specific therapy. Thyroid nodules are evaluated in order to see if the lesion is benign or malignant, or, in a patient with hyperthyroidism, to see if the nodule is the source of excessive thyroid hormone. In addition to important historical details, neck examination, a serum TSH measurement, and, in some instances, a serum calcitonin measurement, with a thyroid and neck ultrasonography, provide a substantial amount of important information which will direct subsequent evaluation, including the need for a fine-needle-aspiration biopsy (FNAB) of the lesion(s). The management of the nodule is dictated by these findings and subsequent behavior.

Epidemiology of Thyroid Nodules

As part of the Framingham Heart Disease Epidemiological Study, 5,127 members of the community had their thyroid palpated and 4.2% were found to have thyroid nodules [1]. Among women, 6.4% had nodules, in contrast to only 1.5% of the men. These patients were followed up for 15 years and 67 new lesions were found for a 15-year incidence rate of 1.4%, 1.7% in females and 0.9% in males [2]. Neck examination of 2,979 residents of Whickham, England, yielded a nodule prevalence of 3.2% [3], while in 253 Finns 5.1% were found to have palpable nodules [4]. Following the Chernobyl nuclear reactor accident, 2,416 male clean-up workers were carefully examined and 6.9% were found to have nodules [5]. We examined 100 normal hospital workers in Los Angeles and found 21 palpable nodules, including 9 with single nodules and 12 with multiple nodules [6]. Thus, the prevalence of palpable thyroid nodules falls between 3.2 and 21% in various populations.

A number of studies have examined the prevalence of thyroid nodules detected by ultrasonography. The prevalence of thyroid "incidentalomas" accidentally discovered during performance of a carotid ultrasound or for evaluation of hyperparathyroidism ranges from 13 to 46% [7–9]. Multiple prospective studies of the prevalence of thyroid nodules detected by ultrasound have yielded figures that vary from 10 to 67% [5, 6, 10–13]. One of the reasons for the discrepancies between the different studies may be related to the type of transducer used in the studies. The range in nodule prevalence for those studies that used 5.5–7.5-MHz transducers was 10–27% [4, 5, 7, 10, 11], whereas those that used 10–15-MHz transducers reported a prevalence of 34.7–67% [6, 8, 9, 13].

G.D. Braunstein (✉) • W. Sacks
Divison of Endocrinology, Diabetes, and Metabolism,
Department of Medicine, Cedars-Sinai Medical Center,
8700 Beverly Blvd Room 2119, Plaza Level,
Los Angeles, CA 90048, USA
e-mail: braunstein@cshs.org

G.D. Braunstein (ed.), *Thyroid Cancer*, Endocrine Updates 30,
DOI 10.1007/978-1-4614-0875-8_3, © Springer Science+Business Media, LLC 2012

Therefore, as the sensitivity of the imaging instruments increases, more nodules are detected.

The prevalence of thyroid nodules found at autopsy in patients dying from unrelated conditions is relatively high. In a series of 821 patients who had normal thyroids on clinical examination and died, 49.5% were found to have nodules, with 12.2% having a single nodule and 37.3% with multiple nodules [14]. Another autopsy series of 215 patients reported a 60% prevalence of nodules in patients who had had normal thyroids reported on clinical examination [15]. Other studies have reported prevalences that range from 8.2 to 64.6% [16–20]. These data suggest that with the use of sensitive 10–15-MHz ultrasound transducers, most thyroid nodules will be detected.

The differences between the prevalence of thyroid nodules found on clinical examination and those found on ultrasound or at autopsy relate to the skill of the individual performing the neck examination, the size of the nodule, and the location of the nodule, with small posterior nodules being more difficult to feel than the same-sized nodule located in a more anterior position. Takahashi and co-workers examined the relationship between the ability to palpate a nodule and the nodule size. They found that nodules under 5 mm were not palpable, about 35% of 1 cm nodules were detected, 80% of 1.5-cm nodules were palpated, and close to 100% of 2.0-cm nodules could be felt [21]. Indeed, in one study of thyroid incidentalomas picked up by palpation and/or ultrasound, 63% of the nodules were less than 1 cm, accounting for the discrepancy between nodules detected by palpation and those detected by ultrasonography [6].

Malignancy Rate of Thyroid Nodules

The percentage of thyroid nodules that are malignant in unselected populations is low. In the Framingham Heart Disease Epidemiological Study, none of the 218 original patients with nodules or the 67 who developed nodules during the 15-year follow-up was found to have thyroid cancer [1, 2]. In contrast, numerous other studies have documented a 5–17% risk of malignancy in patients with thyroid nodules, whether detected by palpation or ultrasonography [22–30].

The size of the thyroid nodule does not predict the likelihood of differentiated thyroid carcinoma. In 494 patients with nonpalpable nodules, Papini and colleagues found that 7% of nodules measuring 8–10 mm were cancer, while 9.1% of 11–15-mm nodules had cancer [27]. Nam-Goong et al. noted that 8% of the 25 patients with incidentally found thyroid nodules <5 mm, 15% of the 153 patients with nodules measuring 5–10 mm, and 13% of the 139 patients with 10–15-mm nodules had cancer [30]. In addition, the cancer rates for patients with solitary nodules and those with multiple thyroid nodules are virtually identical, as shown by numerous groups [22–29].

Autopsy studies have found that 0.5–35.6% of populations from the US, Japan, Canada, Poland, Portugal, Sweden, Italy, Chile, Finland, Germany, and Argentina have at least microscopic thyroid cancer [31–44]. The differences between studies relate in part to the thinness of the microscopic sections that were made from the thyroid, the diligence of the pathologists, the diagnostic criteria applied to very small lesions or lesions with a few features of papillary carcinoma, and the population studied. The median prevalence from these studies is 6.5%. The majority of the tumors found at autopsy are microcarcinomas, measuring less than a centimeter.

Evaluation of the Patient with Thyroid Nodules

Most thyroid nodules are benign and represent hyperplastic multinodular goiter, colloid nodules, Hashimoto's thyroiditis, simple or hemorrhagic cysts, or follicular adenomas (Fig. 3.1). They need to be differentiated from thyroid malignancies, which include papillary, follicular, Hürthle cell, medullary and anaplastic carcinomas, as well as primary thyroid lymphomas and metastatic lesions to the thyroid. In most instances, the combination of history, physical examination, blood tests, ultrasonography, and fine-needle aspiration allows a diagnosis to be made with a reasonable degree of confidence.

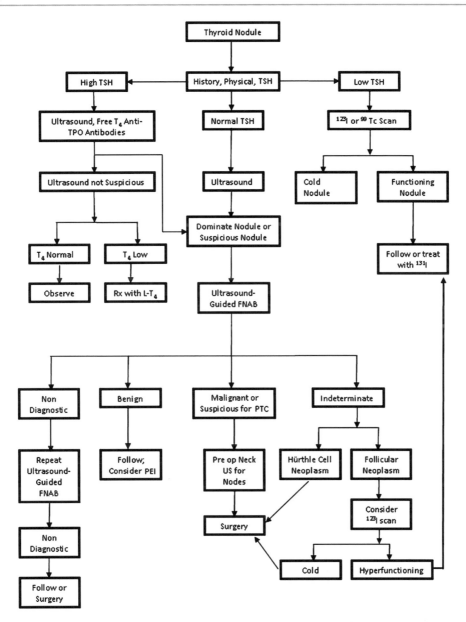

Fig. 3.1 Algorithm of diagnostic and therapeutic management of patients with thyroid nodules. *TSH* thyroid stimulating hormone; *Anti-TPO Antibodies* antithyroid peroxidase antibodies; ^{123}I ^{123}Iodine; ^{99}Tc Technetium ^{99}Tc pertechnetate; ^{131}I ^{131}Iodine; T_4 thyroxine; *L-T_4*levothyroxine; *Rx* treatment; *PTC* papillary thyroid carcinoma; *FNAB* fine needle aspiration biopsy; *PEI* percutaneous ethanol injection; *US* ultrasound

History and Physical Examination

About 5% of papillary thyroid carcinomas are familial, and there is an increased risk of developing a thyroid carcinoma with several complex familial syndromes if first-degree relatives are involved [45]. These include familial polyposis coli (multiple colonic polyps, skin epidermoid cysts, and desmoid tumors of the abdominal wall), Gardner's syndrome (familial polyposis coli with osteomas of the bones), Cowden disease (hamartomas of the skin and tumors of the breast, colon, brain, and endometrium), and Carney complex (skin and mucosal lentigines, cardiac myxomas, adrenal, pituitary and testicular neoplasms) [45]. A family history of isolated medullary carcinoma of the thyroid or multiple endocrine neoplasia type 2A (medullary carcinoma of the thyroid, pheochromocytomas, and hyperparathyroidism) or 2B (medullary carcinoma of the thyroid, pheochromocytomas, mucosal neuromas, and a "marfanoid" habitus) also raises the risk for thyroid cancer, especially if the nodule is discovered in a young individual.

External beam radiation was used in the past to shrink the thymus glands in infants with respiratory symptoms, to treat birthmarks, ringworm, and scrofula in children, and to treat acne in adolescents [46]. In addition, radium implants were used to shrink tonsils and adenoids in childhood [46]. Following a lag period of 15 to about 40 years, this radiation to the head and neck led to the development of benign and malignant thyroid nodules, hyperparathyroidism, skin cancers, salivary gland neoplasms, and, depending on the site of treatment and dose, brain tumors [46]. The risk of a malignancy in thyroids exposed to such irradiation in which a nodule is detected is about 33%, although this figure includes incidentally discovered carcinomas in thyroids removed because of the history of radiation and the presence of a nodule, which was found to be benign following removal [47]. An increased risk of thyroid cancer has also been found in children and adolescents exposed to ionizing radiation from nuclear fallout, and following total-body radiation in preparation for bone marrow transplantation [48, 49].

Thyroid nodules in patients under the age of 20 or over 70 years have an increased risk of malignancy, as does male gender [23, 50–53]. A history of persistent hoarseness, dysphagia, or dyspnea also increases the risk, although these symptoms also can occur with benign nodular goiters. Rapid growth of a nodule most often occurs because of bleeding inside of a benign nodule, which then undergoes cystic degeneration. This is often accompanied by pain and tenderness that resolves over a few days to weeks. On the other hand, rapid, painless growth of a solid nodule is of more concern and raises the suspicion for carcinoma,

especially if there has been growth while the patient was receiving levothyroxine treatment. A thyroid nodule that is metabolically active on a [^{18}F] fluorodeoxyglucose positron emission tomography scan performed for non-thyroid-related reasons has an approximately 30% chance of being malignant [53]

Symptoms of hyperthyroidism, such as weight loss, tremor, palpitations, increased sweating, heat intolerance, insomnia, and hyperdefecation, should be sought, as their presence suggests that the nodule may be a functioning, toxic nodule that is causing hyperthyroidism. Functioning nodules are usually follicular adenomas and have a 1% or less risk of being malignant [50].

On physical examination, a nodule that is firm or hard, fixed to the adjacent structures in the neck, or is associated with cervical lymphadenopathy in the lateral compartments (II–IV especially), or paralysis of the vocal cords should be considered highly suspicious for thyroid carcinoma [50, 51]. Signs of hyperthyroidism, including tremor, tachycardia, lid lag, and rapid return phase to the deep tendon reflexes, should be sought, and, if present, suggest that the patient may have a functioning, toxic nodule. However, nodules do occur in patients with a diffuse toxic goiter from Graves' disease, and about 9% of such nodules are malignant [54]. Similarly, patients with hyperthyroidism from one or more toxic nodules in a multinodular thyroid may also have nonfunctioning nodules in their gland which are malignant. Thus, although the presence of hyperthyroidism in a patient with thyroid nodule(s) reduces the risk that the patient is harboring a carcinoma, it does not eliminate the risk; hence, additional studies such as a thyroid scan and possibly a biopsy should be performed.

Laboratory Tests

The most important blood test is a measurement of serum thyroid-stimulating hormone (thyrotropin; TSH). A low level indicates hyperthyroidism, and is found in about 10% of patients with a solitary nodule [50]. This should be followed up with a measurement of free thyroxine and free triiodothyronine. A normal thyroxine and triiodothyronine indicate that the patient has subclinical hyper-thyroidism, while an elevation of thyroxine or triiodothyronine or both is diagnostic of hyper-thyroidism. Conversely, an elevated TSH level indicates hypothyroidism. In addition to measurement of a free thyroxine level to differentiate between subclinical hypothyroidism (high TSH, normal free thyroxine) and hypothyroidism (high TSH, low free thyroxine), a serum antithyroid peroxidase antibody should be measured to determine if the patient has Hashimoto's thyroiditis [55]. Most patients with thyroid cancer have TSH levels within the normal range. However, the risk of thyroid cancer increases with increasing TSH levels starting with those in the normal range [53]. Boelaert and colleagues calculated the odds ratio for thyroid malignancy based upon TSH levels. They used patients with a TSH below the normal range (<0.4 mU/L) as the reference group and their malignancy rate was 2.8%. Patients with a TSH level between 0.4 and 0.9 mU/L had an odds ratio of 1.31 (95% confidence limits of 0.45–3.81; $p = 0.622$; malignancy rate = 3.7%); those with a TSH between 1.0 and 1.7 mU/L had an odds ratio of 2.72 (1.02–7.27; $p = 0.046$; malignancy rate = 8.3%); those with a TSH between 1.8 and 5.5 mU/L had an odds ratio of 3.88 (1.48–10.19; $p = 0.006$; malignancy rate = 12.3%); and those with a TSH >5.5 mU/L had an odds ratio of 11.18 (3.23–38.63; $p < 0.001$; malignancy rate = 29.6%) [53].

The most controversial laboratory test concerns the measurement of serum calcitonin to detect medullary thyroid carcinoma. Clearly this test, along with an *RET* protooncogene mutation analysis, is indicated for patients with a single or multiple nodules and family members with hereditary medullary thyroid carcinoma or multiple endocrine neoplasia, type IIA or B, which accounts for 25% of the cases of medullary carcinoma[56]. The controversy surrounds its measurement in patients without a family history of medullary carcinoma who present with one or more thyroid nodules in order to detect the 75% of patients with nonfamilial medullary thyroid carcinoma.

In a series of studies that involved over 40,000 patients, several European investigators screened all patients with a basal serum calcitonin measure-ment and either sent patients to surgery if the calcitonin was above a certain level (usually 100 pg/mL) or performed a pentagastrin-stimulation test if the basal calcitonin level was elevated, but not diagnostic for medullary carcinoma [57–65]. These studies found a prevalence of medullary carcinoma to be between 0.18 and 1.37% of patients with nodules, with a median of 0.57%. The detection of an elevated basal serum calcitonin followed by a pentagastrin-stimulation test was more sensitive in detecting medullary carcinoma than a FNAB which has up to a 50% false-negative rate for this tumor [57–60, 64, 66]. The only definitive therapy for medullary thyroid cancer is total removal of the tumor, which can be achieved if it is localized to the thyroid or involves only a few lymph nodes [56]. This has been achieved in many patients with familial medullary carcinoma or the MEN 2 syndromes whose tumors (or precursor C-cell hyperplasia) are detected by routine screening. However, sporadic medullary thyroid carcinoma is often metastatic to local lymph nodes or distant sites at the time of diagnosis [56]. Therefore, the rationale for screening patients with nodules is to detect medullary carcinoma at a stage when it can be cured. Indeed, Elisei and co-workers, using a screening protocol, found patients with medullary carcinoma at a lower stage of disease than a group of patients previously detected by standard techniques prior to calcitonin screening, and, following surgery, patients detected by calcitonin screening normalized their serum calcitonin more frequently than did the historical controls and had improved survival [63]. These data led the European Thyroid Association and Cancer Research Network to recommend the use of calcitonin measurements in the initial diagnostic evaluation of thyroid nodules [67].

In contrast, in their most recent guidelines, the American Thyroid Association's expert panel "cannot recommend either for or against the routine measurement of serum calcitonin." [68]. There are a number of conditions other than medullary carcinoma and C-cell hyperplasia thst may result in hypercalcitoninemia, which reduces the specificity of calcitonin measurements for medullary carcinoma. These include chronic renal insufficiency, neuroendocrine tumors, pancreatitis, pernicious anemia, proton pump inhibitors, sepsis, inflammation, and Hashimoto's thyroiditis [69]. The European endocrinologists use pentagastrin stimulation as part of the diagnostic protocols to increase the specificity of calcitonin testing as the stimulated levels of calcitonin in patients with medullary carcinoma far exceed those of the other conditions. However, pentagastrin is no longer available in the U.S., and other secretagogs such as calcium do not result in as robust stimulation of calcitonin. In addition, there have been issues with the performance of the various calcitonin immunoassays, although many of the issues dealing with cross-reaction with calcitonin precursors and nonspecific assay interference have been overcome with the newer two-site immunomimetric assays [69]. These transatlantic differences in societal recommendations are reflected in actual practice by clinicians as assessed by a series of surveys carried out between 1999 and 2002 [70–73]. When asked whether a calcitonin level is routinely ordered in the diagnostic evaluation of a nontoxic solitary nodule or a nontoxic multinodular goiter with no suspicion of malignancy, 5 and 4% of members of the American Thyroid Association answered "yes" for the two conditions, while 43 and 32% of the members of the European Thyroid Association indicated that they measured calcitonin routinely for these two scenarios [55, 70–73]. To make matters even more complicated, a recent cost effectiveness and decision analysis of calcitonin measurements in the evaluation of thyroid nodules in the U.S. concluded that such measurements were as cost effective as routine TSH measurements, colonoscopy, and mammography screening [74]. However, the prevalence estimates used in that analysis included patients with C-cell hyperplasia and micromedullary carcinoma, the clinical significance of which is uncertain [68].

Ultrasonography

Ultrasound evaluation of the thyroid and surrounding neck structures provides a great deal of information including the number and size of the nodules, demonstrating nodules that were not detected by palpation, the morphologic features of the nodule(s), nodular blood flow pattern, and whether there are abnormal-appearing cervical lymph nodes. The American Thyroid Association recommends that "thyroid sonography should be performed in all patients with known or suspected thyroid nodules" [68]. In many respects, this procedure is an ideal method to examine nodules in that it is readily available, does not expose the patient to radiation, provides high resolution, and can be performed in the physician's office at the time of initial evaluation. In addition, it is useful for guiding fine-needle-aspiration biopsies of the thyroid or lymph nodes, and is useful for serial measurements for monitoring nodule size during observation or following treatment.

Multiple studies have examined the sensitivity and specificity of various features of thyroid nodules for distinguishing malignant from benign thyroid nodules [27, 30, 75–86]. Features suggesting malignancy include solid, rather than cystic, hypoechogenicity in comparison to the surrounding thyroid tissue, microcalcifications representing calcified psammoma bodies, dystrophic calcification, a surrounding halo that is thick, irregular, or absent, irregular or microlobulated margins, invasion into the surrounding tissue, being taller in anterior–posterior dimensions than wide in the transverse dimension, intranodular vascularity rather than peripheral vascularity, and regional lymphadenopathy, especially if the lymph nodes have malignant characteristics such as being round, have cystic degeneration, punctate calcifications, loss of a hilus, and increased intranodal blood flow. Table 3.1 provides the ranges of sensitivity, specificity, and positive and negative predictive values for several of these features [87]. When more than one of these features is present, the specificity for thyroid carcinoma increases to 87–93% [51].

Tables 3.2–3.4 summarize the consensus recommendations from three professional organizations – the American Thyroid Association, the American Association of Clinical Endocrinologists, and the Society of Radiologists in Ultrasound – concerning the criteria for choosing which nodules on which a FNAB should be performed [51, 68, 87]. Although there are some differences between these guidelines,

Table 3.1 Ultrasound features associated with thyroid cancer. From Frates et al. [87]. Used with permission

Ultrasound Feature	Sensitivity	Specificity	PPV	NPV
Microcalcifications	26.1–59.1	85.8–95.0	24.3–70.7	41.8–94.2
Hypoechogenicity	26.5–87.1	43.4–94.3	11.4–68.4	73.5–93.8
Irregular margins or no halo	17.4–77.5	38.9–85.0	9.3–60.0	38.9–97.8
Solid	69.0–75.0	52.5–55.9	15.6–27.0	88.0–92.1
Intranodule vascularity	54.3–74.2	78.6–80.8	24.0–41.9	85.7–97.4
More tall than wide	32.7	92.5	66.7	74.8

Table 3.2 The American Thyroid Association's recommendations for FNAB. Based on sonographic and clinical features of thyroid nodules [68]

Nodule sonographic or clinical features	Recommended nodule	Strength of threshold size for FNAB recommendation[a]
High-risk history[b]		
Nodule WITH suspicious sonographic features[c]	>5 mm	A
Nodule WITHOUT suspicious sonographic features[c]	>5 mm	I
Abnormal cervical lymph nodes	All[d]	A
Microcalcifications present in nodule	≥1 cm	B
Solid nodule		
AND hypoechoic	>1 cm	B
AND iso- or hyperechoic	≥1–1.5 cm	C
Mixed cystic–solid nodule		
WITH any suspicious ultrasound features[c]	≥1.5–2.0 cm	B
WITHOUT suspicious ultrasound features	≥2.0 cm	C
Spongiform nodule	≥2.0 cm[e]	C
Purely cystic nodule	FNA not indicated[f]	E

[a]Strength of Recommendation: A = Strongly recommends based on good evidence; B = Recommends based on fair evidence; C = Recommends based on expert opinion; E = Recommends against based on fair evidence; I = Recommends neither for or against – evidence insufficient

[b]High-risk history: History of thyroid cancer in one or more first degree relatives; history of external beam radiation as a child; exposure to ionizing radiation in childhood or adolescence; prior hemithyroidectomy with discovery of thyroid cancer; [18]FDG avidity on PET scanning; MEN2/FMTC-associated RET protooncogene mutation, calcitonin >100 pg/mL. *MEN* multiple endocrine neoplasia; *FMTC* familial medullary thyroid cancer; [18]*FDG* [18]flurodeoxyglucose; *PET* positron emission tomography

[c]Suspicious features: microcalcifications; hypoechoic; increased nodular vascularity; infiltrative margins; taller than wide on transverse view

[d]FNAB cytology may be obtained from the abnormal lymph node in lieu of the thyroid nodule

[e]Sonographic monitoring without biopsy may be an acceptable alternative

[f]Unless indicated as therapeutic modality

all agree that lesions that are suspicious for cancer based upon ultrasound criteria should be biopsied rather than just performing a biopsy on the largest lesion in a gland with multiple nodules.

Radioisotope Thyroid Scan

Radioiodine scans, preferably using ^{123}I, are useful for determining whether or not a thyroid nodule is autonomous in a patient with a suppressed TSH. A "hot" nodule, which suppresses the surrounding normal thyroid tissue, or a "warm" nodule, which is functioning but has not suppressed the surrounding tissue, has a <1% chance of being malignant. These findings obviate the need for a FNAB. A "cold" nodule, which is hypofunctioning in comparison to the surrounding tissue and accounts for 77–94% of nodules, has an 8% or higher chance of being malignant [51, 55]. Thyroid scans are also

Table 3.3 The American Association of Clinical Endocrinologists and Associazione Medici Endocrinologi recommendations for ultrasound-guided FNAB of thyroid nodules with strength of recommendation [51]. Used with permission

No US-FNAB of nodules <1 cm unless suspicious US findings or high-risk history (grade C)
US-FNAB of nodules of any size in patients with history of neck irradiation or family History of MTC or MEN2 (grade C)
US-FNAB should be based on US features (grade B)
US-FNAB should be performed on all hypoechoic nodules ≥1 cm with irregular margins, chaotic intranodular vascular spots, a more-tall-than-wide shape, or microcalcifications (grade B)
US findings suggestive of extracapsular growth or metastatic cervical lymph nodes warrant an immediate cytologic evaluation, no matter the size of the lesion (grade B)
In complex thyroid nodules, obtain US–FNAB sampling of the solid component of the lesion before fluid drainage (grade C)

Grading Recommendations: B=evidence from at least one large well-designed clinical trial, cohort or case-controlled analytic study, or meta-analysis; C=evidence based on clinical experience, descriptive studies, or expert consensus opinion

MTC medullary thyroid carcinoma; *MEN2* multiple endocrine neoplasia type 2; *US* ultrasonography

Table 3.4 The Society of Radiologists in Ultrasound consensus recommendation for ultrasound-guided FNAB of thyroid nodules [87]. Used with Permission

US feature	Recommendation
Solitary nodule	
Microcalcifications	Strongly consider if ≥1 cm
Solid (or almost entirely solid) or coarse calcifications	Strongly consider if ≥1.5 cm
Mixed solid and cystic or almost entirely cystic with solid mural component	Consider if ≥2 cm
None of the above but substantial growth since prior US exam	Consider US-guided FNAB
Almost entirely cystic and none of the above and no substantial growth	FNAB probably unnecessary
Multiple nodules	Consider FNAB of one or more nodules, with selection prioritized on basis of criteria (in order listed) for solitary nodule[a]

[a]Panel had two opinions regarding selection of nodules for FNAB. The majority opinion is stated here
Note: FNAB is likely unnecessary in diffusely enlarged gland with multiple nodules of similar US appearance without intervening parenchyma. Presence of abnormal lymph nodes overrides ultrasound features of thyroid nodule(s) and should prompt US-guided FNAB or biopsy of lymph node and/or ipsilateral nodule

useful for examining substernal extension of a multinodular goiter, for identifying a cold nodule in a patient with Graves' disease with otherwise diffuse isotope increased uptake, or for identifying ectopic thyroid tissue. The resolution of scans is inferior to that of ultrasound, as they generally are unable to detect lesions <1 cm. Technetium ^{99m}Tc pertechnetate is also used for thyroid scintigraphy, but unlike ^{123}I, is trapped but not organified, and may lead to a false-positive appearance of a functioning nodule.

Other Imaging Modalities

Neither magnetic resonance imaging nor computed tomography scanning is recommended as part of the initial evaluation of thyroid nodules as they add little information over that obtained by ultrasonography [51]. They may provide detail about substernal extension of a goiter, as well as additional detail about cervical and mediastinal lymphadenopathy. If iodinated contrast is administered for the computed tomography scan, the large iodine load may

Table 3.5 Tiered classification scheme for thyroid fine-needle-aspiration biopsies from the 2008 National Cancer Institute Thyroid Fine Needle Aspiration State of the Science Conference [100]. Used with Permission

Suggested categories	Alternate category (s) terms	Risk of malignancy
Benign		<1%
Follicular lesion of undetermined significance	Atypia of undetermined significance	5–10%
	R/O Neoplasm	
	Atypical follicular lesion	
	Cellular Follicular Lesion	
Follicular Neoplasm	Suspicious for follicular neoplasm	20–30%
Suspicious for Malignancy		50–75%
Malignant		100%
Non-diagnostic	Unsatisfactory	

preclude the administration of radioactive iodine either diagnostically or therapeutically for multiple months. [^{18}F]-fluorodeoxyglucose positron emission tomography should not be used to screen patients for thyroid nodules. If this scan is done for other reasons and a thyroid nodule is positive, then the risk of malignancy in the nodule increases to about 30% [88].

Fine-Needle-Aspiration Biopsy (FNAB)

FNAB is the most useful test for establishing the diagnosis of a thyroid nodule, and its use has decreased the number of patients undergoing thyroid surgery by 35–75%, while increasing the number of thyroid cancers found at surgery by two- to threefold [89–91]. From a compilation of many series, about 80–90% of FNAB are satisfactory for interpretation, showing six or more follicular cell groups, each containing 10–15 well-preserved cells derived from at least two aspirates [68, 92]. Several studies have shown that the rate of nondiagnostic or unsatisfactory due to insufficient number of cells can be reduced by half or more with the use of ultrasound-guided FNAB, as this reduces sampling error and allows biopsy of the solid portions of mixed solid–cystic lesions [93–97]. Rebiopsy of a nodule whose initial biopsy was classified as insufficient, yields a sufficient number of cells in about 50% of the patients with cystic lesions and up to 75% of patients with solid nodules, further reducing the number of inadequate biopsies [92, 98, 99]. Based upon an analy-sis of several series, the mean sensitivity of FNAB is 83%, the mean specificity is 92%, the positive predictive value is 75%, the false-negative rate is 5%, and the false-positive rate averages 5% [51].

Until recently, about 70% of the results were reported as benign (no evidence of malignancy, usually colloid nodules, thyroiditis, or cysts), about 10–20% as suspicious or indeterminate (primarily representing follicular neoplasms, follicular variant of papillary carcinoma, Hurthle-cell neoplasms, and lymphomas), about 5% as malignant, and the remainder as nondiagnostic [51, 55]. In 2008, new reporting recommendations were made following a National Cancer Institute consensus conference [100]. These guidelines added new categories and provide the clinician with risk estimates for malignancy (Table 3.5).

From a clinical standpoint, the most vexing groups of FNAB results deal with are the indeterminate group classified as "follicular neoplasm, suspicious for follicular neoplasm," which carry a 20–30% risk of malignancy, and the "follicular lesion, atypia of undetermined significance" which has a 5–10% risk of malignancy [68, 100]. In these groups, the cellular morphology cannot reliably distinguish between benign and malignant behavior of the cells. Such differentiation has relied upon the histologic examination of the lesion after it has been surgically removed. There are a number of molecular and protein markers that may be applied to the FNAB specimens that have the potential to improve the diagnostic specificity for this indeterminate group. These include HBME-1, galectin-3, cytokeratin, and mutations of the BRAF, Ras, and RET/PTC genes [68, 101–103]. It is likely that a combination of these and other markers will allow a more precise diagnosis to be made on this group of lesions.

Management of Patients with Thyroid Nodules

Figure 3.1 provides an algorithm for the evaluation and treatment of patients with thyroid nodule(s) which mostly conforms to several published algorithms including those generated by expert committees of the American Association of Clinical Endocrinologists, Associazione Medici Endocrinologi, and the American Thyroid Association [50, 51, 68]. As detailed above, the first step is to perform a history and physical examination and obtain a serum TSH. A low TSH indicating hyperthyroidism should be followed up with a thyroid scan. A functioning "warm" or "hot" nodule has such a low risk of thyroid cancer that an FNAB is not required, and the patient can be either followed or treated with radioactive iodine. If a "cold" nodule is found on thyroid scan, then an ultrasound should be performed. The finding of an elevated TSH indicates that the patient has hypothyroidism, most often due to autoimmune (Hashimoto's) thyroiditis. This does not preclude the diagnosis of cancer, and there is an increased risk of cancer in a thyroid nodule associated with an elevated TSH [53]. Therefore, in addition to measurement of free thyroxine to determine whether the patient has subclinical hypothyroidism or clinical hypothyroidism and measurement of antithyroid peroxidase antibodies to see if the patient has Hashimoto's thyroiditis, a thyroid ultrasound should be performed. Similarly, an ultrasound should be performed in patients with a normal TSH. If no nodule is seen (i.e., the palpable nodule was a false-positive finding), no further action is necessary. If one or more nodules are present, then each needs to be evaluated for size, morphology, and vascular pattern. Each nodule with suspicious features for thyroid carcinoma should undergo ultrasound-guided FNAB, and, in the absence of specific features for thyroid cancer, the dominant nodule should be biopsied according to the recommendations outlined in Tables 3.2–3.4. Further evaluation and treatment depend upon the results of the FNAB. The various options will be discussed in more detail in the sections to follow.

Observation

Nonfunctioning, benign nodules can be followed up at 6–18-month intervals to monitor the lesions for changes in size and morphology, as there is a 5% false-negative rate on FNAB [68, 94, 104]. Growth of nodules is very common, and most solid nodules that grow are benign [105–108]. In fact, Alexander and colleagues demonstrated that 89% of benign solid nodules had a ≥15% increase in volume over 5 years [107]. The rate of tumor growth does not distinguish between benign and malignant tumors [108]. The American Thyroid Association recommends that a repeat FNAB of a lesion should be performed if there is a "20% increase in nodule diameter with a minimum increase in two or more dimensions or at least 2 mm" as this corresponds to an approximately 50% increase in nodule volume, which is the minimally significant reproducible change in recorded nodule size [68, 109]. Cystic nodules may be drained at the time of initial biopsy, but there is a high rate of fluid reaccumulation, often from recurrent hemorrhage into the lesion. With such lesions, it is important to monitor the size of the solid portion of the lesion for growth, which should prompt an ultrasound-guided FNAB.

Levothyroxine Suppressive Therapy

On theoretical grounds, since TSH is a growth factor for thyroid follicular cells, depressing TSH levels below the normal range should result in a decrease in the size of both normal and abnormal thyroid cells. Such treatment does decrease the normal thyroid tissue surrounding thyroid nodules, but may not decrease the size of the nodule. Multiple studies have reported a statistically significant decrease in nodule size with suppressive therapy [110–116], while others have not shown a significant decrease [117, 118]. There appears to be a greater likelihood of shrinkage when the TSH level is suppressed to a level <0.1 mU/L in comparison to suppression to <0.3 mU/L [114, 116, 119]. Suppression appears to work better on small colloid nodules and in regions of borderline iodine deficiency [120]. Several meta-analyses have been performed to resolve the conflicts but have not been conclusive, with most showing a nonsignificant trend toward reduction in volume [114, 119, 121, 122]. Levothyroxine suppressive therapy does appear to diminish growth of nodules and can prevent new nodules from developing [116, 121–123]. The difficulty in interpreting the data is due to multiple factors, including small numbers of subjects, lack of control groups, lack of randomization, mixtures of patients with single nodules and multiple nodules, variable doses of levothyroxine, variable degrees of TSH suppression, variable duration of treatment, and different criteria to define response in the various studies [91].

Although the authors of the various studies of levothyroxine suppression generally have not reported adverse effects of levothyroxine suppression, long-term suppression of TSH is a risk factor for decreasing bone mineral density and increasing the risk of atrial fibrillation [124–128]. Based upon these considerations, neither the American Thyroid Association nor the American Association of Clinical Endocrinologists recommends routine suppression therapy in iodine-sufficient populations [51, 68].

Surgery

Surgery is indicated for malignant, suspicious for malignancy, and for most patients with follicular neoplasms that are cold, especially if the nodule is >4 cm in an older male patient and has atypical features [68, 129–131]. For patients with lesions compatible with or suspicious for papillary thyroid cancer, a total thyroidectomy should be performed, preferably with a central compartment dissection for adequate staging and to reduce recurrences [132, 133]. Small papillary carcinomas that are confined to the thyroid may be treated

with a total or near-total thyroidectomy without lymph node dissection, although some patients with tumors <1 cm, which are unifocal and confined to the thyroid and without a history of head and neck irradiation, may be cured with a thyroid lobectomy alone [68]. Patients with small follicular neoplasms, which carry a 20–30% risk of malignancy, or with a follicular lesion with atypia of undetermined significance, which carries a 5–10% risk of malignancy, may undergo a lobectomy, with the understanding that a complete thyroidectomy may be necessary should the pathology show an invasive follicular carcinoma or a follicular variant of papillary carcinoma.

Surgery should also be considered for patients with large nodules or a multinodular goiter that causes symptoms such as dysphagia, choking, dysphonia, shortness of breath in the supine position or dyspnea on exertion, and neck pressure or neck pain [51]. Continued growth of a thyroid nodule is another indication to consider surgery.

Radioactive Iodine

^{131}I therapy is primarily used to treat toxic nodules. Generally, higher doses are required than needed to effectively treat Graves' disease as nodules are relatively radioresistant [134]. The therapy is successful in controlling hyperthyroidism in over 75% of patients and leads to a reduction of nodule volume of 35–45% at two years [134–136]. The major side effect is hypothyroidism that occurs in about 10% of patients by 5 years, especially those whose non-nodular portion of the thyroid was not suppressed and those with antithyroid peroxidase antibodies [135–138].

Percutaneous Ethanol Injection

Ultrasound-guided percutaneous ethanol injection, which causes coagulation necrosis and thrombosis in small vessels, has been used to treat benign simple and complex cysts and toxic and nontoxic thyroid nodules [139–153]. About 75–85% of patients with thyroid cysts have a >50% reduction in cyst volume, with a very low recurrence rate at one year [145–149]. Autonomously functioning nodules respond well initially to percutaneous ethanol injections with an increase in TSH and a 60–75% reduction in nodule volume, but there is a high relapse rate due to regrowth of the residual tissue [145, 150–152]. The therapy works best in nodules <15 ml [139, 153, 154]. In patients with solid benign cold nodules, there is also a significant decrease in nodule size but may require multiple treatments with the potential for an increase in the complication rate [155, 156]. Complications include pain at the site of injection, radiating cervical pain, fever, flushing, transient dysphonia due to ethanol-induced damage to the recurrent laryngeal nerve, and hematoma [139].

Future Developments

As noted above, there is great interest in developing a panel of molecular and protein markers that can be applied to FNAB samples and which can differentiate benign from malignant lesions. A number of candidate markers have been identified in research settings, but it remains to be seen if one or more of these markers will be sensitive and specific enough to enhance clinical decision making over and above the currently available information gained from history and physical examination, a TSH, and ultrasound characteristics [68, 101–103].

Ultrasound elastography is a new technique that measures the change of the ultrasound beam that occurs when pressure is applied to a thyroid nodule. Since thyroid carcinomas tend to be firmer than benign lesions, the external pressure will distort carcinomas less than it would for benign nodules [157–161]. In several early studies, this technique had an 82–97% sensitivity and a 77–100% specificity for predicting malignancy [157–161].

Percutaneous laser ablation or photocoagulation is performed under ultrasound guidance in which a 300–400-μm optical fiber is inserted through an 18–21-gauge needle that is placed into the nodule. The needle is withdrawn and the lesion undergoes thermal necrosis using a laser source [51, 162, 163]. Several treatments are usually required and may result in an approximately 50% reduction in the size of the nodule and relief of pretreatment local discomfort symptoms. Neck pain and tenderness are the most frequent side effects of this experimental therapy [51, 162, 163].

References

1. Vander JB, Gaston EA, Dawber TR. Significance of solitary nontoxic nodules; preliminary report. New Engl J Med. 1954;251:970–3.
2. Vander JB, Gaston EA, Dawber TR. The significance of nontoxic thyroid nodules. Final report of a 15 year study of the incidence of thyroid malignancy. Ann Intern Med. 1968;69:537–40.
3. Turnbridge WMG, Evered DC, Hall R, et al. The spectrum of thyroid disease in a community: the Whickham Survey. Clin Endocrinol (Oxf). 1977;7:481–93.
4. Brader A, Viikinkiski P, Nickels J, et al. Thyroid gland: US screening in a random adult population. Radiology. 1991;181:683–7.
5. Wiest PW, Hartshorne MF, Inskip PD, et al. Thyroid palpation versus high-resolution thyroid ultrasonography in the detection of nodules. J Ultrasound Med. 1998;17:487–96.
6. Ezzat S, Sarti DA, Cain DR, et al. Thyroid incidentalomas. Prevalence by palpation and ultrasonography. Arch Intern Med. 1994;154:1838–40.
7. Carroll BA. Asymptomatic thyroid nodules: incidental sonographic detection. Am J Roentgenol. 1982;138:499–501.
8. Horlocker TT, Hay ID. Prevalence of incidental nodular thyroid disease detected during high-resolution parathyroid sonography. In: Medeiros-Neto G, Gaitan E, editors. Frontiers in thyroidology, vol. 2. New York, NY: Plenum; 1985. p. 1309–12.
9. Stark DD, Clark OH, Gooding GAW, et al. High-resolution ultrasonography and computed tomography of thyroid lesions in patients with hyperparathyroidism. Surgery. 1983;94:863–8.
10. Woestyn J, Afschrift M, Schelstraete K, et al. Demonstration of nodules in the normal thyroid by echography. Br J Radiol. 1985;58:1179–82.
11. Tomimori E, Pedrinola F, Cavaliere H, et al. Prevalence of incidental thyroid disease in a relatively low iodine intake area. Thyroid. 1995;5:273–6.
12. Struve C, Hinrichs J. Schilddrusenvolumina und Haufigkeit herdformiger Veranderungen bei schilddrusengesunden Mannern und Frauen verschiedener Altersklassen. Dtsch Med Wochenschr. 1989;114:283–7.
13. Bruneton JN, Balu-Maestro C, Marcy PY, et al. Very high frequency (13 MHz) ultrasonographic examination of the normal neck: detection of normal lymph nodes and thyroid nodules. J Ultrasound Med. 1994;13:87–90.

14. Mortenson JD, Woolner LB, Bennett WA. Gross and microscopic findings in clinically normal thyroid glands. J Clin Endocrinol Metab. 1955;15:1270–80.
15. Furmanchuk AW, Roussak N, Ruchti C. Occult thyroid carcinoma in the region of Minsk, Belarus. An autopsy study of 215 patients. Histopathology. 1993;23:319–25.
16. Rice CO. Incidence of nodules in the thyroid: a comparative study of symptomless thyroid glands removed at autopsy and hyperfunctioning goiters operatively removed. Arch Surg. 1932;24:505–15.
17. Hellwig CA. The thyroid gland in Kansas. Am J Clin Pathol. 1935;5:103–11.
18. Schlesinger MJ, Gargill SL, Saxe IH. Studies in nodular goiter: incidence of thyroid nodules in routine necropsies in a nongoitrous region. JAMA. 1938;110:1638–41.
19. Hull OH. Critical analysis of two hundred twenty-one thyroid glands: study of thyroid glands obtained at necropsy in Colorado. Arch Pathol. 1955;59:291–311.
20. Ortel JE, Klinck GH. Structural changes in the thyroid glands of healthy young men. Med Ann Dist Columbia. 1965;34:75–7.
21. Takahashi T, Trott KR, Fujimori K, et al. An investigation into the prevalence of thyroid disease on Kwajalein Atoll, Marshall Islands. Health Phys. 1997;73:199–213.
22. McCall A, Jarosz H, Lawrence AM, et al. The incidence of thyroid carcinoma in solitary cold nodules and in multinodular goiters. Surgery. 1986;100:1128–32.
23. Belfiore A, La Rosa GL, La Porta GA, et al. Cancer risk in patients with cold nodules: relevance of iodine intake, sex, age and multinodularity. Am J Med. 1992;93:363–9.
24. Cochand-Priollet B, Guillausseau PJ, Chagnon S, et al. The diagnostic value of fine-needle aspiration biopsy under ultrasonography in nonfunctional thyroid nodules: a prospective study comparing cytologic and histologic findings. Am J Med. 1994;97:152–7.
25. Sachmechi I, Miller E, Varatharajah R, et al. Thyroid carcinoma in single cold nodules and in cold nodules of multinodular goiters. Endocr Pract. 2000;6:5–7.
26. Marqusee E, Benson CB, Frates MC, et al. Usefulness of ultrasonography in the management of nodular thyroid disease. Ann Intern Med. 2000;133:696–700.
27. Papini E, Guglielmi R, Bianchini A, et al. Risk of malignancy in nonpalpable thyroid nodules: predictive value of ultrasound and color-Doppler features. J Clin Endocrinol Metab. 2002;87:1941–6.
28. Deandrea M, Mormile A, Veglio M, et al. Fine-needle aspiration biopsy of the thyroid: comparison between thyroid palpation and ultrasonography. Endocr Pract. 2002;8:282–6.
29. Frates MC, Benson CB, Doubilet PM, et al. Prevalence and distribution of carcinoma in patients with solitary and multiple thyroid nodules on sonography. J Clin Endocrinol Metab. 2006;91:3411–7.
30. Nam-Goong IS, Kim HY, Gong G, et al. Ultrasonography-guided fine-needle aspiration of thyroid incidentaloma: correlation with pathological findings. Clin Endocrinol. 2004;60:21–8.

31. Silverberg SG, Vidone RA. Carcinoma of the thyroid in surgical and postmortem material. Analysis of 300 cases at autopsy and literature review. Ann Surg. 1966;164:291–2.
32. Farooki MA. Epidemiology and pathology of cancer of the thyroid. Int Surg. 1969;51:232–43.
33. Sampson RJ, Key CR, Buncher CR, et al. Thyroid carcinoma in Hiroshima and Nagasaki. I. Prevalence of thyroid carcinoma at autopsy. JAMA. 1969;209:65–70.
34. Sampson RJ, Woolner LB, Bahn RC, et al. Occult thyroid carcinoma in Olmstead County, Minnesota: prevalence at autopsy compared with that in Hiroshima and Nagasaki, Japan. Cancer. 1974;34:2072–6.
35. Fukunaga FH, Yatani R. Geographic pathology of occult thyroid carcinoma. Cancer. 1975;36:1095–9.
36. Sobrinho-Simoes MA, Sambade MC, Goncalves V. Latent thyroid carcinoma at autopsy. Cancer. 1979;43:1702–6.
37. Bondeson L, Ljungberg O. Occult thyroid carcinoma at autopsy in Malmo, Sweden. Cancer. 1981;47:319–23.
38. Pingitore R. Rilievi morfologici autopsicisu 111 tiroidi clinicamente normali in un`area italiana senza edemia gozzigena. Pathologica. 1982;74:545–52.
39. Arellano L, Ibarra A. Occult carcinoma of the thyroid gland. Pathol Res Pract. 1984;179:88–91.
40. Harach HR, Franssila KO, Wasenius VM. Occult papillary carcinoma of the thyroid. A "normal" finding in Finland. A systematic autopsy study. Cancer. 1985;56:531–8.
41. Franssila KO, Harach HR. Occult papillary carcinoma of the thyroid in children and young adults. A systemic autopsy study in Finland. Cancer. 1986;58:715–9.
42. Lang W, Borrusch H, Bauer L. Occult carcinomas of the thyroid. Evaluation of 1020 sequential autopsies. Am J Clin Pathol. 1988;90:72–6.
43. Ottino A, Pianzola HM, Castelletto RH. Occult papillary thyroid carcinoma at autopsy in La Plata, Argentina. Cancer. 1989;64:547–51.
44. Yamamoto Y. Occult papillary carcinoma of the thyroid. A study of 408 autopsy cases. Cancer. 1990;65:1173–9.
45. Loh KC. Familial nonmedullary thyroid carcinoma: a meta-review of case series. Thyroid. 1997;7:107–13.
46. DeGroot LJ, Frohman LA, Kaplan EL, et al. Radiation-associated thyroid carcinoma. New York: Gruene & Stratton; 1977.
47. Mihailescu DV, Schneider AB. Size, number, and distribution of thyroid nodules and the risk of malignancy in radiation-exposed patients who underwent surgery. J Clin Endocrinol Metab. 2008;93:2188–93.
48. Pacini F, Vorontsova T, Demidchik E, et al. Post-Chernobyl thyroid carcinoma in Belarus children and adolescents: comparison with naturally occuring thyroid carcinoma in Italy and France. J Clin Endocrinol Metab. 1997;81:3563–9.
49. Curtis RE, Rowlings PA, Deeg HJ, et al. Solid cancers after bone marrow transplantation. N Engl J Med. 1997;336:897–904.

50. Hegedüs L. The thyroid nodule. N Engl J Med. 2004;351:1764–71.

51. Gharib H, Papini E, Valcavi R, Baskin HJ, Crescenzi A, Dottorini ME. American Association of Clinical Endocrinologists and Associazione Medici Endocrinologi medical guidelines for clinical practice for the diagnosis and management of thyroid nodules. Endocr Pract. 2006;12:63–102.

52. Niedziela M. Pathogenesis, diagnosis and management of thyroid nodules in children. Endocr Relat Cancer. 2006;13:427–53.

53. Boelaert K, Horacek J, Holder RL, et al. Serum thyrotropin concentration as a novel predictor of malignancy in thyroid nodules investigated by fine-needle aspiration. J Clin Endocrinol Metab. 2006;91: 4295–301.

54. Kim WB, Han SM, Kim TY, et al. Ultrasonographic screening for detection of thyroid cancer in patients with Graves' disease. Clin Endocrinol (Oxf). 2004;60:719–25.

55. Hegedüs L, Bonnema SJ, Bennedbæk FN. Management of simple nodular goiter: current status and future prospectives. Endocr Rev. 2003;24:102–32.

56. Kloos RT, Eng C, Evans DB, et al. Medullary thyroid cancer: management guidelines of the American Thyroid Association. Thyroid. 2009;19:565–612.

57. Pacini F, Fontanelli M, Fugazzola L, et al. Routine measurement of serum calcitonin in nodular thyroid disease allows the preoperative diagnosis of unsuspected sporadic medullary thyroid carcinoma. J Clin Endocrinol Metab. 1994;78:826–9.

58. Rieu M, Lame MC, Richard A, et al. Prevalence of sporadic medullary thyroid carcinoma: the importance of routine measurement of serum calcitonin in the diagnostic evaluation of thyroid nodules. Clin Endocrinol (Oxf). 1995;42:453–60.

59. Niccoli P, Wion-Barbot N, Caron P, et al. Interest of routine measurement of serum calcitonin: study in a large series of thyroidectomized patients. The French Medullary Study Group. J Clin Endocrinol Metab. 1997;82:338–41.

60. Vierhapper H, Reber W, Bieglmayer C, et al. Routine measurement of plasma calcitonin in nodular thyroid diseases. J Clin Endocrinol Metab. 1997;82: 1589–93.

61. Ozgen AG, Hamulu F, Bayraktar F, et al. Evaluation of routine basal serum calcitonin measurement for early diagnosis of medullary thyroid carcinoma in seven hundred seventy-three patients wih nodular goiter. Thyroid. 1999;9:579–82.

62. Hahm JR, Lee MS, Min YK, et al. Routine measurement of serum calcitonin is useful for early detection of medullary thyroid carcinoma in patients with nodular thyroid diseases. Thyroid. 2001;11:73–80.

63. Elisei R, Bottici V, Luchetti F, et al. Impact of routine measurement of serum calcitonin on the diagnosis and outcome of medullary thyroid cancer: experience in 10,864 patients with nodular thyroid disorders. J Clin Endocrinol Metab. 2004;89:163–8.

64. Costante G, Meringolo D, Durante C, et al. Predictive value of serum calcitonin levels for preoperative diagnosis of medullary thyroid carcinoma in a cohort of 5817 consecutive patients with thyroid nodules. J Clin Endocrinol Metab. 2007;92:450–5.

65. Rink T, Truong P-N, Schroth H-J, et al. Calculation and validation of a plasma calcitonin limit for early detection of medullary thyroid carcinoma in nodular thyroid disease. Thyroid. 2009;19:327–32.

66. Bugalho MJ, Santos JR, Sobrinho L. Preoperative diagnosis of medullary thyroid carcinoma: fine needle aspiration cytology as compared with serum calcitonin measurement. J Surg Oncol. 2005;91:56–60.

67. Pacini F, Schlumberger M, Dralle H, et al. European consensus for the management of patients with differentiated thyroid carcinoma of the follicular epithelium. Eur J Endocrinol. 2006;154:787–803 [Erratum (2006) 155:385].

68. Cooper DS, Doherty GM, Haugen BR, et al. Revised American Thyroid Association management guidelines for patients with thyroid nodules and differentiated thyroid cancer. Thyroid. 2009;19:1167–215.

69. Elisei R. Routine serum calcitonin measurement in the evaluation of thyroid nodules. Best Pract Res Clin Endocrinol Metab. 2008;22:941–53.

70. Bennedbæk FN, Perrild H, Hegedüs L. Diagnosis and treatment of the solitary thyroid nodule. Results of a European survey. Clin Endocrinol (Oxf). 1999;50: 357–63.

71. Bennedbæk FN, Hegedüs L. Management of the solitary thyroid nodule: results of a North American survey. J Clin Endocrinol Metab. 2000;85:2493–8.

72. Bonnema SJ, Bennedbæk FN, Wiersinga WM, et al. Management of the nontoxic multinodular goitre: a European questionnaire study. Clin Endocrinol (Oxf). 2000;53:5–12.

73. Bonnema SJ, Bennedbæk FN, Ladenson PW, et al. Management of the nontoxic multinodular goiter: a North American survey. J Clin Endocrinol Metab. 2002;87:112–7.

74. Cheung K, Roman SA, Wang TS, et al. Calcitonin measurement in the evaluation of thyroid nodules in the United States: a cost-effectiveness and decision analysis. J Clin Endocrinol Metab. 2008;93:2173–80.

75. Khoo ML, Asa SL, Witterick IJ, et al. Thyroid calcification and its association with thyroid carcinoma. Head Neck. 2002;24:651–5.

76. Kim EK, Park CS, Chung WY, et al. New sonographic criteria for recommending fine-needle aspiration biopsy of nonpalpable solid nodules of the thyroid. Am J Roentgenol. 2002;178:687–91.

77. Peccin S, de Castro JA, Furlanetto TW, et al. Ultrasonography: is it useful in the diagnosis of cancer in thyroid nodules? J Endocrinol Invest. 2002;25:39–43.

78. Frates MC, Benson CB, Doubilet PM, et al. Can color Doppler sonography aid in the prediction of malignancy of thyroid nodules? J Ultrasound Med. 2003;22:127–31.

79. Leenhardt L, Hejblum G, Franc B, et al. Indications and limits of ultrasound-guided cytology in the management of nonpalpable thyroid nodules. J Clin Endocrinol Metab. 1999;84:24–8.

80. Cappelli C, Castellano M, Pirola I, et al. The predictive value of ultrasound findings in the managment of thryoid nodules. QJM. 2007;100:29–35.

81. Moon WJ, Jung SL, Lee JH, et al. Benign and malignant thyroid nodules: US differentiation – multicenter retrospective study. Radiology. 2008;247:762–70.

82. Kang HW, No JH, Chung JH, et al. Prevalence, clinical and ultrasonographic characteristics of thyroid incidentalomas. Thyroid. 2004;14:29–33.

83. Shimura H, Haraguchi K, Hiejima Y, et al. Distinct diagnostic criteria for ultrasonographic examination of papillary thyroid carcinoma: a multicenter study. Thyroid. 2005;15:251–8.

84. Ito Y, Amino N, Yokozawa T, et al. Ultrasonographic evaluation of thyroid nodules in 900 patients: comparison among ultrasonographic, cytological, and histological findings. Thyroid. 2007;17:1269–76.

85. Park J-Y, Lee HJ, Jang HW, et al. A proposal for a thyroid imaging reporting and data system for ultrasound features of thryoid carcinoma. Thyroid. 2009;19:1257–64.

86. Horvath E, Majlis S, Rossi R, et al. An ultrasound reporting system for thyroid nodules stratifying cancer risk for clinical management. J Clin Endocrinol Metab. 2009;90:1748–51.

87. Frates MC, Benson CB, Charboneau JW, et al. Management of thyroid nodules detected at US: Society of Radiologists in Ultrasound Consensus Conference Statement. Radiology. 2005;237:794–800.

88. Kim TY, Kim WB, Ryu JS, et al. 18 F-fluorodeoxyglucose uptake in thyroid from positron emission tomogram (PET) for evaluation in cancer patients: high prevalence of malignancy in thyroid PET incidentaloma. Laryngoscope. 2005;115:1074–8.

89. Korun N, Asci C, Yilmazlar T, et al. Total thyroidectomy or lobectomy in benign nodular disease of the thyroid: changing trends in surgery. Int Surg. 1997;82:417–9.

90. Mazzaferri EL. Management of a solitary thyroid nodule. N Engl J Med. 1993;328:553–9.

91. Castro MR, Gharib H. Continuing controversies in the management of thyroid nodules. Ann Intern Med. 2005;142:926–31.

92. Goellner JR, Gharib H, Grant CS, et al. Fine needle aspiration cytology of the thyroid, 1980 to 1986. Acta Cytol. 1987;31:587–90.

93. Takashima S, Fukuda H, Kobayashi T. Thyroid nodules: clinical effect of ultrasound-guided fine-needle aspiration biopsy. J Clin Ultrasound. 1994;22:535–42.

94. Carmeci C, Jeffrey RB, McDougall IR, et al. Ultrasound-guided fine-needle aspiration biopsy of thyroid masses. Thyroid. 1998;8:283–9.

95. Danese D, Sciacchitano S, Farsetti A, et al. Diagnostic accuracy of conventional versus sonography-guided fine-needle aspiration biopsy of thyroid nodules. Thyroid. 1998;8:15–21.

96. Hatada T, Okada K, Ishii H, et al. Evaluation of ultrasound-guided fine-needle aspiration biopsy for thyroid nodules. Am J Surg. 1998;175:133–6.

97. Cochand-Priollet B, Guillausseau PJ, Chagnon S, et al. The diagnostic value of fine-needle aspiration biopsy under ultrasonography in nonfunctional thyroid nodules: a prospective study comparing cytologic and histologic findings. Am J Med. 1994;97:152–7.

98. Gharib H, Goellner JR. Fine-needle aspiration biopsy of the thyroid: an appraisal. Ann Intern Med. 1993;118:282–9.

99. Alexander EK, Heering JP, Benson CB, et al. Assessment of nondiagnostic ultrasound-guided fine needle aspiration of thyroid nodules. J Clin Endocrinol Metab. 2002;87:4924–7.

100. Baloch ZW, Cibas ES, Clark DP, et al. The National Cancer Institute thyroid fine needle aspiration state of the science conference: a summation. Cytojournal. 2008;5:6.

101. Haugen BR, Woodmansee WW, McDermott MT. Towards improving the utility of fine-needle aspiration biopsy for the diagnosis of thyroid tumors. Clin Endocrinol (Oxf). 2002;56:281–90.

102. Sapio MR, Posca D, Raggioli A, et al. Detection of RET/PTC, TRK and BRAF mutations in preoperative diagnosis of thyroid nodules with indeterminate cytological findings. Clin Endocrinol (Oxf). 2007;66:678–83.

103. Nikiforov YE, Nikiforov YE, Steward DL, et al. Molecular testing for mutations in improving the fine-needle aspiration diagnosis of thyroid nodules. J Clin Endocrinol Metab. 2009;94:2092–8.

104. Ylagan LR, Farkas T, Dehner LP. Fine needle aspiration of the thyroid: a cytohistologic correlation and study of discrepant cases. Thyroid. 2004;14:35–41.

105. Kuma K, Matsuzuka F, Kibayashi A, et al. Outcome of long standing solitary thyroid nodules. World J Surg. 1992;16:583–7.

106. Bennedbæk FN, Nielsen LK, Hegedüs L. Effect of percutaneous ethanol injection therapy vs. suppressive doses of L-thyroxine on benign solitary solid cold thyroid nodules: a randomized trial. J Clin Endocrinol Metab. 1998;83:30–5.

107. Alexander EK, Hurwitz S, Heering JP, et al. Natural history of benign solid and cystic thyroid nodules. Ann Intern Med. 2003;138:315–8.

108. Asanuma K, Kobayashi S, Shingu K, et al. The rate of tumour growth does not distinguish between malignant and benign thyroid nodules. Eur J Surg. 2001;167:102–5.

109. Brauer VF, Eder P, Miehle K, et al. Interobserver variation for ultrasound determination of thyroid nodule volumes. Thyroid. 2005;15:1169–75.

110. Shimoaka K, Sokal JE. Suppressive therapy of nontoxic goiter. Am J Med. 1974;57:576–83.

111. Celani MF, Mariani M, Mariani G. On the usefulness of levothyroxine suppressive therapy in the medical treatment of benign solitary, solid or predominantly solid, thyroid nodules. Acta Endocrinol (Copenh). 1990;123:603–8.

112. Lima N, Knobel M, Cavaliere H, et al. Levothyroxine suppressive therapy is partially effective in treating patients with benign, solid thyroid nodules and multinodular goiters. Thyroid. 1997;7:691–7.

113. La Rosa GL, Lupo I, Giuffrida D, et al. Levothyroxine and potassium iodide are both effective in treating benign solitary solid cold nodules of the thyroid. Ann Intern Med. 1995;122:1–8.

114. Zelmanovitz F, Genro S, Gross JL. Suppressive therapy with levothyroxine for solitary thyroid nodules: a double-blind controlled clinical study and cumulative meta-analysis. J Clin Endocrinol Metab. 1998;83:3881–5.

115. Wémeau JL, Caron P, Schvartz C, et al. Effects of thyroid-stimulating hormone suppression with levothyroxine in reducing the volume of solitary thyroid nodules and improving extranodular nonpalpable changes: a randomized, double-blind, placebo-controlled trial by the French Thyroid Research Group. J Clin Endocrinol Metab. 2002;87:4928–34.

116. Papini E, Petrucci L, Guglielmi R, et al. Long-term changes in nodular goiter: a 5-year prospective randomised trial of levothyroxine suppressive therapy for benign cold thyroid nodules. J Clin Endocrinol Metab. 1998;83:780–3.

117. Gharib H, James EM, Charboneau JW, et al. Suppressive therapy with levothyroxine for solitary thyroid nodules. A double-blind controlled clinical study. N Engl J Med. 1987;317:70–5.

118. Larijani B, Pajouhi M, Bastanhagh MH, et al. Evaluation of suppressive therapy for cold thyroid nodules with levothyroxine: double-blind, placebo-controlled clinical trial. Endocr Pract. 1999;5:251–6.

119. Castro MR, Caraballo PJ, Morris JC. Effectiveness of thyroid hormone suppressive therapy in benign solitary thyroid nodules: a meta-analysis. J Clin Endocrinol Metab. 2002;87:4154–9.

120. La Rosa GL, Ippolito AM, Lupo L, et al. Cold thyroid nodule reduction with L-thyroxine can be predicted by initial nodule volume and cytological characteristics. J Clin Endocrinol Metab. 1996;81:4385–7.

121. Csako G, Byrd D, Wesley RA, et al. Assessing the effects of thyroid suppression on benign solitary thyroid nodules. A model for using quantitative research synthesis. Medicine (Baltimore). 2000;79:9–26.

122. Richter B, Neises G, Clar C. Pharmacotherapy for thyroid nodules. A systemic review and meta-analysis. Endocrinol Metab Clin. 2002;31:699–722.

123. Subbiah S, Collins BJ, Schneider AB. Factors related to the recurrence of thyroid nodules after surgery for benign radiation-related nodules. Thyroid. 2007;17:41–7.

124. Gharib H, Mazzaferri EL. Thyroxine suppressive therapy in patients with nodular thyroid disease. Ann Intern Med. 1998;128:386–94.

125. Faber J, Galloe AM. Changes in bone mass during prolonged subclinical hyperthyroidism due to L-thyroxine treatment: a meta-analysis. Eur J Endocrinol. 1994;130:350–6.

126. Uzzan B, Campos J, Cucherat M, et al. Effects on bone mass of long term treatment with thyroid hormones: a meta-analysis. J Clin Endocrinol Metab. 1996;81:4278–89.

127. Sawin CT, Geller A, Wolf PA, et al. Low serum thyrotropin concentrations as a risk factor for atrial fibrillation in older persons. N Engl J Med. 1994;331:1249–52.

128. Perle JV, Maisonneuve P, Sheppard MC, et al. Prediction of all-cause and cardiovascular mortality in elderly people from one low serum thyrotropin result: a 10 year cohort study. Lancet. 2001;358:861–5.

129. Tuttle RM, Lemar H, Burch HB. Cinical features associated with an increased risk of thyroid malignancy in patients with follicular neoplasia by fine-needle aspiration. Thyroid. 1998;8:377–83.

130. Tyler DS, Winchester DJ, Caraway NP, et al. Indeterminate fine-needle aspiration biopsy of the thyroid: identification of subgroups at high risk for invasive carcinoma. Surgery. 1994;116:1054–60.

131. Kelman AS, Rathan A, Leibowitz J, et al. Thyroid cytology and the risk of malignancy in thyroid nodules: importance of nuclear atypia in indeterminate specimens. Thyroid. 2001;11:271–7.

132. Tisell LE, Nilsson B, Molne J, et al. Improved survival of patients with papillary thyroid cancer after surgical microdissection. World J Surg. 1996;20:854–9.

133. Sywak M, Cornford L, Roach P, et al. Routine ipsilateral level VI lymphadenectomy reduces postoperative thyroglobulin levels in papillary thyroid cancer. Surgery. 2006;140:1000–7.

134. Moser E. Radioiodine treatment of Plummer's disease. Exp Clin Endocrinol Diabetes. 1998;106 Suppl 4:S63–5.

135. Nygaard B, Hegedüs L, Nielsen KG, et al. Long-term effect of radioactive iodine on thyroid function and size in patients with solitary autonomously functioning toxic thyroid nodules. Clin Endocrinol (Oxf). 1999;50:197–202.

136. Ferrari C, Reschini E, Paracchi A. Treatment of the autonomous thyroid nodule: a review. Eur J Endocrinol. 1996;135:383–90.

137. Mariotti S, Martino E, Francesconi M, et al. Serum thyroid autoantibodies as a risk factor for development of hypothyroidism after radioactive iodine therapy for single thyroid 'hot' nodule. Acta Endocrinol (Copenh). 1986;113:500–7.

138. Goldstein R, Hart IR. Follow-up of solitary autonomous thyroid nodules treated with [131]I. N Engl J Med. 1983;309:1473–6.

139. Lippi F, Ferrari C, Manetti L, et al. Treatment of solitary autonomous thyroid nodules by percutaneous ethanol injection: results of an Italian multicenter study. J Clin Endocrinol Metab. 1996;81:3261–4.

140. Verde G, Papini E, Pacella CM, et al. Ultrasound guided percutaneous ethanol injection in the treatment of cystic thyroid nodules. Clin Endocrinol (Oxf). 1994;41:719–24.

141. Bennedbæk FN, Karstrup S, Hegedüs L. Percutaneous ethanol injection therapy in the treatment of thyroid and parathyroid diseases. Eur J Endocrinol. 1997;136:240–50.

142. Livraghi T, Paracchi A, Ferrari C, et al. Treatment of autonomous thyroid nodules with percutaneous ethanol injection: preliminary results: work in progress. Radiology. 1990;175:827–9.

143. Papini E, Pacella CM, Verde G. Percutaneous ethanol injection (PEI): what is its role in the treatment of benign thyroid nodules? Thyroid. 1995;5:147–50.

144. Valcavi R, Frasoldati A. Ultrasound-guided percutaneous ethanol injection therapy in thyroid cystic nodules. Endocr Pract. 2004;10:269–75.

145. Guglielmi R, Pacella CM, Bianchini A, et al. Percutaneous ethanol injection treatment in benign thyroid lesions: role and efficacy. Thyroid. 2004;14:125–31.

146. Kim JH, Lee HK, Lee JH, et al. Efficacy of sonographically guided percutaneous ethanol injection for treatment of thyroid cysts versus solid thyroid nodules. Am J Roentgenol. 2003;180:1723–6.

147. Zingrillo M, Torlontano M, Chiarella R, et al. Percutaneous ethanol injection may be a definitive treatment for symptomatic thyroid cystic nodules not treatable by surgery: five-year follow-up study. Thyroid. 1999;9:763–7.

148. Bennedbæk FN, Hegedüs L. Treatment of recurrent thyroid cysts with ethanol: a randomized double-blind controlled trial. J Clin Endocrinol Metab. 2003;88:5773–7.

149. Monzani F, Lippi F, Goletti O, et al. Percutaneous aspiration and ethanol scelerotherapy for thyroid cysts. J Clin Endocrinol Metab. 1994;78:800–2.

150. Monzani F, Goletti O, Caraccio N, et al. Percutaneous ethanol injection treatment of autonomous thyroid adenoma: hormonal and clinical evaluation. Clin Endocrinol (Oxf). 1992;36:491–7.

151. Papini E, Panunzi C, Pacella CM, et al. Percutaneous ultrasound-guided ethanol injection: a new treatment of toxic autonomously functioning thyroid nodules? J Clin Endocrinol Metab. 1993;76:411–6.

152. Livraghi T, Paracchi A, Ferrari C, et al. Treatment of autonomous thyroid nodules with percutaneous ethanol injection: 4-year experience. Radiology. 1994;190:529–33.

153. Di Lelio A, Rivolta M, Casati M, et al. Treatment of autonomous thyroid nodules: value of percutaneous ethanol injection. Am J Roentgenol. 1995;164:207–13.

154. Mazzeo S, Toni MG, DeGaudio C, et al. Percutaneous injection of ethanol to treat autonomous thyroid nodules. Am J Roentgenol. 1993;161:871–6.

155. Goletti O, Monzani F, Lenziardi M, et al. Cold thyroid nodules: a new application of percutaneous ethanol injection treatment. J Clin Ultrasound. 1994;22:175–8.

156. Zingrillo M, Collura D, Chiggi MR, et al. Treatment of large cold benign thyroid nodules not eligible for surgery with percutaneous ethanol injection. J Clin Endocrinol Metab. 1998;83:3905–7.

157. Lyshchik A, Higashi T, Asato R, et al. Thyroid gland tumor diagnosis at US elastography. Radiology. 2005;237:202–11.

158. Rago T, Santini F, Scutari M, et al. Elastography: new developments in ultrasound for predicting malignancy in thyroid nodules. J Clin Endocrinol Metab. 2007;92:2917–22.

159. Dighe M, Bae U, Richardson ML, et al. Differential diagnosis of thyroid nodules with US elastography using carotid artery pulsation. Radiology. 2008;248:662–9.

160. Rago T, Vitti P. Role of thyroid ultrasound in the diagnostic evaluation of thyroid nodules. Best Pract Res Clin Endocrinol Metab. 2008;22:913–28.

161. Hong Y, Liu X, Li Z, et al. Real-time ultrasound elastography in the differential diagnosis of benign and malignant thyroid nodules. J Ultrasound Med. 2009;28:861–7.

162. Dossing H, Bennedbæk FN, Hegedüs L, et al. Effect of ultrasound-guided interstitial laser photocoagulation on benign solitary solid cold thyroid nodules: one versus three treatments. Thyroid. 2006;16:763–8.

163. Cakir B, Ugras NS, Gul K, et al. Initial report of the results of percutaneous laser ablation of benign cold thyroid nodules: evaluation of histopathological changes after 2 years. Endocr Pathol. 2009;20:170–6.

Ultrasound Imaging of Thyroid Cancer

4

Michelle Melany

Introduction

Ultrasound is an ideal imaging modality for detection and assessment of thyroid cancer because it is widely available and is highly sensitive for both detection and characterization of thyroid nodules due to improvements in transducer technology. In addition, it does not involve ionizing radiation and can be combined with fine-needle-aspiration biopsy. Recent consensus guidelines from the American Thyroid Association highlight the importance of ultrasound and state that thyroid ultrasound should be performed in all patients with a suspected thyroid nodule, nodular goiter, or radiographic thyroid abnormality; e.g., a nodule found incidentally on CT, PET, MRI, carotid Doppler, or other radiographic examinations [1].

The role of ultrasound in thyroid cancer imaging includes detection and characterization of thyroid cancer. Ultrasound is also used to detect cervical lymph node metastases prior to surgery for thyroid cancer. At our institution, ultrasound "lymph node mapping" refers to a detailed ultrasound examination, performed by an experienced sonographer prior to treatment for thyroid cancer, in an effort to detect nodal metastatic disease. Ultrasound in experienced hands is more

accurate than other imaging modalities, including whole-body iodine scan, MR, CT, and PET/CT, in detecting cervical metastases from thyroid cancer [2]. Therefore, preoperative neck ultrasound to evaluate the contralateral lobe and cervical lymph nodes (central and lateral compartments) is recommended for all patients undergoing thyroidectomy for malignancy [1]. Additional uses of ultrasound include routine follow-up of thyroid cancer patients after initial treatment in order to identify early local recurrence in the thyroid bed or cervical nodal metastases. Neck ultrasound is more sensitive than whole-body iodine scans and serum thyroglobulin levels in detecting cervical recurrence and should be a first-line test in the follow-up of all differentiated thyroid cancer patients [3].

Ultrasound guidance may be used for fine-needle-aspiration biopsy of thyroid nodules, morphologically abnormal cervical lymph nodes prior to or after treatment, and masses in the postoperative bed that may represent recurrent thyroid cancer or central compartment nodal metastases. Ultrasound guidance is occasionally used for other interventional procedures such as needle localization of nodes or other masses with methylene blue dye prior to surgical excision, radiofrequency ablation, and percutaneous ethanol injection treatment of local recurrence or neck metastases [4, 5].

Ultrasound elastography is a relatively new diagnostic technique that assesses stiffness of a lesion as an indicator of malignancy and this technique has been recently applied to nodular

M. Melany (✉)
Department of Imaging, Cedars-Sinai Medical Center,
8700 Beverly Blvd, M-335, Los Angeles,
CA 90048, USA
e-mail: melanym@cshs.org

G.D. Braunstein (ed.), *Thyroid Cancer*, Endocrine Updates 30,
DOI 10.1007/978-1-4614-0875-8_4, © Springer Science+Business Media, LLC 2012

thyroid disease. A firm or hard consistency is associated with an increased risk of malignancy in thyroid nodules. An ultrasound elastogram is displayed over the B-mode image in a color scale that corresponds to tissue elasticity. Conventional ultrasound is used to determine which lesions are suitable for elastographic evaluation. Cystic and rim-calcified nodules and coalescent nodules seen in multinodular goiters are not suitable for elastography [6]. Although some studies report promising results with high sensitivity and specificity for papillary thyroid cancer [6–8], other investigators note unreliable inter-observer agreement with ultrasound elastography for the diagnosis of malignant thyroid nodules [9].

Computed tomography (CT) and magnetic resonance imaging (MRI) of the neck have a limited role in the initial investigation of a patient presenting with a thyroid nodule. Similarly, routine use of neck imaging studies other than ultrasound (CT, MR, and PET) is not recommended in patients diagnosed with differentiated thyroid cancer. In invasive thyroid malignancy with gross extension outside of the gland, these modalities can be helpful to evaluate extra-thyroidal spread to adjacent structures such as the larynx, trachea, carotid, and jugular vein. These modalities can also provide evidence of regional or distant metastases [1, 10].

Technique/Equipment Specifications

Ultrasound of the thyroid gland is typically performed from the patient's right side with the neck in slight hyperextension. If possible, a towel or pillow under the shoulders may be used to increase the degree of neck extension. Thyroid ultrasound can be limited in patients who are obese, who cannot hyperextend their neck (due to cervical stenosis or degenerative disc disease) and in patients with prior extensive radical neck surgery in whom incomplete contact of the ultrasound transducer with the neck can limit evaluation [11].

Thyroid ultrasound examinations should be performed with a high-frequency linear or curved linear transducer. Thyroid sonography is performed with mean frequencies of 10–14 MHz and higher; however, some patients may require a lower-frequency transducer in order to penetrate thicker neck soft tissues or to better evaluate extension of large goiters into the subclavicular or substernal region. We have found that smaller-footprint, lower-frequency curved transducers (such as those used to evaluate the neonatal brain through an open fontanelle) can be useful for ultrasound evaluation and fine-needle-aspiration biopsy of thyroid nodules and nodes, the postoperative thyroid bed, supraclavicular and central compartment nodes, and even masses extending toward the superior mediastinum.

The thyroid ultrasound examination should be performed at the highest clinically appropriate frequency. The examiner performing the examination should recognize that there is a tradeoff between resolution and penetration such that higher-frequency transducers produce higher-resolution images, especially in the near field, but may not provide sufficient penetration. Conversely, lower-frequency transducers may penetrate the gland but provide less morphologic detail. High-resolution ultrasound provides the basis for characterization of benign and malignant nodules.

Spectral, color, and/or power Doppler evaluation may be useful to determine overall vascularity of the gland and of individual nodules. Color Doppler frequencies should be set in order to optimize detection of blood flow. Power Doppler imaging is especially useful in low-flow states.

Both lobes should be evaluated in two dimensions and the isthmus imaged at least in the transverse imaging plane. When identified, abnormalities in thyroid gland and the adjacent soft tissues, such as nodes and thrombosed vessels, should be documented [12].

Ultrasound Features of Thyroid Nodules

A thyroid nodule is a discrete lesion within the thyroid gland that is radiographically distinguishable from the adjacent thyroid tissue (Fig. 4.1).

Fig. 4.1 Two hypoechoic rounded nodules are distinct from the uniform-appearing adjacent thyroid tissue

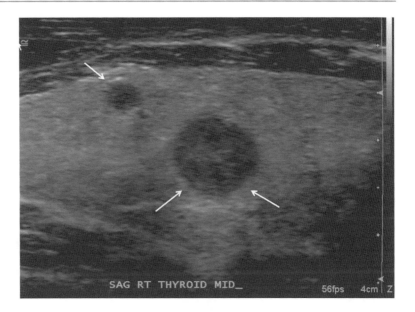

The expanded use of CT, MR, US, and PET for neck imaging has fueled a dramatic increase in US-guided FNA of "incidentalomas" or nonpalpable thyroid nodules. The incidence of thyroid cancer has more than doubled in the ultrasound era since about 1973. However, there has been no change in the mortality of thyroid cancer. Some authors feel that the increased incidence is due, in part, to the increase in detection of "subclinical" papillary cancer with US-guided FNA [13, 14].

Other investigators feel that increased diagnostic scrutiny leading to US-guided FNA is not the sole explanation and that other influences should be investigated [15]. Our goal as thyroid ultrasound imagers is to maximize the detection of clinically relevant thyroid cancers and minimize the number of benign US-guided fine-needle-aspiration biopsies. One of the confounding variables is that the major clinical societies dealing with thyroid disease disagree about guidelines for US-guided FNA in nonpalpable nodules [16].

Topics for discussion in this chapter include ultrasound features that suggest benign versus malignant thyroid lesions and also pattern recognition, particularly recognition of "low yield for biopsy" nodules. It is a challenge to determine how to reliably sort out the large number of patients with benign nodules from the relatively small number with carcinoma. Because thyroid nodules are so prevalent and because relatively few are malignant, a method of distinguishing nodules that require further evaluation with FNA is critical to improve the utilization of medical resources. Ultrasound features of thyroid nodules influencing biopsy include size, grayscale features, grayscale pattern, and color Doppler findings.

Ultrasound Features of Thyroid Cancer

Ultrasound features of thyroid malignancy include predominately solid, hypoechoic, intranodular vascularity, the presence of calcifications, the absence of a well-defined halo, spiculated and ill-defined margins, and a taller-than-wide shape. Sensitivities, specificities, and positive and negative predictive values for these features are, however, highly variable from study to study such that no isolated ultrasound feature of thyroid nodules is sufficiently sensitive or specific to diagnose or exclude malignancy.

Combinations of ultrasound features have been used by many authors to stratify nodules into high and low risk for malignancy. Nodules without any suspicious features have a <2% risk

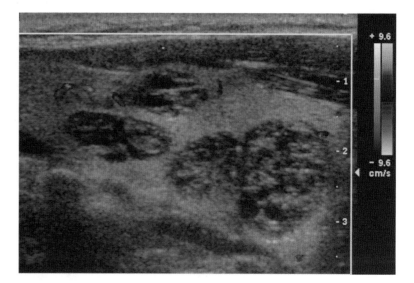

Fig. 4.2 Three spongiform or honeycomb nodules are made up of multiple adjacent avascular septations that form tiny elongated cysts

of malignancy, whereas nodules with at least two suspicious features have much higher malignancy rates [17]. The presence of multiple criteria increases the specificity for thyroid cancer; however, decreases the sensitivity [18–20].

Pattern recognition (grouping nodules into reproducible patterns of morphology) rather than analysis of individual sonographic features has been proposed as an accurate method to predict *benignity* of thyroid nodules. Four patterns have been described to have 100% specificity for benign lesions: (1) avascular or iso-vascular spongiform or honeycomb configuration with>50% diffuse internal linear cysts (Fig. 4.2), (2) cyst with central avascular colloid clot, (3) giraffe pattern (alternating blocks of hyperechogenicity surrounded by thin areas of hypoechogenicity, and (4) diffuse hyperechogenicity [21].

Various authors have proposed a thyroid imaging reporting and data system for thyroid nodules similar to the American College of Radiology's Breast Imaging Reporting And Data System (BIRADS), developed and utilized by radiologists for mammography and breast ultrasound [22]. "TIRADS" or "THIRADS" will hopefully be a cost-effective future strategy that not only improves patient management but also reduces the number of unnecessary thyroid biopsies [23, 24].

It is important to remember that the most common sonographic appearances of papillary and follicular thyroid cancer differ. Papillary

thyroid cancer is typically predominantly solid, hypoechoic, and often with increased vascularity and irregular margins. Microcalcifications are specific for papillary thyroid cancer but can be difficult to distinguish from colloid and are not seen in follicular carcinoma. Follicular carcinoma is more often iso- to hyperechoic, and can have a thick irregular halo. Papillary thyroid cancers more often conform to the current ultrasound criteria for malignant nodules; however, if these criteria are strictly applied to guide decision for FNA, follicular carcinomas may be missed [25].

Calcifications

Thyroid calcifications occur in both benign and malignant diseases. Calcifications in thyroid nodules are the most reproducible sonographic feature with excellent interobserver reliability [26]. Thyroid calcifications can be classified as microcalcifications, macrocalcifications, or peripheral calcifications (Fig. 4.3). The presence of any calcification in a nodule has been reported to increase the chance of malignancy [27, 28].

Microcalcifications typically appear as punctate echogenic foci (Fig. 4.3a) that, individually, do not cast an acoustic shadow; however, a conglomerate of multiple microcalcifications may shadow. Microcalcifications correspond histologically to calcified psammoma bodies (infarcted

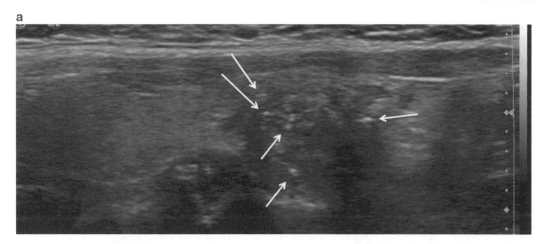

Fig. 4.3 (a) A hypoechoic, nodule with poorly defined anterior margins. *Arrows* mark multiple punctate microcalcifications that represent calcified psammoma bodies. (b) A macrocalcification with *straight arrows* marking posterior acoustic shadowing distal to the coarse calcification. *Curved arrow* demonstrates disorganized flow pattern also seen in this papillary thyroid malignancy. (c) Smooth, curvilinear, peripheral (eggshell) calcification is marked by *arrows* in this benign thyroid nodule (d) Interrupted peripheral calcification (*straight arrows*) more typical of a malignant nodule. An adjacent nodule containing microcalcifications (*curved arrow*) is also present in this patient with papillary thyroid cancer

papillae) that are typical of papillary cancer [28]. The presence of microcalcifications in a solid nodule has been reported to increase the risk of cancer threefold. Thyroid microcalcification is the feature with the highest positive predictive value; however, it has low sensitivity and is seen in only 26–59% of cancers [17].

Unfortunately, colloid crystals and microcalcifications can occasionally be difficult to distinguish. Comet-tail artifacts (Fig. 4.4) are posterior "ring down" artifacts or triangular-shaped posterior acoustic enhancement distal to echogenic foci seen in cystic and partially cystic colloid lesions. These artifacts are caused by reverberation of the colloid crystals when they encounter the ultrasound beam. When thyroid lesions with the comet-tail artifact undergo FNA, abundant colloid is seen in the specimen in 85% of cases. In one study, none of the lesions with the comet-tail artifact were associated with malignancy [29]. Because of the overlap between the appearance of colloid and microcalcification, when considering the risk of malignancy, punctate echogenic foci in a thyroid nodule should be assumed to represent microcalcifications if comet-tail artifacts are not present [17].

Macrocalcifications (Fig. 4.3b) are coarse aggregates of calcification that often cast an acoustic shadow. These calcifications are thought to represent tissue fibrosis and degeneration [28]. Large, irregularly shaped macrocalcifications have been reported to be associated with long-standing benign thyroid lesions and Hashimoto's thyroiditis [30]. However, it is widely recognized that coarse macrocalcifications can be seen in malignant thyroid lesions. The presence of macrocalcification in a solid nodule has been reported to increase the risk of cancer twofold [17]. The risk of malignancy increases when coarse calcifications are associated with additional suspicious ultrasound features such as marked hypoechogenicity, irregular or microlobulated margins, and a taller-than-wide shape [31].

Peripheral or eggshell calcifications (Fig. 4.3c) have also previously been reported to be a feature that suggests a thyroid nodule is more likely to be benign. A recent literature report recommended FNA for lesions with peripheral eggshell calcification based on the relatively high prevalence of malignancy in these lesions (up to 18.5%) [32]. Other authors specify interrupted (Fig. 4.3d) or disrupted and thickened (>5 mm) peripheral calcifications as being more highly associated with malignancy [33–35].

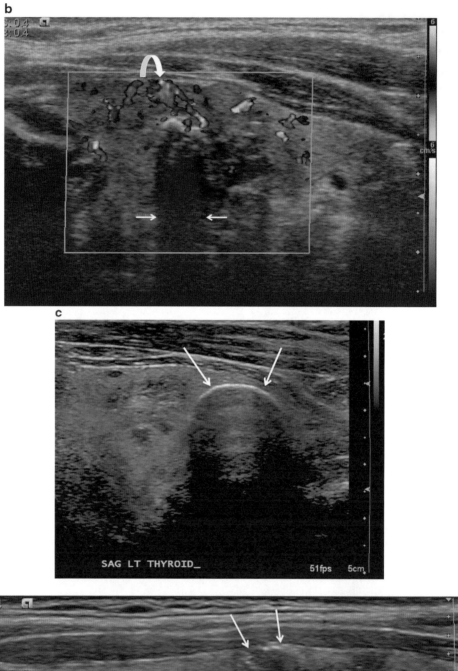

Fig. 4.3 (continued)

Fig. 4.4 (**a**) A cystic lesion with low-level internal echoes has echogenic foci floating in the complex fluid. The echogenic foci represent crystals that demonstrate posterior triangular-shaped "ring down" artifact (*arrows*) characteristic of colloid. (**b**) Two, avascular cystic lesions are seen, one of which contains colloid crystals floating in the cyst fluid. The colloid crystals demonstrate classic "comet tail" or ring down artifact (*arrows*)

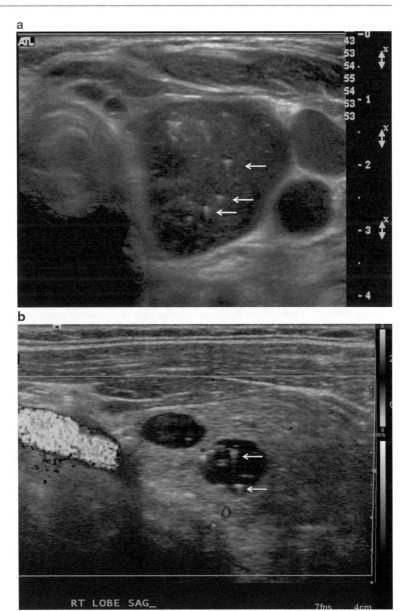

Margins

Thyroid nodules follow the imaging trends of tumors in other organs in that benign thyroid nodules tend to have sharp, well-defined margins and malignant lesions tend to have poorly defined margins. Margins of thyroid lesions have been described as well-defined smooth, spiculated, or ill-defined [17, 28] (Fig. 4.5). Spiculated and ill-defined margins suggest malignant infiltration into adjacent parenchyma. A thyroid nodule is considered ill-defined if more than 50% of its border is not clearly demarcated. The reported sensitivity of ill-defined margins varies widely. Up to 47% of papillary cancers have well-defined margins and many of these are encapsulated at histology [36]. The specificity of ill-defined margins is also variable and 15–59% of benign nodules have ill-defined margins [19, 26]. Therefore, because of variable specificity and sensitivity, the

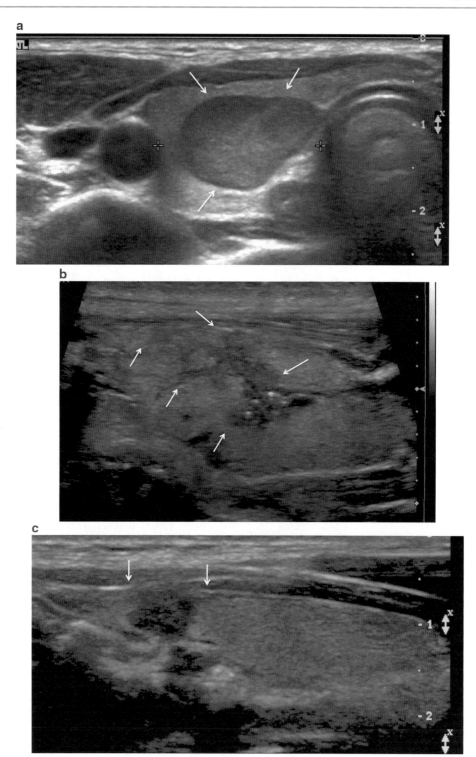

Fig. 4.5 (a) *Arrows* point to a well-defined nodule with smooth margins. This lesion, a follicular adenoma, also demonstrates a hypoechoic halo. (b) *Arrows* denote a nodule with spiculated or angular margins rendering it suspicious for malignancy. Additional suspicious features include hypoechoic echotexture and echogenic foci that likely represent microcalcifications. (c) More than 50% of the border of this hypoechoic nodule with ill-defined margins is not clearly demarcated. Arrows depict interruption of the thyroid capsular margin by the nodule compatible with frank invasion beyond the thyroid capsule

ultrasound appearance of nodular margin alone is unreliable in determining malignancy unless frank invasion beyond the thyroid capsule is identified [37].

Halo

The halo or hypoechoic rim surrounding a thyroid nodule is produced by a pseudocapsule of fibrous connective tissue or blood vessels coursing around the periphery of a lesion or compressed thyroid tissue or chronic inflammatory infiltrates [37–39] (Fig. 4.6). A completely uniform halo around a nodule is highly suggestive of benignity with a specificity of 95%. However a halo is absent in more than half of all benign thyroid nodules. Ten to twenty-four percent of papillary thyroid cancers have either a complete or an incomplete halo [36, 37]. Thick irregular, hypovascular or avascular halos are seen in rapidly growing malignant thyroid nodules and the halo is thought to represent compressed adjacent thyroid parenchyma [38] (Fig. 4.6c).

Shape

The shape of a thyroid nodule is considered a potentially useful feature when predicting the

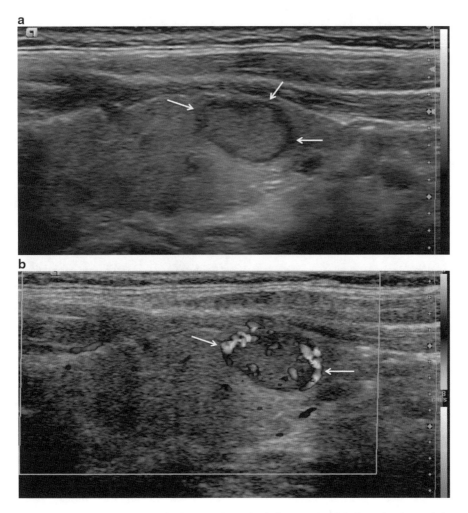

Fig. 4.6 (a) *Arrows* point to a hypoechoic rim or halo completely surrounding this isoechoic benign nodule. (b) Color Doppler image demonstrates portions of the halo to represent blood vessels coursing around the periphery of the lesion. (c) A thick, irregular, hypoechoic, avascular halo is seen surrounding this malignant thyroid nodule. Small amounts of perinodular and central blood flow in the lesion do not correspond to the thick halo

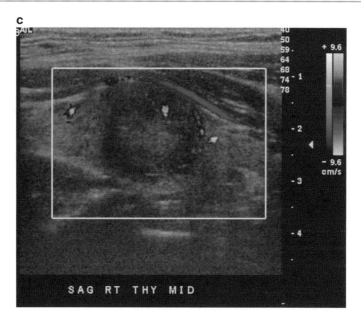

Fig. 4.6 (continued)

risk of malignancy. A solid nodule that is "taller than wide" (greater in its anterior–posterior dimension than its transverse dimension) has been correlated with an increased risk of malignancy [28, 40, 41] (Fig. 4.7). The "taller-than-wide" appearance is thought to be due to the fact that malignant nodules grow across normal tissue planes, whereas benign nodules grow parallel to normal tissue planes [28]. Similar characteristics have been used to distinguish malignant from benign breast masses.

Nodule Composition: Solid Versus Cystic

Solid composition is the ultrasound feature with the highest sensitivity for malignancy, in the range of 69–86%. Malignant thyroid nodules tend to be solid [42]. However, the fact that a nodule is solid has a low positive predictive value in that a solid nodule has only a 15–27% chance of being malignant. Several studies have demonstrated an inverse relationship between the cystic component of a nodule and the risk of malignancy. A simple thyroid cyst has high specificity for benignity; however, less than

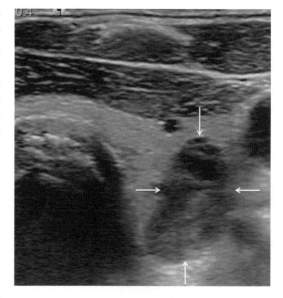

Fig. 4.7 This papillary thyroid cancer is "taller than wide." It is greater in its AP dimension than its transverse dimension. As noted with this case, this "taller than wide" distinction must be made when evaluating the transverse view of the nodule rather than the sagittal view

1–2% of thyroid lesions are simple cysts [1, 18]. In a mixed echogenicity (solid and cystic) lesion, the risk of malignancy is greater if more than 50% of the lesion is solid. There is also an increased risk of malignancy in mixed lesions if the solid component is eccentric and if microcalcifications are present [43] (Fig. 4.8). In multiple series, the so-called "spongiform" appearance of a nodule was >99% specific for benignity. In a recent article, spongiform lesions that were avascular or isovascular compared to adjacent thyroid tissue were always benign. A single case of a spongiform lesion that was hypervascular on color Doppler examination was malignant [28, 43, 44].

Cystic papillary carcinoma is rare and accounts for approximately 5–7% of partially cystic nodules. All of these lesions have a vascular solid component [36]. A solid component in a cyst with multiple punctate echogenic foci (representing microcalcifications) protruding into the cyst suggests a cystic papillary cancer (Fig. 4.9). Needle

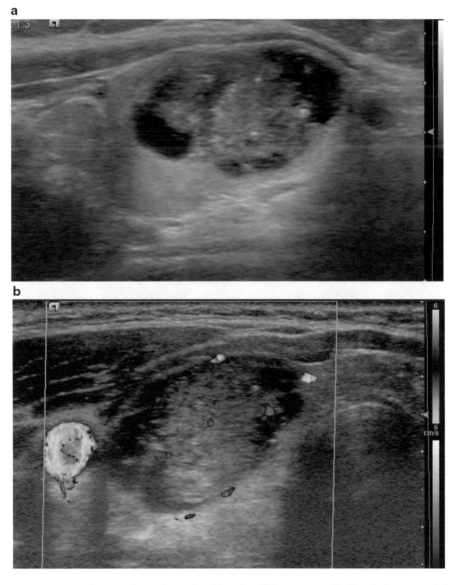

a

b

Fig. 4.8 (**a**) A mixed solid and cystic papillary thyroid cancer demonstrates >50% solid component. Additional features increasing the risk of malignancy include the presence of microcalcifications and eccentric location of the solid component. (**b**) Flow in the nonanechoic component of the nodule confirms this portion of the lesion is solid tissue rather than avascular clot

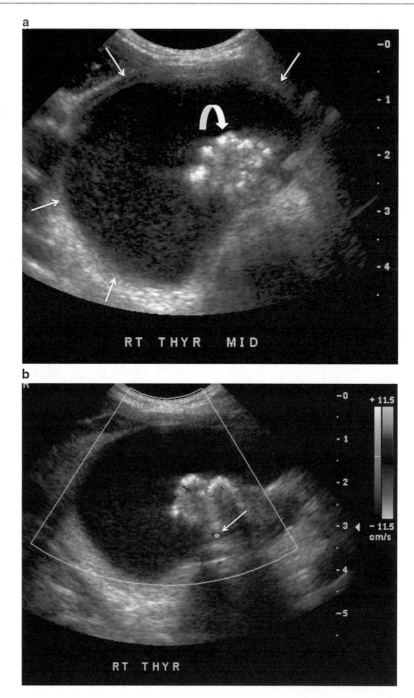

Fig. 4.9 (a) *Straight arrows* point to the margins of a cystic papillary cancer, while the curved arrow denotes the solid component of the lesion that contains micro-calcifications. (b) In this color Doppler image of the same lesion, the arrow points to vascularity in the solid component of the nodule. (c) This image was obtained during ultrasound-guided FNA of this cystic papillary cancer with the needle directed toward the solid component of the lesion, ensuring an adequate cytologic result

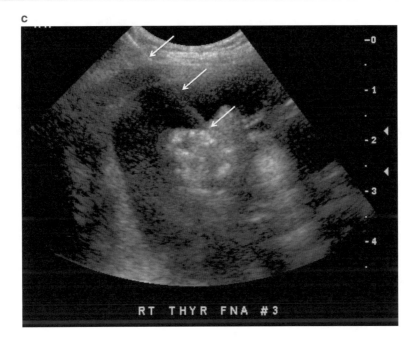

Fig. 4.9 (continued)

biopsy of these lesions should be performed under ultrasound guidance with the needle tip directed toward the solid component to obtain an adequate cytologic result.

Echogenicity

Malignant thyroid nodules, including carcinomas and lymphomas, are typically solid and appear hypoechoic compared to the adjacent thyroid parenchyma (Fig. 4.10). The combination of these two sonographic features has been reported to have a sensitivity of 87% for detection of thyroid malignancy [19]. Benign thyroid nodules were solid and hypoechoic in up to 55% in the same series. This combination of features has low specificity (15–27%) and low positive predictive value [17, 37]. When the solid component of a nodule is classified as *markedly* hypoechoic (the echotexture of the nodule is compared to the strap muscles rather than the adjacent thyroid parenchyma), there is increased specificity for malignancy up to 94%; however, sensitivity is reduced to 12% [40] (Fig. 4.6).

Multinodularity

Patients with multiple nodules have the same risk of malignancy (approximately 14%) as patients with solitary nodules [18, 30]. In the case of multiple discrete nodules, FNA is typically performed on those lesions with suspicious morphology rather than on the dominant lesion. If no suspicious features are seen, biopsy of the dominant nodule may be performed. In the case of a diffusely enlarged gland with multiple nodules with similar ultrasound appearance and without intervening normal parenchyma, FNA is likely not necessary [1, 17].

Color Doppler Imaging

Vascularity in a thyroid nodule is determined with color or power Doppler. Three different patterns have been described, including complete absence of flow, exclusive perinodular flow, and intranodular flow, with chaotically arranged vessels with or without perinodular vessels (Fig. 4.11). The pattern of vascularity is another sonographic feature of thyroid nodules that has been used to

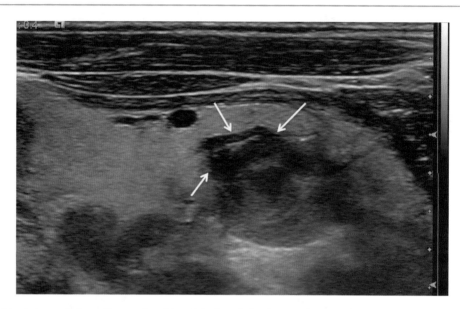

Fig. 4.10 A hypoechoic malignant thyroid nodule is shown with the majority of the lesion more hypoechoic than the background thyroid parenchyma. A portion of the lesion (*arrows*) is *markedly* hypoechoic – more hypoechoic than the adjacent strap muscle

predict malignancy. However, as with other individual ultrasound features, the range of sensitivity and specificity for this finding is quite broad with reported high interobserver variability.

The most common vascular pattern in thyroid malignancy, central hypervascularity (defined as flow in the central portion of the nodule greater than the surrounding thyroid parenchyma), occurs in 69–74% of all thyroid malignancies [19, 36]. However, more than 50% of solid, hypervascular lesions are benign and intrinsic thyroid nodule vascularity is not specific for malignancy [45].

Perinodular flow is defined as vascularity around at least 25% of thyroid nodule circumference and is more characteristic of benign lesions. However, this vascular flow pattern has been reported in up to 22% of thyroid malignancies [10, 36, 37]. Completely avascularity is a useful feature and is typical of hyperplastic lesions. Thyroid nodules without any flow are unlikely to be carcinomas [10, 36].

Size

The size of a lesion is not helpful for predicting or excluding malignancy. There is significant discrepancy between consensus guidelines about which size nodules and associated features for malignancy require FNA. Recent ATA consensus guidelines suggest that nodules <1 cm should not routinely undergo FNA. The reason is not because larger lesions are more likely to harbor malignancy, but rather because clinically significant cancers are more likely to be present in nodules larger than 1 cm [1, 30]. Smaller lesions < 1 cm may undergo FNA if suspicious ultrasound features are present and if the patient has a high-risk history or if suspicious cervical nodes are identified. High-risk history includes patients with a family history of thyroid malignancy, personal history of radiation exposure in childhood – either external beam or ionizing radiation – prior history of partial thyroidectomy with known or incidental discovery of thyroid cancer, or nodules that are PET positive. The ATA guidelines define suspicious features as nodules with the following: microcalcifications, increased intranodular vascularity, hypoechoic, irregular infiltrative margins, absent halo, and a taller-than-wide shape.

When ultrasound features of malignancy are applied to subcentimeter nodules (<1 cm), the same sensitivity, specificity, and positive and negative predictive values are achieved as when the criteria are applied to lesions >1 cm [46]. Some authors feel that subcentimeter nodules

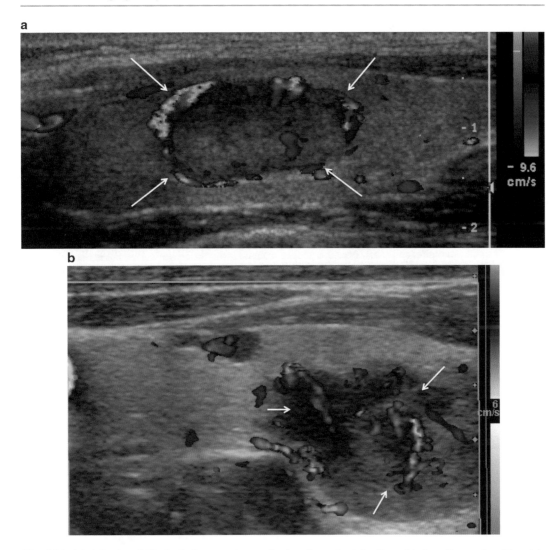

Fig. 4.11 (**a**) A benign follicular lesion contains predominantly perinodular flow. (**b**) A malignant thyroid nodule demonstrates chaotically arranged intranodular flow

that are <5 mm have a high rate of false-positive ultrasound findings and often yield inadequate cytology on fine-needle-aspiration biopsy. They conclude that thyroid nodules of this size should not undergo routine FNA, even if they appear sonographically suspicious. [47]

Ultrasound Features of Follicular Lesions

Follicular thyroid lesions include follicular adenomas and follicular carcinomas and the two can only be distinguished on histology of the surgical specimen by the presence or absence of vascular and capsular invasion. Therefore, it is often not possible to differentiate benign from malignant follicular lesions on FNA or even core biopsy and the collective term "follicular lesion" is used.

Follicular carcinomas account for 5–15% of all thyroid cancers and are more prevalent in iodine-deficient areas [10]. Follicular cancer is thought to develop in a pre-existing adenoma and has the potential to develop hematogenous metastases to lung, liver, bone, and brain. Nodal metastases to the neck are less common.

Sonographic differentiation of follicular carcinomas from benign follicular neoplasms is difficult because follicular cancers usually lack the ultrasound features seen in papillary cancers.

Follicular carcinomas are predominantly solid and homogeneous in 70% of cases [48]. Follicular cancers are more often iso to hyperechoic and have a thick and irregular halo, but do not have microcalcifications [25] (Fig. 4.12). In large nodules with benign sonographic features, the absence of cystic degeneration is suggestive of follicular cancer but not definitive [11]. Malignant follicular lesions typically have intranodular flow with multiple vascular poles, chaotically arranged, with or without perinodular flow, whereas benign lesions are more likely to have exclusively perinodular flow [10, 38] (Fig. 4.12b). Follicular cancers that are < 2 cm in diameter reportedly are not associated with metastatic disease [49].

Ultrasound Features of Medullary Cancer

Medullary carcinoma represents approximately 5% of malignant thyroid lesions. Medullary lesions arise from the parafollicular C cells that secrete calcitonin, a useful tumor marker for the disease. Recurrence in the neck and mediastinum is common in medullary carcinoma and typically causes an increase in serum calcitonin. When patients present, 50% of them have nodal metastases and 15–25% have distant metastases to liver, lung, and bone. Medullary cancer is familial in 20% of cases and it is associated with MEN II syndrome and these patients have more aggressive tumors and worse prognosis with approximately 55% 5-year survival [10, 38].

Sonographically, medullary cancer may present as a solid, hypoechoic mass with internal vascularity. Punctate echogenic foci are seen in 80–90% of cases due to amyloid deposition and associated calcification (Fig. 4.13). The echogenic foci are also seen in 50–60% of associated nodal metastases from medullary cancer. The findings in medullary carcinoma of the thyroid do no differ greatly from papillary carcinoma, except that medullary cancers tend to have round to ovoid shape [50].

Ultrasound Features of Lymphoma

Lymphoma represents 1–4% of all thyroid malignancies and is most often the non-Hodgkin's type. In 70–80% of cases, lymphoma arises in the setting of Hashimoto's thyroiditis. Patients may present with a rapidly growing mass that may lead to obstructive symptoms such as dyspnea and dyphagia [51]. The prognosis depends on the stage of the disease at presentation. The 5-year survival may range from 90% in early stages to 5% in advanced disease.

Sonographically, thyroid lymphoma is hypoechoic, lobulated, and often hypovascular (Fig. 4.14). The lesions may appear pseudocystic with posterior acoustic enhancement or may be heterogeneous. If the entire gland is involved, the gland may be heterogeneous or diffusely enlarged and hypoechoic. Large areas of cystic necrosis may occur and lymphoma, if it presents late, may encase adjacent vessels and structures. Rounded hypoechoic cervical lymph nodes with or without reticulation may be present. The adjacent, uninvolved thyroid parenchyma may be heterogeneous with fine echogenic fibrous linear strands due to underlying chronic thyroiditis [10, 38, 52] (Fig. 4.14). Flow cytometry is needed to diagnose lymphoma. For this reason, core biopsies of the thyroid may sometimes be performed in suspected cases of thyroid lymphoma.

Ultrasound Features of Anaplastic Cancer

Anaplastic thyroid carcinoma accounts for less than 5% of all thyroid cancer and is one of the most aggressive head and neck cancers. It carries the worst prognosis of all thyroid cancers with a 5-year mortality rate of greater than 95% and typically occurs in the elderly. The diagnosis is suspected clinically with rapid growth of a neck mass that invades adjacent structures. These lesions are often associated with papillary or follicular carcinomas and they presumably represent

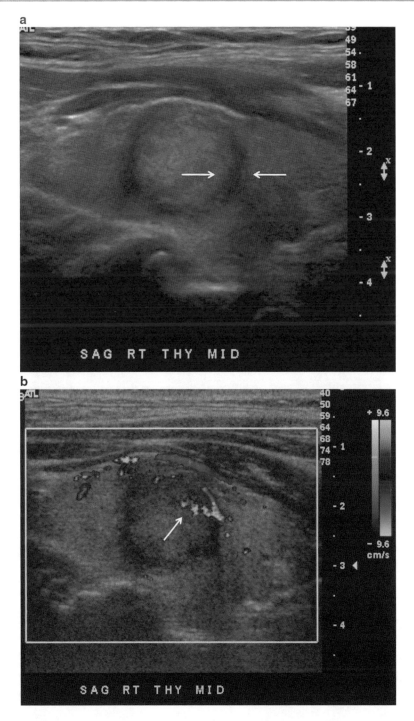

Fig. 4.12 (a) This follicular carcinoma is isoechoic compared to the surrounding thyroid parenchyma and has a thick irregular halo (*arrows*) and does not contain microcalcifications. (b) Color Doppler image shows both peripheral and perinodular flow and also an irregular intranodular vascular pole

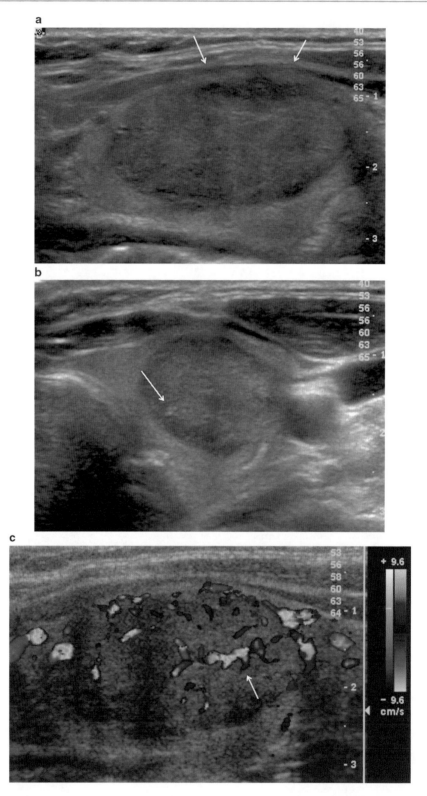

Fig. 4.13 (a) A hypoechoic, solid, oval-shaped medullary cancer has ill-defined anterior margins. (b) The medullary carcinoma contains tiny echogenic foci which represent microcalcifications. (c) Color Doppler image demonstrates internal vascularity in the lesion

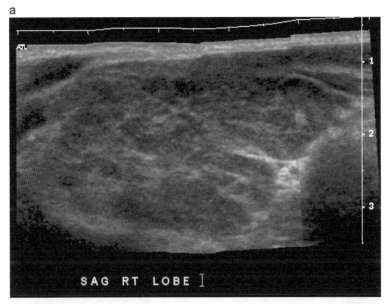

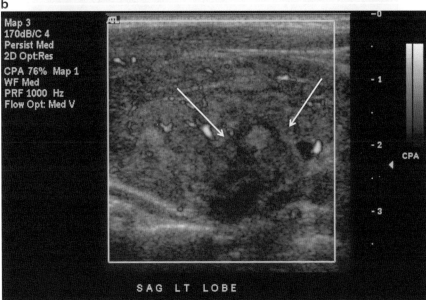

Fig. 4.14 (a) Right lobe of the thyroid shows classic features of Hashimoto's disease with heterogeneous parenchyma with fine echogenic linear fibrous strands. (b) Left lobe of the thyroid in the same patient reveals the background thyroid parenchyma has features of Hashimoto's disease. Arrows point to a hypoechoic, irregular-shaped, avascular, heterogeneous mass. FNA with flow cytometry demonstrated the lesion to represent lymphoma

dedifferentiation of a pre-existing neoplasm. Patients may present with signs and symptoms of airway compression and the patients are usually inoperable at the time of presentation.

Ultrasound features of anaplastic thyroid cancer include a hypoechoic mass diffusely involving the entire lobe or gland with ill-defined margins and areas of necrosis. Patients typically have nodal or distant metastases with the involved nodes demonstrating necrosis about half of the time. Multiple intra-nodular vessels are seen on color Doppler imaging and the lesions demonstrate aggressive local invasion with extra-capsular spread, leading to invasion of neck muscles and vascular invasion or encasement (Fig. 4.15). Often, these tumors cannot be adequately imaged

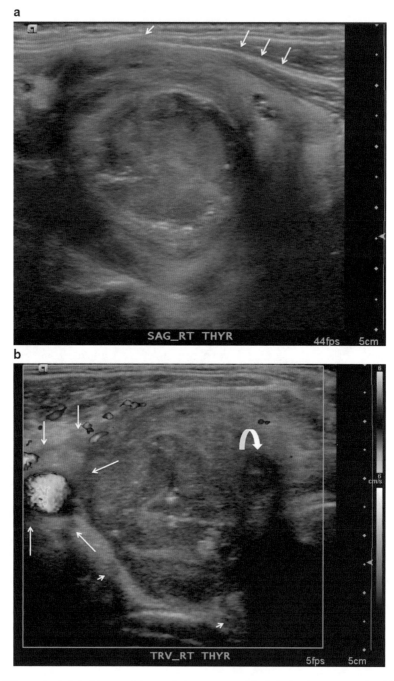

Fig. 4.15 (a) This anaplastic thyroid cancer is hypoechoic and heterogeneous with microcalcifications and completely replaces the right lobe. The mass has ill-defined margins and invades the anterior strap muscles. The three adjacent *arrows* delineate intact segment of strap muscle while the short single *arrow* points to the anterior margin of the mass which has invaded through the entire thickness of the muscle into the subcutaneous tissues. (b) The same anaplastic lesion demonstrates local invasion beyond the thyroid capsule that encases the carotid artery (*straight arrows*). The *curved arrow* highlights an area of focal necrosis. *Short arrows* highlight additional foci of extracapsular tumor spread. (c) A necrotic jugular chain metastatic lymph node from anaplastic cancer partially encases/invades the jugular vein

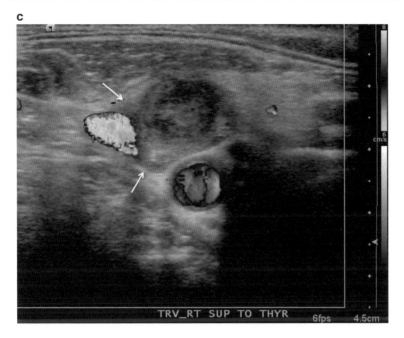

Fig. 4.15 (continued)

Ultrasound Features of Recurrent Thyroid Cancer

with ultrasound because of their large size relative to the field of view of the transducer. CT and MRI of the neck usually more accurately demonstrate the extent of disease [10, 38, 53].

Recurrent thyroid cancer in the postoperative bed is typically circumscribed, hypoechoic, and smoothly marginated. Differential diagnosis includes postoperative change due to suture granulomas. Color flow in a thyroid bed lesion suggests recurrence or central compartment metastatic disease rather than postoperative change (Fig. 4.16a, b). Calcifications and cystic change in a thyroid bed lesion postoperatively is worrisome for metastatic or recurrent disease. In postoperative suture granulomas, echogenic foci from suture material can mimic microcalcifications but they are typically are more irregular in shape, > 1 mm in diameter and have echogenic foci with a paired appearance clustered centrally or paracentrally [54] (Fig. 4.16 c, d).

Ultrasound Features of Lymph Node Metastases

Ultrasound is accurate in preoperative evaluation for extra-thyroidal tumor extension and lateral lymph node (level 2–5) metastases and is now used as a guide for surgery. CT has been reported to have greater sensitivity than US in the detection of central node metastases [2].

Macroscopic lymph node involvement impacts recurrence and may influence survival. Therefore, preoperative ultrasound "mapping" of the neck prior to surgical intervention is now part of published treatment guidelines for cases of newly diagnosed papillary thyroid cancer [55]. If pathologic nodes are identified in either the central or lateral compartment, they are removed at the time of the initial surgery [56].

Several ultrasound criteria have been described to help distinguish malignant from benign lymph nodes, including absent fatty hilum, cystic change, calcification, rounded shape, abnormal color Doppler pattern, and hyperechoic changes in the node (Fig. 4.17). Absent fatty hilum has been reported by some to be the least accurate of

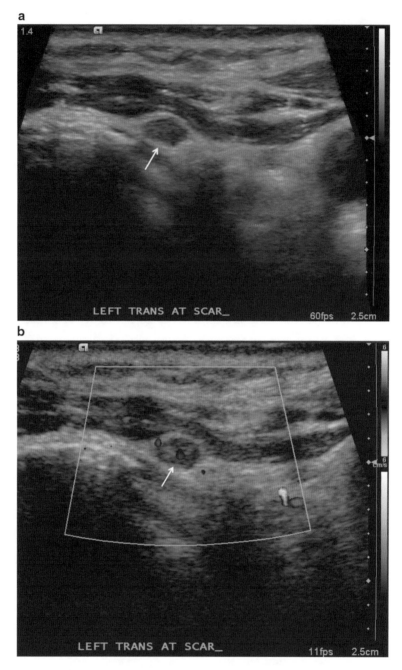

Fig. 4.16 (a) A circumscribed, hypoechoic, smoothly marginated mass in the thyroid bed is suspicious for recurrent papillary thyroid cancer. (b) Color Doppler imaging demonstrates blood flow in the lesion and eliminates postoperative change from the differential diagnosis. (c) The same patient has an additional ipsilateral, hypoechoic, smoothly marginated nodule in the thyroid bed with paired, central, linear, echogenic foci suspicious for suture granuloma. (d) Color Doppler imaging demonstrates no flow in this lesion supporting the suspicion that this lesion represents postoperative change

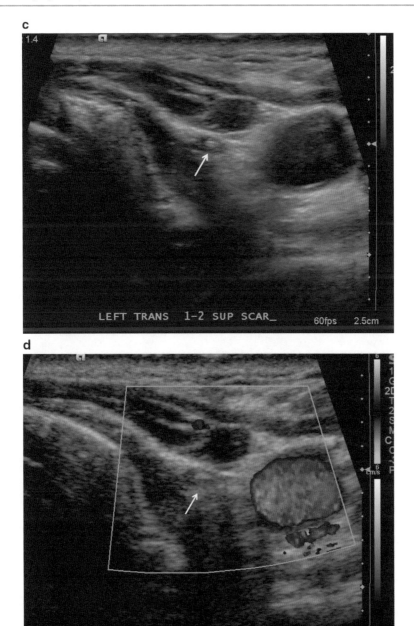

Fig. 4.16 (continued)

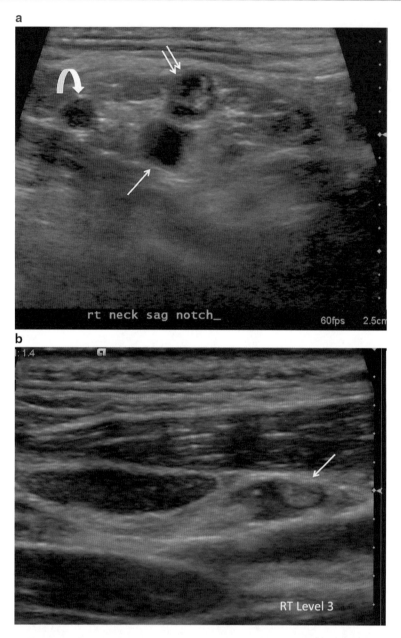

Fig. 4.17 (**a**) Multiple abnormal central compartment nodes are seen in the sternal notch in this patient with a history of papillary thyroid cancer. The curved area depicts an abnormal rounded hypoechoic node. The single *straight arrow* demonstrates a node with cystic change and the paired arrows point to a node with both cystic change and microcalcifications. (**b**) Two adjacent jugular chain nodes are seen, one of which is elongated and hypoechoic with absent fatty hilum and proved to be a benign node. An adjacent node is also elongated and hypoechoic but contains oval-shaped hyperechoic change (*arrow*) that represents deposits of metastatic disease. (**c**) Two adjacent metastatic nodes in a patient with papillary thyroid cancer, one of which contains a small focus of hyperechoic change (*curved arrow*) and an adjacent node contains calcifications (*straight arrows*). (**d**) A large cervical node demonstrates cystic change (*curved arrow*) and disorganized vessels and hypervascularity

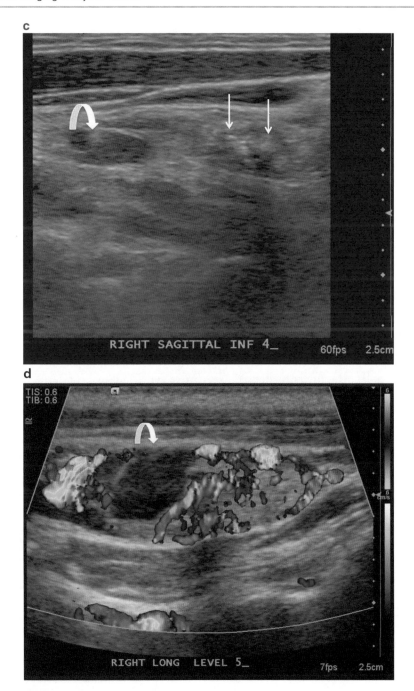

Fig. 4.17 (continued)

the above features in predicting that a node is malignant. Furthermore, even if positive cytology is not obtained, nodes with the above-described malignant features could still represent malignant nodes [57]. Other investigators have reported that only two of the above criteria – calcification and abnormal Doppler pattern – accurately predict the presence of metastases in the central compartment lymph nodes, whereas all six features of malignant nodes have been described in lateral compartment nodal metastases [58]. Preoperative ultrasound of cervical lymph nodes is used to determine the necessity and extent of neck dissection in thyroid cancer patients [59].

If positive cytology is not obtained when morphologically abnormal nodes are sampled, it is possible to assess the thyroglobulin content of the node by performing wash-out on one or more of the aspirates (see section on FNA). Another differential diagnostic consideration in patients who present with thyroid nodules and cervical lymphadenopathy includes Hashimoto's thyroiditis. Lymph nodes in these patients are often enlarged and rounded and hypoechoic. Gray-scale abnormalities in the nodes in this population that suggest metastatic diseases include cystic change and calcification [60].

Ultrasound-Guided FNA in Thyroid Cancer

Despite the many ultrasound findings that suggest that a lesion is malignant, FNA remains the gold standard for diagnosis of thyroid nodules and lymph nodes [1]. Several studies have shown that US-guided FNA is more sensitive than palpation-guided FNA with a decreased rate of insufficient or inadequate cytology specimens. Ultrasound allows for sampling of nonpalpable nodules and improves cytologic adequacy by allowing aspiration of the solid component of partially cystic nodules [61]. In addition, ultrasound-guided FNA has a 1% false-negative rate compared to 2.3% with palpation-guided FNA [62].

Although controversy exists among different clinical societies about size criteria and thresholds for recommending biopsy of a nodule, FNA

of nodules <1 cm appears to be a useful diagnostic tool and unsatisfactory results in these cases have been reported to be unrelated to the size of the nodule [63]. Furthermore, US-guided FNA of thyroid nodules smaller than 5 mm in maximum diameter has been reported to be an effective diagnostic procedure with reported accuracy of 92% and false-negative rate of 8% [64].

Thyroglobulin (Tg) assay of material aspirated from neck masses can help distinguish those of thyroid origin from other masses. This assay can be used to further evaluate whether masses in the thyroid bed or abnormal nodes represent recurrent or metastatic thyroid cancer [65]. The role of this assay in patients who have not been previously ablated is limited because, in these patients, lesions in the thyroid bed could represent normal regenerated thyroid tissue. Typically, FNA is performed and, for one or more of the needle passes, after the initial aspirate is placed on a slide for cytology specimen, the needle tip is then rinsed in one to two milliliters of sterile saline for subsequent Tg analysis should the cytology be nondiagnostic or negative. Combined FNAB-Tg/FNAB cytology is more sensitive and accurate at detecting metastatic nodes than FNAB cytology alone. Furthermore, FNAB-Tg has been reported to be better at diagnosing metastases in small lymph nodes [66].

Conclusion

Thyroid ultrasound is essential in the diagnosis and management of thyroid cancer. All patients with thyroid nodules detected by palpation or imaging should undergo diagnostic ultrasound to further characterize the nodules and determine whether FNA is indicated based on imaging features that suggest an increased risk of malignancy. Ultrasound is also used to detect cervical lymph node metastases preoperatively in patients with known differentiated thyroid malignancy. Neck ultrasound is used to follow thyroid cancer patients postoperatively in an effort to detect local recurrence or residual disease in the postoperative bed and to monitor patients for development of cervical lymph node metastases.

Ultrasound-guided intervention in thyroid cancer diagnosis and management includes ultrasound-guided FNA of suspicious thyroid nodules, lymph nodes, or thyroid bed masses in postoperative patients. Other applications of ultrasound-guided intervention in thyroid cancer include localization of recurrent disease or cervical nodal metastases prior to surgical excision, percutaneous ethanol injection and radiofrequency ablation of malignant thyroid nodules, local thyroid cancer recurrence, and cervical nodal metastases.

References

1. Cooper DS, Doherty GM, Haugen BR, Kloos RT, Lee SL, Mandel SJ, et al. 2009 Revised American Thyroid Association management guidelines for patients with thyroid nodules and differentiated thyroid cancer. Thyroid. 2009;19(11):1167–214.
2. Choi JS, Kim J, Kwak JY, Kim MJ, Chang HS, Kim EK. Preoperative staging of papillary thyroid carcinoma: comparison of ultrasound imaging and CT. Am J Roentgenol. 2009;193(3):871–8.
3. Frasoldati A, Presenti M, Gallo M, Caroggio A, Salvo D, Valcavi R. Diagnosis of neck recurrences in patients with differentiated thyroid carcinoma. Cancer. 2003;97(1):90–6.
4. Monchik JM, Donatini G, Iannuccilli J, Dupuy DE. Radiofrequency ablation and percutaneous ethanol injection treatment for recurrent local and distant well-differentiated thyroid carcinoma. Ann Surg. 2006;244(2):296–304.
5. Sippel RS, Elaraj DM, Poder L, Duh QY, Kenebew E, Clark OH. Localization of recurrent thyroid cancer using intraoperative ultrasound-guided dye injection. World J Surg. 2009;33:434–9.
6. Rago T, Vitti P. Potential value of elastography in the diagnosis of malignancy in thyroid nodules. Q J Nucl Med Mol Imaging. 2009;53(5):455–63.
7. Friedrich-Rust M, Sperber A, Holzer K, Diener J, Grunwald F, Badenhoop K, et al. Real-time elastography and contrast-enhanced ultrasound for the assessment of thyroid nodules. Exp Clin Endocrinol Diabetes. 2009;118:602–9.
8. Hong Y, Liu X, Li Z, Zhang X, Chen M, Luo Z. Real-time ultrasound elastography in the differential diagnosis of benign and malignant thyroid nodules. J Ultrasound Med. 2009;28:861–7.
9. Park SH, Kim SJ, Ek K, Son EJ, Kwak JY. Interobserver agreement in assessing the sonographic and elastographic features of malignant thyroid nodules. Am J Roentgenol. 2009;193(5):W416–23.
10. Wong KT, Ahuja AT. Ultrasound of thyroid cancer. Cancer Imaging. 2005;5(1):157–66.
11. Murakami T. Ultrasonography. In: Clark OH, Noguchi S, editors. Thyroid cancer diagnosis and treatment. St. Louis, Mo: Quality Medical Publishing; 2000. p. 209–25.
12. ACR practice Guidelines for the Performance of Thyroid and Parathyroid Ultrasound Examinations, revised 2007. http://www.acr.org/SecondaryMain MenuCategories/quality_safety/guidelines/us/us_thyroid_parathyroid.aspx. Accessed June 10, 2010
13. Davies L, Welch HG. Increasing incidence of thyroid cancer in the United States, 1973–2002. JAMA. 2006; 295:2164–7.
14. Hall SF, Walker H, Siemens R, Schneeberg A. Increasing detection and increasing incidence in thyroid cancer. World J Surg. 2009;33:2567–71.
15. Chen AY, Jemal A, Ward EM. Increasing incidence of differentiated thyroid cancer in the United States, 1988–2005. Cancer. 2009;115(16):3801–7.
16. Frates MC, Benson CB, Charboneau JW, et al. Management of thyroid nodules detected at US: Society of Radiologists in Ultrasound consensus conference statement. Ultrasound Q. 2006;22:231–40.
17. Bastin S et al. Role of ultrasound in the assessment of nodular thyroid disease. J Med Imaging Radiat Oncol. 2009;53(2):177–87.
18. Frates MC, Benson CB, Doubilet PM, Kunreunther E, Contreras M, Bibas ES, et al. Prevalence and distribution of carcinoma in patients with solitary and multiple thyroid nodules on sonography. J Clin Endocrinol Metab. 2006;91:3411–7.
19. Papini E, Guglielmi R, Bianchini A, Crescenzi A, Taccogna S, Nardi F, et al. Risk of malignancy in nonpalpable thyroid nodules: predictive value of ultrasound and color Doppler features. J Clin Endocrinol Metab. 2002;87:1941–6.
20. Capelli C, Castellano M, Pirola I, Gandossi E, De Martino E, Cumetti D, et al. Thyroid shape suggests malignancy. Eur J Endocrinol. 2006;155:27–31.
21. Bonavita JA, Mayo J, Babb J, Bennett G, Oweity T, Macari M, et al. Pattern recognition of benign thyroid nodules at ultrasound: which nodules can be left alone? Am J Roentgenol. 2009;193(1):207–13.
22. Park JY, Lee HJ, Jang HW, Kim HK, Yi JH, Lee W, et al. A proposal for a thyroid imaging reporting and data system for ultrasound features of thyroid nodules. Thyroid. 2009;19(11):1257–64.
23. Horvath E, Majlis S, Rossi R, Franco C, Niedman JP, Castro A, et al. An ultrasonogram reporting system for thyroid nodules stratifying cancer risk for clinical management. J Clin Endocrinol Metab. 2009;94(5): 1748–51.
24. Liu YI, Kamaya A, Desser TS, et al. A Bayesian classifier for differentiating benign versus malignant thyroid nodules using sonographic features. AMIA Annu Symp Proc. 2008;6:419–23.
25. Jeh SK, Jung SL, Kim BS, Lee YS. 2007 Evaluating the degree of conformity of papillary carcinoma and follicular carcinoma to the reported ultrasonographic findings of malignant thyroid tumor. Korean J Radiol. 2007;8:192–7.

26. Wienke JR, Chong WK, Fielding JR, Zhou KH, Mittelstaedt CA. Sonographic features of benign thyroid nodules: interobserver reliability and overlap with malignancy. J Ultrasound Med. 2003;22:1027–31.

27. Moon WJ, Jung SL, Lee JH, Na DG, Baek JH, Lee YH, et al. Benign and malignant thyroid nodules: US differentiation – multicenter retrospective study. Radiology. 2008;247(3):602–4.

28. Wang N, Xu Y, Ge C, Guo R, Guo K. Association of sonographically detected calcification with thyroid carcinoma. Head Neck. 2006;28:1077–83.

29. Ahuja A, Chick W, King W, Metreweli C. Clinical significance of the comet-tail artifact in thyroid ultrasound. J Clin Ultrasound. 1996;24:129–33.

30. Sipos JA. Advances in ultrasound for the diagnosis and management of thyroid cancer. Thyroid. 2009;19(12):1363–72.

31. Kim MJ, Kim EK, Kwak JY, Park CS, Chung WY, Nam KH, et al. Differentiation of thyroid nodules with macrocalcifications: role of suspicious sonographic findings. J Ultrasound Med. 2008;27(8):1179–84.

32. Yoon DY, Lee JW, Chang SK, Choi CS, Yun EJ, Seo YL, et al. Peripheral calcification in thyroid nodules: ultrasonographic features and prediction of malignancy. J Ultrasound Med. 2007;26:1349–55.

33. Lee SK, Rho BH. Follicular thyroid carcinoma with an eggshell calcification: report of 3 cases. J Ultrasound Med. 2009;28(6):801–6.

34. Park M, Shin JH, Han BK, et al. Sonography of thyroid nodules with peripheral calcifications. J Clin Ultrasound. 2009;37(6):324–8.

35. Kim BM, Kim MJ, Kim EK, Kwak JY, Hong SW, Son EJ, et al. Sonographic differentiation of thyroid nodules with eggshell calcifications. J Ultrasound Med. 2008;27(10):1425–30.

36. Chan BK, Desser TS, McDougall IR, Weigel RJ, Jeffrey RB. Common and uncommon sonographic features of papillary thyroid carcinoma. J Ultrasound Med. 2003;22(10):1083–90.

37. Hoang JK, Lee WK, Lee M, Johnson D, Farrell S. Ultrasound features of thyroid malignancy: pearls and pitfalls. Radiographics. 2007;27:847–65.

38. Solbiati L, Charnoneau JW, James EM, Hay ID. The thyroid gland. In: Rumack CM, Wilson SR, Charboneau JW, editors. Diagnostic ultrasound. St. Louis, MO: Mosby-Yearbook; 1998. p. 713–4.

39. Propper RA, Skolnick ML, Weinstein BJ, Dekker A. The nonspecificity of the thyroid halo sign. J Clin Ultrasound. 1980;8(2):129–32.

40. Kim EK et al. New sonographic criteria for recommending fine-needle aspiration biopsy of nonpalpable solid nodules of the thyroid. Am J Roentgenol. 2002;178:687–91.

41. Alexander EK, Marqusee E, Orcutt J, Benson CB, Frates MC, Doubilet PM, et al. Thyroid nodule shape and prediction of malignancy. Thyroid. 2004;14:953–8.

42. Baier ND, Hahn PF, Gervais DA, Samir A, Halpern EF, Mueller PR, et al. Fine-needle aspiration biopsy of thyroid nodules: experience in a cohort of 944 patients. Am J Roentgenol. 2009;193(4):1175–9.

43. Lee MJ, Kim EK, Kwak JY, Kim MJ. Partially cystic thyroid nodules on ultrasound: probability of malignancy and sonographic differentiation. Thyroid. 2009;19(4):341–6.

44. Reading CC, Charboneau JW, Hay ID, Sebo TJ. Sonography of thyroid nodules: a "classic pattern" diagnostic approach. Ultrasound Q. 2005;21:157–65.

45. Frates MC, Benson CB, Doubilet PM, Cibas ES, Marqusee E. Can color Doppler sonography aid in the prediction of malignancy of thyroid nodules? J Ultrasound Med. 2003;22(2):127–31.

46. Kwak JY, Kim EK, Kim MJ, Son EJ. Significance of sonographic characterization for managing subcentimeter thyroid nodules. Acta Radiol. 2009;50(8):917–23.

47. Mazzeferri EL, Sipos J. Should all patients with subcentimeter thyroid nodules undergo fine-needle aspiration biopsy and preoperative neck ultrasonography to define the extent of tumor invasion? Thyroid. 2008;18(6):597–602.

48. Lin JD, Hsueh C, Chao TC, Wneg HF, Huang BY. Thyroid follicular neoplasms diagnosed by high-resolution ultrasonography with fine needle aspiration cytology. Acta Cytol. 1997;41:687–91.

49. Machens A, Holzhausen HJ, Dralle H. The prognostic value of primary tumor size in papillary and follicular thyroid carcinoma. Cancer. 2005;103:2269–73.

50. Kim SH, Kim BS, Jung SL, et al. Ultrasonographic findings of medullary thyroid carcinoma: a comparison with papillary thyroid carcinoma. Korean J Radiol. 2009;10(2):101–5.

51. Ruggiero FP, Frauenhoffer E, Stack Jr BC. Thyroid lymphoma: a single institution's experience. Otolaryngol Head Neck Surg. 2005;133:888–96.

52. Kasagi K, Hatabu H, Tokuda Y, et al. Lymphoproliferative disorders of the thyroid gland: radiological appearances. Br J Radiol. 1991;64:569–75.

53. Nel CJC, Van Heerden JA, James EM, et al. Anaplastic carcinoma of the thyroid: a clinicopathologic study of 82 cases. Mayo Clin Proc. 1985;60:51–8.

54. Kim JH, Lee JH, Shong YK, Hong SJ, Ko MS, Lee DH, et al. Ultrasound features of suture granulomas in the thyroid bed after thyroidectomy for papillary thyroid carcinoma with an emphasis on their differentiation from locally recurrent thyroid carcinoma. Ultrasound Med Biol. 2009;35(9):1452–7.

55. Marshall CL, Lee JE, Xing Y, Perrier ND, Edeiken BS, Evans BS, et al. Routine pre-operative ultrasonography for papillary thyroid cancer: effects on cervical recurrence. Surgery. 2009;146(6):1063–72.

56. Sippel RS, Chen H. Controversies in the surgical management of newly diagnosed and recurrent/residual thyroid cancer. Thyroid. 2009;19(12):1373–80.

57. Sohn YM, Kwak JY, Kim EK, Moon HJ, Kim SJ, Kim MJ. Diagnostic approach for evaluation of lymph node metastasis from thyroid cancer using ultrasound and fine-needle aspiration. Am J Roentgenol. 2010;194(1):38–43.

58. Park J, Son KR, Na DG, Kim E, Kim S. Performance of preoperative sonographic staging of papillary thyroid carcinoma based on sixth edition AJCC/UICC

TNM classification system. Am J Roentgenol. 2009; 192(3):66–72.

59. Roh JL, Park JY, Kim JM, Song CJ. Use of preoperative ultra sonography as guidance for neck dissection in patients with papillary thyroid carcinoma. J Surg Oncol. 2009;99(1):28–31.

60. Paksoy N, Yazal K. Cervical lymphadenopathy associated with Hashimoto's thyroiditis: an analysis if 22 cases by fine needle aspiration cytology. Acta Cytol. 2009;53(5):491–6.

61. Cesur M, Corapcioglu D, Bulut S, et al. Comparison of palpation-guided fine needle aspiration biopsy to ultrasound-guided fine needle aspiration biopsy in the evaluation of thyroid nodules. Thyroid. 2006;16(6):555–61.

62. Danese D, Sciacchitano S, Farsetti A, Andreoli M, Pontecorvi A. Diagnostic accuracy of conventional versus sonography guided fine needle aspiration biopsy of thyroid nodules. Thyroid. 1998;8:15–21.

63. Accurso A, Rocco N, Palumbo A, Feleppa C. Usefulness of ultrasound-guided fine-needle aspiration cytology in the diagnosis of non-palpable small thyroid nodules: our growing experience. J Endocrinol Invest. 2009;32(2):156–9.

64. Kim DW, Park AW, Lee EJ, Choo HJ, Kim SH, Lee SH, et al. Ultrasound-guided fine-needle aspiration biopsy of thyroid nodules smaller than 5 mm in the maximum diameter: assessment of efficacy and pathological findings. Korean J Radiol. 2009;10(5):4333–40.

65. Bruno R, Giannasio P, Chiarella R, et al. Identification of a neck lump as a lymph node metastasis from an occult contralateral papillary microcarcinoma. Thyroid. 2009;19(5):531–3.

66. Jeon SJ, Kim E, Park JS. Diagnostic benefit of thyroglobulin measurement in fine needle aspiration for diagnosing metastatic cervical lymph nodes from papillary thyroid cancer: correlations with US features. Korean J Radiol. 2009;10(2):106–11.

Fine Needle Aspiration of the Thyroid

5

Shikha Bose

Introduction

Fine needle aspiration biopsy (FNAB) is a safe and inexpensive procedure that is easily performed with minimal patient discomfort. It has become the cornerstone in the management of patients with thyroid nodules; its main purpose is to provide a rational approach to management, to triage individuals for surgical management, and to determine the correct surgical procedure – lobectomy versus total thyroidectomy [1–3]. FNAB has successfully reduced the number of patients requiring surgery by 50%, has increased the yield of thyroid malignancy at surgery by two to three times, and has decreased the cost of managing thyroid nodules by 25% [4, 5].

The Indications

FNAB is commonly performed on thyroid nodules (>1.0–1.5 cm) with suspicious clinical/sonographic features.

The Training

Appropriate training in specimen collection and smear preparation is essential for obtaining adequate diagnostic material and results in increased accuracy. Reports in literature have demonstrated that the root cause of about half of the diagnostic failures was unsatisfactory samples. The remaining were due to either short comings in interpretation of adequate samples or pathologists rendering diagnoses on samples with inadequate material [6–8], thus emphasizing the need for adequate samples. One of the most important factors for mastering the procedure is focused training with appropriate feedback by expert practitioners [9].

FNAB: The Technique

The FNAB is best performed using 27–25 gauge needles, starting with the smallest diameter needle and increasing the needle size as required; the larger diameter needles is reserved for drainage of viscous colloid filled cysts [10]. The use of topical anesthesia is variable among practitioners and is left to individual preference [11]. Sufficient anesthesia is obtained by injecting between 0.5 and 1.5 cc of 2% lidocaine with or without epinephrine (1:100,000) into the subcutaneous fat (not the reticular dermis) using a 30–32 gauge needle to minimize discomfort during the initial skin puncture. The needle is inserted into the lesion by manual or

S. Bose (✉)
Department of Pathology and Lab Medicine,
Cedars-Sinai Medical Center, 8700 Beverly Blvd,
Room 8732, Los Angeles, CA 90048, USA
e-mail: Shikha.bose@cshs.org

G.D. Braunstein (ed.), *Thyroid Cancer*, Endocrine Updates 30,
DOI 10.1007/978-1-4614-0875-8_5, © Springer Science+Business Media, LLC 2012

ultrasound guidance. Ultrasound guidance has been shown to significantly improve the sensitivity and specificity of the FNA procedure. It should be utilized for aspirations of nonpalpable nodules, difficult-to-palpate nodules that are located posteriorly, suspicious nodules within a multinodular goiter, or nodules with a cystic component. Previously unsuccessful thyroid FNAs may also benefit from ultrasound guidance [12]. Negative suction is generally unnecessary and may only be needed for drainage of cyst contents [6, 13]. As a starting point, a dwell time of 2–5 s within the nodule with three forward and back oscillations per second maximizes cellular yield, minimizes blood, and produces cellular material sufficient for one to two slides per biopsy pass [14]. Review of literature suggests that there is only a small increment in adequacy beyond five passes and therefore it is felt that additional passes do not justify the potential increased morbidity and trauma associated with additional passes [15]. Adequate postbiopsy care to prevent and monitor any intranodular bleeding should be provided.

Smearing techniques should be mastered to allow the best presentation of the aspirated material on the slides for optimal fixation, staining, and microscopic assessment. Failure in the smearing process can limit microscopic evaluation, irrespective of the amount of material obtained during the FNA procedure. Material should be submitted to the laboratory as air-dried and alcohol-fixed smears for Romanowsky (Diff-Quik, May Grunwald Geimsa, or Wright) stains and Papanicolaou stains, respectively. Additional material should be submitted in the liquid medium either by rinsing the needle off in liquid medium to capture any residual material remaining after preparation of smears or by submitting material obtained from a separate pass. This is particularly useful in the preparation of concentrated smears and/or cell blocks, which can be a valuable complement to direct smears particularly when special studies (immunostains) are required. Should a lymphoma be suspected, material should be submitted in RPMI for flow cytometry studies. In the event that a cyst fluid is aspirated, it is preferable to submit all of the material in fixative for lab processing.

On-site evaluation for specimen adequacy, if available, is reported to lessen the number of unsatisfactory specimens, limit the number of passes required for obtaining diagnostic material, and provide an opportunity for triaging material for special studies if required [16, 17], although it is felt by some that that this is useful only for less experienced radiologists [18].

Complications of FNA

Potential side effects include pain, swelling, hematoma, and acute infection. Tissue disruption is an infrequent occurrence after FNA; however, a wide range of morphologic changes have been reported ranging from granulation tissue formation to partial or complete infarction of neoplasms [19–21]. Reported incidence of infarction varies from 1.4 to 10% and is noted commonly in papillary carcinomas or Hurthle cell tumors [22, 23]. Seeding of the needle tract with tumor cells particularly in cases with papillary carcinoma is also described [24], although these are rare occurrences.

Accuracy and Limitation of FNA

Thyroid FNA is widely accepted as an accurate means of evaluating a thyroid nodule and is considered by some to be the most sensitive and specific nonsurgical thyroid cancer test available with diagnostic accuracy varying between 90 and 100% [25]. False-positive diagnoses make up less than 1% of cases, and result from overinterpretation of reparative and reactive nuclear changes as papillary thyroid carcinoma. False-negative rates range from 1 to 11%, and are mostly due to unsatisfactory specimens [26]. Sampling errors, interpretation errors, and cystic neoplasms, especially papillary carcinomas, account for the remainder of cases [27]. The major limitation of thyroid FNA is its inability to distinguish hypercellular non-neoplastic nodules from follicular adenomas or carcinomas [28].

The Pathology Requisition

In addition to patient identification information, it is important to provide the pathologist with location and size of the nodule. This is particularly useful since it allows correlation with sonographic findings and subsequent surgical excisions. Additionally, in patients with multiple nodules, it allows appropriate follow-up over time. Additional available clinical information regarding the presence of autoimmune (Hashimoto's) thyroiditis and history of I-131 therapy or external radiation [29, 30] is helpful, as these conditions may mimic malignancy resulting in misdiagnosis [31, 32]. A prior FNA causes morphologic alterations that can affect cytologic interpretation [19, 20]. Likewise, it is important to note a personal history of malignancy since metastatic tumors to the thyroid may mimic the appearance of primary thyroid neoplasms. Metastatic renal cell carcinomas and lung cancers may resemble follicular neoplasms or anaplastic thyroid carcinomas while malignant melanomas are known to mimic medullary carcinomas. Knowledge of family history can alert the pathologist to the possibility of hereditary syndromes.

The Cytologic Evaluation

The pathologist assesses the adequacy of the sample, presence and relative amounts of colloid and epithelium, architectural patterns of tissue fragments, and the cytomorphology of the cellular material on the slides to arrive at the diagnosis.

Specimen Adequacy

The precise criteria for thyroid FNA adequacy is much debated and variably used. An FNA specimen must be of good quality and with sufficient material that is well preserved so that an accurate interpretation is rendered. However, the number of follicular cells required for an adequate smear varies from five to six groups with 10–15 cells each to eight to ten tissue fragments with 20 cells each [33–36]. Review of the literature determines that the minimum criteria for adequacy should be five to six follicle groups each with at least 10 cells [14]. It is imperative that each case be evaluated in the context of the available clinical and radiological information. Moreover, it has been demonstrated that under certain situations strict application of the required number of follicular cells is inappropriate. Studies have determined that aspirates with abundant inflammatory cells suggestive of thyroiditis [37] and aspirates with abundant colloid [38–40] but lacking follicular epithelium do not require the presence of strict numbers of follicular epithelial cells for accurate cytologic diagnoses. Additionally, smears with any cytological atypia irrespective of the adequacy require a diagnostic interpretation of at least atypia [41]. FNAs from thyroid cysts with little to no follicular cells also require special consideration. In most instances, these lesions do not yield sufficient numbers of follicular cells but are benign. It is therefore appropriate to label these as "cyst fluid only" under the heading "nondiagnostic" and not "unsatisfactory" [14]. An optional disclaimer that a cystic carcinoma cannot be entirely excluded may be added with a recommendation for correlation with the cyst size and complexity.

The Reporting System

A tiered system for classifying thyroid FNA is favored [42, 43]. The following is the scheme proposed at the recently held The Bethesda Conference [14]. FNA diagnoses are grouped into six categories – benign, follicular lesion (atypia) of undetermined significance, follicular neoplasm, suspicious, malignant, and unsatisfactory. Risk of malignancy estimates is provided for each of the diagnostic categories; however, inclusion in reports is optional.

Suggested categories	Alternate category(s) terms	Risk of malignancy
Benign		<1%
Follicular lesion of undetermined significance	Atypia of undetermined significance	5–10%
	R/O neoplasm	
	Atypical follicular lesion	
	Cellular follicular lesion	
Neoplasm	Suspicious for neoplasm	20–30%
Suspicious for malignancy		50–75%
Malignant		100%
Nondiagnostic	Unsatisfactory	

Inflammatory Lesions

Autoimmune Thyroiditis (Fig. 5.1)

Synonyms. Chronic lymphocytic thyroiditis and Hashimoto's thyroiditis

This is the most frequently encountered form of thyroiditis and a major cause of goiter and hypothyroidism in the US. Due to the associated increased risk of developing malignant lymphoma and papillary carcinoma, FNA may be performed in patients with chronic lymphocytic thyroiditis to evaluate dominant nodules that are cold on thyroid scan [44, 45].

Cytomorphology. Characteristic cytologic features include a cellular smear consisting predominantly of an inflammatory infiltrate with scant colloid. The inflammatory infiltrate consists of a mixed population of lymphocytes, plasma cells, and aggregates of lymphocytes and histiocytes, many of which contain pyknotic nuclear material (tingible bodies). Epithelial component is generally sparse and consists of follicular cells with Hurthle cell metaplasia and variable degrees of nuclear atypia [46, 47].

Differential diagnosis and pitfalls
1. Malignant lymphoma: A prominent monomorphic lymphoid infiltrate may give rise to

this possibility. Additional testing by flow cytometry will be confirmatory [48].
2. Papillary carcinoma: The presence of nuclear atypia is common and Hurthle cells may on occasion develop nuclear clearing and nuclear grooves, thus mimicking a papillary carcinoma [49, 50].
3. Hurthle cell neoplasm: Lymphocytic thyroiditis is associated with hyperplastic Hurthle cell nodules. An aspirate from such a nodule will consist of a predominant population of Hurthle cells, thus resulting in an erroneous diagnosis of Hurthle cell neoplasm [31, 49, 50].

Subacute Thyroiditis (Fig. 5.2)

Synonyms. de Quervain's thyroiditis, giant cell thyroiditis, and subacute granulomatous thyroiditisRarely, this painful thyroid disease may present with a discrete nodule when it may be sampled.

Cytomorphology. Smears are hypocellular containing a mixed population of inflammatory cells consisting of lymphocytes, plasma cells, eosinophils, and neutrophils, and associated with multinucleated giant cells and loose clusters of epithelioid cells forming granulomas. Follicular cells with reactive nuclear changes are also present [5, 47].

Differential diagnosis and pitfalls. Prominence of giant cells may be observed in FNAs from cases of chronic lymphocytic thyroiditis, adenomatous goiter, papillary carcinoma with degenerative and cystic changes, sarcoidosis, or tuberculosis, thus raising the possibilities of any of these conditions [50].

Reidel's Thyroiditis

FNA usually yields scant cellular material and is often unsatisfactory. Fragment of collagenous tissue containing plump fibroblasts and scattered inflammatory cells may be seen [5, 47].

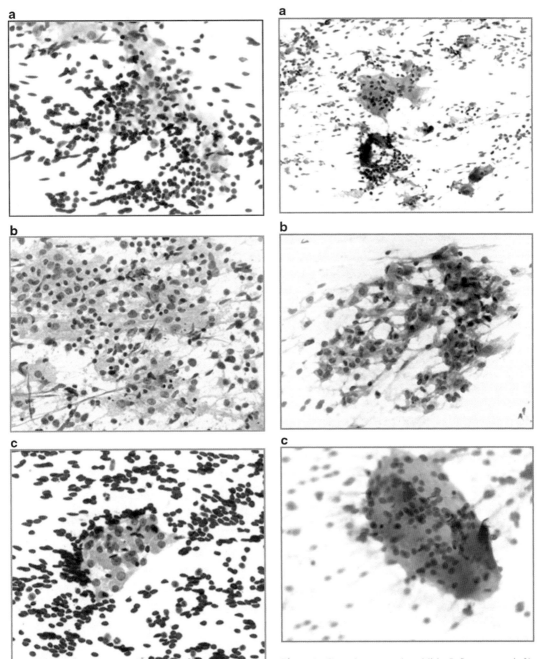

Fig. 5.1 Hashimoto's thyroiditis. Lymphoplasma-cytic infiltrate (**a**) is interspersed by lymphohistiocytic aggregates (**b**) and oncocytes (**c**)

Fig. 5.2 Granulomatous thyroiditis. Inflammatory infiltrate comprising lymphocytes, histiocytes, and multinucleated giant cells with occasional cluster of follicular cells (**a**), ill-defined granuloma (**b**), and multinucleated giant cells (**c**)

Diffuse Toxic Goiter (Graves' Disease)

Graves' disease usually presents with diffuse enlargement of thyroid gland and hence is not subject to FNA. It is only patients with solitary nodules, which are cold on radioiodine scan, who are selected for FNA.

Cytomorphology. Aspirates are cellular and show similar features to hyperplastic goiter. Lymphocytes and oncocytic cells may also be observed [5, 47].

Differential diagnosis and pitfalls. Follicular cells in Graves' disease may show variable grades of atypia, particularly after treatment with antithyroid therapies [29], and on occasion may display focal nuclear chromatin clearing and rare intranuclear grooves; however, other diagnostic nuclear features of papillary carcinoma are absent [51].

Nodular Goiter (Fig. 5.3)

Synonyms. Colloid nodule/goiter, adenomatous/adenomatoid nodule, benign thyroid nodule, and nodular hyperplasia

Cytomorphology. Characteristic features include background colloid with variable numbers of interspersed follicular epithelial cells present as monolayered honeycomb sheets. Hurthle cell metaplasia, histiocytes with or without hemosiderin, multinucleated giant cells, and calcific debris suggest degenerative changes. Hyperplastic nodules show cellular aspirates consisting of tissue fragments of bland follicular cells with and without a follicular pattern [5, 47, 52–54].

Differential diagnosis and pitfalls

1. Follicular adenoma or carcinoma: Cellular aspirates from hyperplastic nodules may mimic the cytologic features of follicular neoplasm or in instances of goiters with prominent Hurthle cell metaplasia, a Hurthle cell neoplasm. The architectural pattern of the follicular cells (monolayering of sheets with regular follicles in honeycomb arrangement) is supportive of a hyperplastic nodule.

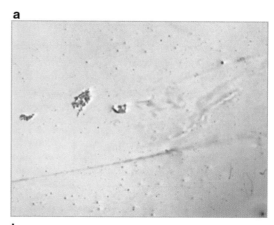

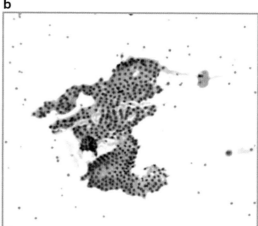

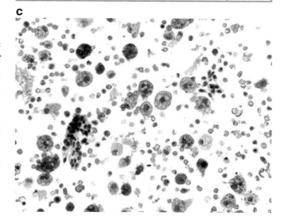

Fig. 5.3 Nodular goiter with abundant colloid (**a**), bland follicular cells (**b**), and cystic degeneration (**c**)

2. Papillary carcinoma: Hyperplastic nodules and adenomatous nodules with cystic degeneration may mimic cytologic features of papillary carcinoma. The absence of the characteristic nuclear features is the clue [55].

Follicular Neoplasm (Fig. 5.4)

The histologic diagnosis of follicular carcinoma is based strictly upon the presence of invasion of the lesion capsule or invasion into vascular spaces [56–58], features that cannot be determined on cytology material. Hence, differentiating a low-grade follicular carcinoma from a follicular adenoma is impossible and a diagnosis of adenoma or carcinoma is rarely rendered on cytologic material; instead, lesions are lumped together as follicular neoplasm.

Cytomorphology. FNA from a follicular neoplasm is usually hypercellular and characterized by follicular cells present in varying combinations of microfollicular or trabecular patterns or as crowded three-dimensional groups. Colloid is sparse and may be present as dense droplets in the center of microfollicles. Variable degrees of nuclear atypia may be seen in the follicular cells [5, 47, 54].

a

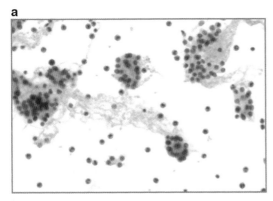

b

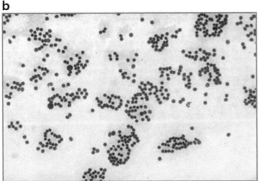

Fig. 5.4 Follicular neoplasm showing prominent micro-follicular pattern in the absence of colloid (**a**) and (**b**)

Differential diagnosis and pitfalls
1. FNAs from hyperplastic nodule/goiter may mimic a microfollicular adenoma, while a colloid nodule may resemble a macrofollicular adenoma with abundant colloid and sparse epithelial cells. The presence of syncytial fragments of follicular epithelium and increased nuclear size and nucleoli are important parameters in differentiating follicular neoplasms from hyperplastic goiters.
2. Follicular variant of papillary carcinoma may be difficult to distinguish from a follicular neoplasm, particularly cases with poorly developed nuclear features. This is a rare pitfall in the diagnosis of follicular neoplasm and a very difficult diagnosis to make cytologically.

Hyalinizing Trabecular Adenoma

Synonym. Paraganglioma-like adenoma of thyroid (PLAT)

This is a distinctive but uncommon subtype of follicular adenoma that is frequently mistaken cytologically for a carcinoma, either papillary or medullary [59–61].

Cytomorphology. Aspirates are cellular and made up of papillary-like branching sheets or trabeculae with central cores of hyaline material. Cells show frequent nuclear inclusions and nuclear grooves. Rare psammoma bodies may be present [62–64].
Differential diagnosis and pitfalls
1. Papillary carcinoma: Cytological features are indistinguishable from those of papillary carcinoma [65]. Strong immunopositivity for MIB-1 (a proliferative marker that stains the nuclei of cells in the late G1, S, G2, and M phases of the cell cycle) localized to the cell membrane and the cytoplasm of hyalinizing trabecular adenomas has been shown to be useful in differentiating this lesion from papillary thyroid carcinoma which shows no cell membrane or cytoplasmic immunoreactivity [66, 67].
2. Medullary carcinoma: Hyaline-like material present in aspirates may be mistaken for amyloid, particularly in the presence of spindle-shaped cells, giving rise to an erroneous diagnosis of medullary carcinoma.

Hurthle Cell Neoplasm (Fig. 5.5)

Synonym. Oncocytic neoplasm, oxyphilic neoplasm

Hurthle cells are not specific to any pathology affecting the thyroid gland and can be found in FNAs from any thyroid lesion – nodular goiter, Hashimoto's thyroiditis, Graves' disease, myxedema, follicular neoplasms, or from aspirates of elderly persons and patients who have received radiation to the head and neck region. In these conditions, they are generally seen admixed with other cytologic components such as follicular cells and inflammatory cells and are felt to represent a metaplastic change. The term Hurthle cell neoplasm refers to a set of tumors, which are composed predominantly of Hurthle cells and, like the follicular neoplasms, the difference between adenoma and carcinoma is based on the histologic presence of transcapsular or vascular invasion and thus these lesions are also lumped together as Hurthle cell neoplasms on FNA [68].

Cytomorphology. Characteristic features observed on the FNA include cellular aspirate comprising of a prominent somewhat uniform population of Hurthle cells in monolayered sheets or as scattered single cells in a background of minimal colloid. Individual cells show abundant densely granular cytoplasm with an enlarged nucleus containing a distinct central nucleolus [5, 47, 69].

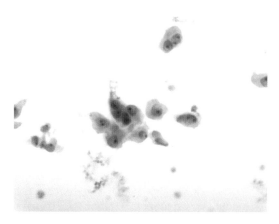

Fig. 5.5 Hurthle cell neoplasm with discohesive cells containing abundant granular cytoplasm, round nuclei, and prominent nucleoli

Differential diagnosis and pitfalls
1. Adenomatous nodule with oncocytic features and Hurthle cell nodules in Hashimoto's thyroiditis are two conditions that may contain a prominent population of Hurthle cells and mimic the cytologic features of Hurthle cell neoplasm [50].
2. Medullary carcinomas and oncocytic and tall cell variants of papillary carcinoma are rarely encountered tumors that share morphologic similarities with Hurthle cell neoplasms. Nuclear features are helpful in the differentiation, in addition to immunostaining with calcitonin, CEA, and thyroglobulin.
3. Metastatic renal cell carcinoma and parathyroid adenomas should also be considered in the differential diagnosis and are easily distinguished by immunohistochemistry for thyroglobulin and thyroid transcription factor (TTF-1), which are positive in Hurthle cell neoplasms but are negative in renal cell carcinoma and parathyroid adenoma.

Papillary Carcinoma (Fig. 5.6)

Papillary carcinoma is the most common form of thyroid malignancy and is diagnosed with a high rate of accuracy (90–94%) on FNAs. However, some variants may pose some diagnostic difficulties [47, 70–72].

Cytomorphology. The diagnosis of papillary carcinoma heavily depends on the presence of characteristic nuclear features (enlarged oval nuclei with powdery chromatin; small, eccentric nucleoli; longitudinal nuclear grooves; and intranuclear cytoplasmic inclusions) regardless of cytoplasmic features or growth pattern. Additional features include hypercellularity, crowded and disorganized monolayered sheets, papillary architecture, cells with squamoid cytoplasm, dense "ropy" colloid, cystic change with multinucleated cells, and psammoma bodies [5, 72–75].

Variants. Several histologic variants of papillary carcinoma have been described based on archi-

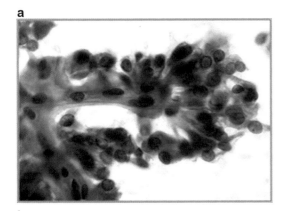

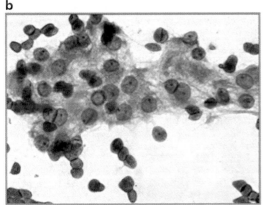

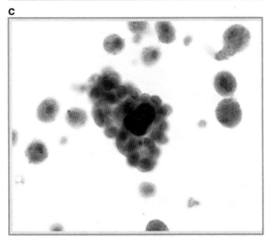

Fig. 5.6 Papillary carcinoma. Papillary clusters (**a**) of atypical cells showing intranuclear inclusions and nuclear grooves (**b**) and associated calcification (**c**)

tectural patterns and cell type. The common denominator for all is the typical nuclear morphology. These variants include *diffuse follicular variant* [76–80], *tall cell variant* [81–84], *columnar cell variant* [85–88], *diffuse sclerosing variant*

[89–91], and *oncocytic variant* [92–94]. The tall cell, columnar cell, oncocytic, and diffuse sclerosing variants are associated with aggressive behavior [95–99]. These variants are rare and often share morphologic similarities with other benign and malignant thyroid neoplasms. Several studies have shown poor correlation between cytologic and histologic subtyping of these variants [84, 100, 101]; identification, therefore, is generally not attempted on cytology.

Differential diagnosis and pitfalls. Although the diagnosis of papillary carcinoma is heavily weighted by nuclear morphology, the nuclear features are not entirely specific and may be seen in other benign and malignant conditions of the thyroid. Nuclear grooves and inclusions can be seen in Hashimoto's thyroiditis, nodular goiter, hyalinizing trabecular adenoma, Hurthle cell neoplasms, and medullary carcinoma. Follicular variants may be mistaken for follicular neoplasms [57], oncocytic variants as Hurthle cell tumors. False-positive diagnoses result from interpretations based on inadequate aspirates and/or due to emphasis on few and not all of the described cytologic features [74, 102].

Medullary Carcinoma (Fig. 5.7)

Medullary carcinoma originates from the C-cells of the thyroid and, unlike other thyroid neoplasms, is a malignancy with neuroendocrine features. Twenty percent cases are associated with familial syndromes; the remainder is sporadic. Medullary carcinomas show a wide range of morphologic patterns and thus constitute a challenging diagnosis that must be confirmed by immunostains or elevated serum calcitonin levels [47, 103–106].

Cytomorphology. Characteristically, FNAs from medullary carcinomas show cellular material consisting predominantly of single plasmacytoid cells with eccentrically situated nuclei and abundant eosinophilic granular cytoplasm, or spindled cells, giving a mesenchymal appearance or polygonal oncocytic appearing cells. The nuclear chromatin is similar to that

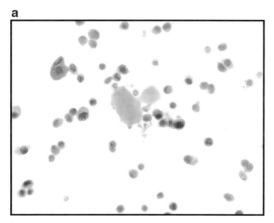

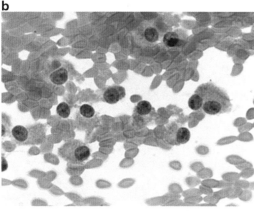

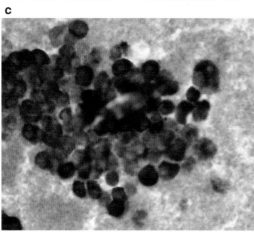

Fig. 5.7 Medullary carcinoma with characteristic plasmacytoid cells and extracellular amyloid (**a**, **b**) staining positive for calcitonin (**c**)

seen in neuroendocrine tumors: salt-and-pepper type with inconspicuous nucleoli. Extracellular amyloid may be observed. Immunostains for

calcitonin, calcitonin gene-related peptide, carcinoembryonic antigen, chromogranin and synaptophysin (all positive), and thyroglobulin (negative) are confirmatory [5, 107–110].

Differential diagnosis and pitfalls

1. Hurthle cell neoplasm is the most common pitfall. The presence of prominent nucleoli and the lack of neuroendocrine chromatin pattern and cytoplasmic granules may help in the differentiation. Positivity for thyroglobulin is confirmatory.

2. Papillary carcinoma arises in the differential diagnosis in cases of medullary carcinoma that exhibit intranuclear cytoplasmic inclusions. However, other classic nuclear features are usually lacking. Immunostaining again is confirmatory (papillary carcinomas are negative for calcitonin and positive for thyroglobulin).

3. Undifferentiated carcinoma: Spindled variants of medullary carcinoma give rise to this possibility and may be confirmed by positivity for calcitonin.

4. Metastatic neuroendocrine tumors, plasmacytomas, malignant melanomas, and small-cell carcinoma are additional differential diagnoses for consideration. Clinical history and immunostains for thyroid transcription factor (positive in medullary carcinoma) are helpful.

Anaplastic Carcinoma (Fig. 5.8)

Anaplastic carcinoma of the thyroid is the most aggressive of thyroid carcinomas. Aspirates from these lesions usually do not pose any diagnostic difficulties due to the presence of obvious malignant features [111].

Cytomorphology. FNAs show markedly pleomorphic and anaplastic cells in a background of inflammation and necrosis. Neoplastic cells may be epithelioid (squamoid) or spindle shaped with multinucleated osteoclast like giant cells. Admixed well-differentiated areas may be seen since these carcinomas frequently originate from pre-existing follicular or papillary carcinomas [5, 47, 112, 113].

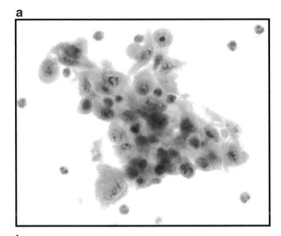

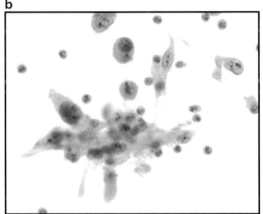

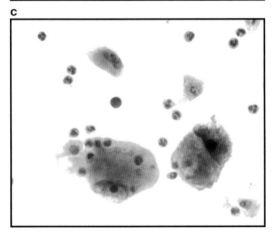

Fig. 5.8 Anaplastic carcinoma showing varied morphology comprising atypical epithelioid cells (**a**), spindle cells (**b**), and bizarre pleomorphic single cells (**c**)

Differential diagnosis and pitfalls

1. Metastatic malignancies from the kidney, lung, breast, head and neck, and skin (including malignant melanomas) may be difficult to

distinguish from anaplastic thyroid carcinomas, as may be the possibility of sarcomas that should be considered in cases with a predominance of spindled cells. Immunohistochemistry for organ-specific markers and correlation with clinical history is most useful in the differentiation. While anaplastic carcinomas are frequently positive for cytokeratin immunostains, they are often negative for thyroglobulin. Other markers that may be used include RCC and CD10 for renal carcinomas, S100, HMB45, and melan A for melanoma, and estrogen receptor for breast carcinoma.

2. Large-cell lymphomas may mimic anaplastic carcinomas due to the presence of single dispersed cells and the presence of abundant necrosis. Immunohistochemistry and/or flow cytometry for lymphoid markers can be used for indentifying lymphomas [114].

3. Medullary carcinomas may on occasion share the single dispersed or spindled cell morphology of anaplastic carcinomas. Positive immunostaining with calcitonin is diagnostic.

Future Developments

Although thyroid FNA is currently the most reliable and commonly used diagnostic test for thyroid nodules and accurately distinguishes a benign from a malignant lesion in the majority of cases, 10–40% of all FNA samples are indeterminate for malignancy resulting in unnecessary diagnostic hemithyroidectomies [43, 115] followed by definitive surgeries. Additionally, 1–3% of nodules are falsely reported as negative on FNA cytology resulting in possible delay in treatment [1]. Recent advances in the molecular genetics of thyroid cancers raise the possibility of utilizing the various known genetic alteration as diagnostic tools. Papillary carcinomas frequently carry mutually exclusive somatic mutations of *BRAF*, *RET/PTC*, or *RAS genes* in more than 70% of cases [116–118], while follicular carcinomas harbor either *RAS* or *PAX8/PPARγ* mutations in approximately 80% cases [119]. Several studies have demonstrated the feasibility of detecting these mutations in thyroid FNA samples and have shown that this improves cytologic diagnosis, allowing better prediction of malignancy in indeterminate nodules [120–122]. Recently, Nikiforov et al [123] used a panel of these mutations on FNA thyroid samples and determined that the presence of any mutation carried a 97% predictive value for carcinoma and resulted in a significant improvement in diagnostic accuracy when a combination of cytology and molecular testing was used.

More recently, analysis of micro-RNAs (miRNAs) has shown some promise. miRNAs are small noncoding RNAs of approximately 21–25 nucleotides that negatively regulate gene expression at the transcriptional level in both plants and animals [124]. They have recently been demonstrated to be important modulators of oncogenesis (onco-MIRs) and are deregulated in various hematological neoplasms and in cancers of prostate, thyroid, lung, pancreas, and colorectum [125]. Early studies demonstrate that evaluation of certain miRNAs may be useful in the diagnosis of thyroid cancers [124, 126, 127].

Conclusion

Overall, thyroid FNA is a sensitive and specific test that is useful in the diagnosis and follow-up of thyroid nodules. Awareness of its shortcomings and pitfalls and correlation of clinical, radiologic, and pathologic features will greatly improve outcome.

References

1. Cooper DS, Doherty GM, Haugen BR, Kloos RT, Lee SL, Mandel SJ, et al. Management guidelines for patients with thyroid nodules and differentiated thyroid cancer. Thyroid. 2006;16:109–42.
2. Yang J, Schnadig V, Logrono R, Wasserman PG. Fine-needle aspiration of thyroid nodules: a study of 4703 patients with histologic and clinical correlations. Cancer. 2007;111:306–15.
3. Goldstein RE, Netterville JL, Burkey B. Johnson JE Implications of follicular neoplasms, atypia, and lesions suspicious for malignancy diagnosed by fine-needle aspiration of thyroid nodules. Ann Surg. 2002;235:656–62. discussion 662–654.
4. Miller JM, Hamburger JI, Kini SR. The impact of needle biopsy on the preoperative diagnosis of thyroid nodules. Henry Ford Hosp Med J. 1980;28:145–8.
5. Clark DPF, Faquin WC. Thyroid cytopathology. Springer: New York; 2005.
6. Pothier DD, Narula AA. Should we apply suction during fine needle cytology of thyroid lesions? A systematic review and meta-analysis. Ann R Coll Surg Engl. 2006;88:643–5.
7. de Vos tot Nederveen Cappel RJ, Bouvy ND, Bonjer HJ, van Muiswinkel JM, Chadha S. Fine needle aspiration cytology of thyroid nodules: how accurate is it and what are the causes of discrepant cases? Cytopathology. 2001;12:399–405.
8. Hall TL, Layfield LJ, Philippe A, Rosenthal DL. Sources of diagnostic error in fine needle aspiration of the thyroid. Cancer. 1989;63:718–25.
9. Ljung BM, Drejet A, Chiampi N, Jeffrey J, Goodson 3 WH, Chew K, et al. Diagnostic accuracy of fine-needle aspiration biopsy is determined by physician training in sampling technique. Cancer. 2001;93:263–8.
10. Unver E, Yilmaz A, Aksoy F, Baysungur V, Celik O, Altinsoy B, et al. Does needle size affect diagnostic yield of transthoracic needle biopsy in malignant pulmonary lesions? Comparison of 18-, 22- and 25-gauge needles in surgical specimens. Respirology. 2006;11:648–51.
11. Zajdela A, de Maublanc MA, Schlienger P, Haye C. Cytologic diagnosis of orbital and periorbital palpable tumors using fine-needle sampling without aspiration. Diagn Cytopathol. 1986;2:17–20.
12. Alexander EK, Heering JP, Benson CB, Frates MC, Doubilet PM, Cibas ES, et al. Assessment of nondiagnostic ultrasound-guided fine needle aspirations of thyroid nodules. J Clin Endocrinol Metab. 2002; 87:4924–7.
13. Cajulis RS, Sneige N. Objective comparison of cellular yield in fine-needle biopsy of lymph nodes with and without aspiration. Diagn Cytopathol. 1993;9:43–5.
14. Cibas ES, Ali SZ. The Bethesda system for reporting thyroid cytopathology. Am J Clin Pathol. 2009;132: 658–65.
15. Redman R, Zalaznick H, Mazzaferri EL, Massoll NA. The impact of assessing specimen adequacy and number of needle passes for fine-needle aspiration biopsy of thyroid nodules. Thyroid. 2006;16:55–60.
16. Zhu W, Michael CW. How important is on-site adequacy assessment for thyroid FNA? An evaluation of 883 cases. Diagn Cytopathol. 2007;35:183–6.
17. Nasuti JF, Gupta PK, Baloch ZW. Diagnostic value and cost-effectiveness of on-site evaluation of fine-needle aspiration specimens: review of 5,688 cases. Diagn Cytopathol. 2002;27:1–4.
18. Ghofrani M, Beckman D, Rimm DL. The value of onsite adequacy assessment of thyroid fine-needle aspirations is a function of operator experience. Cancer. 2006;108:110–3.
19. Baloch ZW, LiVolsi VA. Post fine-needle aspiration histologic alterations of thyroid revisited. Am J Clin Pathol. 1999;112:311–6.
20. Baloch ZW, Wu H, LiVolsi VA. Post-fine-needle aspiration spindle cell nodules of the thyroid (PSCNT). Am J Clin Pathol. 1999;111:70–4.

21. LiVolsi VA, Merino MJ. Worrisome histologic altera-tions following fine-needle aspiration of the thyroid (WHAFFT). Pathol Annu. 1994;29(Pt 2):99–120.

22. Kini SR. Post-fine-needle biopsy infarction of thyroid neoplasms: a review of 28 cases. Diagn Cytopathol. 1996;15:211–20.

23. Gordon DL, Gattuso P, Castelli M, Bayer W, Emanuele MA, Brooks MH. Effect of fine needle aspiration biopsy on the histology of thyroid neoplasms. Acta Cytol. 1993;37:651–4.

24. Karwowski JK, Nowels KW, McDougall IR, Weigel RJ. Needle track seeding of papillary thyroid carci-noma from fine needle aspiration biopsy. A case report. Acta Cytol. 2002;46:591–5.

25. Amrikachi M, Ramzy I, Rubenfeld S, Wheeler TM. Accuracy of fine-needle aspiration of thyroid. Arch Pathol Lab Med. 2001;125:484–8.

26. Gharib H. Fine-needle aspiration biopsy of thyroid nodules: advantages, limitations, and effect. Mayo Clin Proc. 1994;69:44–9.

27. Harvey JN, Parker D, De P, Shrimali RK, Otter M. Sonographically guided core biopsy in the assessment of thyroid nodules. J Clin Ultrasound. 2005;33: 57–62.

28. Baloch ZW, LiVolsi VA. Fine-needle aspiration of thyroid nodules: past, present, and future. Endocr Pract. 2004;10:234–41.

29. Granter SR, Cibas ES. Cytologic findings in thyroid nodules after 131I treatment of hyperthyroidism. Am J Clin Pathol. 1997;107:20–5.

30. Pretorius HT, Katikineni M, Kinsella TJ, Barsky SH, Brennan MF, Chu EW, et al. Thyroid nodules after high-dose external radiotherapy. Fine-needle aspiration cytology in diagnosis and management. JAMA. 1982; 247:3217–20.

31. Kollur SM, El Sayed S, El Hag IA. Follicular thyroid lesions coexisting with Hashimoto's thyroiditis: inci-dence and possible sources of diagnostic errors. Diagn Cytopathol. 2003;28:35–8.

32. Nguyen GK, Ginsberg J, Crockford PM, Villanueva RR. Hashimoto's thyroiditis: cytodiagnostic accuracy and pitfalls. Diagn Cytopathol. 1997;16:531–6.

33. Kini SR, Miller JM, Hamburger JI, Smith-Purslow MJ. Cytopathology of follicular lesions of the thyroid gland. Diagn Cytopathol. 1985;1:123–32.

34. Goellner JR, Gharib H, Grant CS, Johnson DA. Fine needle aspiration cytology of the thyroid, 1980 to 1986. Acta Cytol. 1987;31:587–90.

35. Hamburger JI, Husain M. Semiquantitative criteria for fine-needle biopsy diagnosis: reduced false-negative diagnoses. Diagn Cytopathol. 1988;4:14–7.

36. Nguyen GK, Ginsberg J, Crockford PM. Fine-needle aspiration biopsy cytology of the thyroid. Its value and limitations in the diagnosis and management of solitary thyroid nodules. Pathol Annu. 1991;26(Pt 1):63–91.

37. Shabb NS, Salti I. Subacute thyroiditis: fine-needle aspiration cytology of 14 cases presenting with thyroid nodules. Diagn Cytopathol. 2006;34:18–23.

38. Guidelines of the Papanicolaou Society of Cytopathology for the Examination of Fine-Needle Aspiration Specimens from Thyroid Nodules. The Papanicolaou Society of Cytopathology Task Force on Standards of Practice. Mod Pathol. 1996;9:710–5.

39. Deshpande V, Kapila K, Sai K, Verma K. Follicular neoplasms of the thyroid. Decision tree approach using morphologic and morphometric parameters. Acta Cytol. 1997;41:369–76.

40. Renshaw AA. Accuracy of thyroid fine-needle aspira-tion using receiver operator characteristic curves. Am J Clin Pathol. 2001;116:477–82.

41. Renshaw AA. Evidence-based criteria for adequacy in thyroid fine-needle aspiration. Am J Clin Pathol. 2002;118:518–21.

42. Wang HH. Reporting thyroid fine-needle aspiration: literature review and a proposal. Diagn Cytopathol. 2006;34:67–76.

43. Yassa L, Cibas ES, Benson CB, Frates MC, Doubilet PM, Gawande AA, et al. Long-term assessment of a multidisciplinary approach to thyroid nodule diagnos-tic evaluation. Cancer. 2007;111:508–16.

44. Liu LH, Bakhos R, Wojcik EM. Concomitant papil-lary thyroid carcinoma and Hashimoto's thyroiditis. Semin Diagn Pathol. 2001;18:99–103.

45. Moshynska OV, Saxena A. Clonal relationship between Hashimoto thyroiditis and thyroid lym-phoma. J Clin Pathol. 2008;61:438–44.

46. Kumar N, Ray C, Jain S. Aspiration cytology of Hashimoto's thyroiditis in an endemic area. Cytopathology. 2002;13:31–9.

47. Kini SR. Thyroid cytopathology: an atlas and text. Philadelphia, PA: Lippincott Williams & Wilkins; 2008. A Wolters Kluwer business.

48. Kojima M, Nakamura N, Shimizu K, Segawa A, Kaba S, Masawa N. MALT type lymphoma demonstrating prominent plasma cell differentiation resembling fibrous variant of Hashimoto's thyroiditis: a three case report. Pathol Oncol Res. 2009;15:285–9.

49. MacDonald L, Yazdi HM. Fine needle aspiration biopsy of Hashimoto's thyroiditis. Sources of diag-nostic error. Acta Cytol. 1999;43:400–6.

50. Kumarasinghe MP, De Silva S. Pitfalls in cytological diagnosis of autoimmune thyroiditis. Pathology. 1999; 31:1–7.

51. Anderson SR, Mandel S, LiVolsi VA, Gupta PK, Baloch ZW. Can cytomorphology differentiate between benign nodules and tumors arising in Graves' disease? Diagn Cytopathol. 2004;31:64–7.

52. Harach HR, Zusman SB, Saravia Day E. Nodular goi-ter: a histo-cytological study with some emphasis on pitfalls of fine-needle aspiration cytology. Diagn Cytopathol. 1992;8:409–19.

53. Sidawy MK, Del Vecchio DM, Knoll SM. Fine-needle aspiration of thyroid nodules: correlation between cytology and histology and evaluation of discrepant cases. Cancer. 1997;81:253–9.

54. Busseniers AE, Oertel YC. "Cellular adenomatoid nodules" of the thyroid: review of 219 fine-needle aspirates. Diagn Cytopathol. 1993;9:581–9.

55. Fiorella RM, Isley W, Miller LK, Kragel PJ. Multinodular goiter of the thyroid mimicking malig-

nancy: diagnostic pitfalls in fine-needle aspiration biopsy. Diagn Cytopathol. 1993;9:351–5. discussion 355–57.

56. Thompson LD, Wieneke JA, Paal E, Frommelt RA, Adair CF, Heffess CS. A clinicopathologic study of minimally invasive follicular carcinoma of the thyroid gland with a review of the English literature. Cancer. 2001;91:505–24.

57. Suster S. Thyroid tumors with a follicular growth pattern: problems in differential diagnosis. Arch Pathol Lab Med. 2006;130:984–8.

58. LiVolsi VA, Baloch ZW. Follicular neoplasms of the thyroid: view, biases, and experiences. Adv Anat Pathol. 2004;11:279–87.

59. Evenson A, Mowschenson P, Wang H, Connolly J, Mendrinos S, Parangi S, et al. Hyalinizing trabecular adenoma – an uncommon thyroid tumor frequently misdiagnosed as papillary or medullary thyroid carcinoma. Am J Surg. 2007;193:707–12.

60. Galgano MT, Mills SE, Stelow EB. Hyalinizing trabecular adenoma of the thyroid revisited: a histologic and immunohistochemical study of thyroid lesions with prominent trabecular architecture and sclerosis. Am J Surg Pathol. 2006;30:1269–73.

61. Carney JA, Hirokawa M, Lloyd RV, Papotti M, Sebo TJ. Hyalinizing trabecular tumors of the thyroid gland are almost all benign. Am J Surg Pathol. 2008; 32:1877–89.

62. Casey MB, Sebo TJ, Carney JA. Hyalinizing trabecular adenoma of the thyroid gland: cytologic features in 29 cases. Am J Surg Pathol. 2004;28:859–67.

63. Kuma S, Hirokawa M, Miyauchi A, Kakudo K, Katayama S. Cytologic features of hyalinizing trabecular adenoma of the thyroid. Acta Cytol. 2003; 47:399–404.

64. Jayaram G. Fine needle aspiration cytology of hyalinizing trabecular adenoma of the thyroid. Acta Cytol. 1999;43:978–80.

65. LiVolsi VA, Gupta PK. Thyroid fine-needle aspiration: intranuclear inclusions, nuclear grooves and psammoma bodies – paraganglioma-like adenoma of the thyroid. Diagn Cytopathol. 1992;8:82–3. discussion 83–4.

66. Hirokawa M, Carney JA. Cell membrane and cytoplasmic staining for MIB-1 in hyalinizing trabecular adenoma of the thyroid gland. Am J Surg Pathol. 2000;24:575–8.

67. Hirokawa M, Shimizu M, Manabe T, Kuroda M, Mizoguchi Y. Hyalinizing trabecular adenoma of the thyroid: its unusual cytoplasmic immunopositivity for MIB1. Pathol Int. 1995;45:399–401.

68. Carcangiu ML, Bianchi S, Savino D, Voynick IM, Rosai J. Follicular Hurthle cell tumors of the thyroid gland. Cancer. 1991;68:1944–53.

69. Elliott DD, Pitman MB, Bloom L, Faquin WC. Fine-needle aspiration biopsy of Hurthle cell lesions of the thyroid gland: a cytomorphologic study of 139 cases with statistical analysis. Cancer. 2006;108:102–9.

70. Carcangiu ML, Zampi G, Pupi A, Castagnoli A, Rosai J. Papillary carcinoma of the thyroid. A clinicopathologic study of 241 cases treated at the University of Florence, Italy. Cancer. 1985;55:805–28.

71. Al-Brahim N, Asa SL. Papillary thyroid carcinoma: an overview. Arch Pathol Lab Med. 2006;130:1057–62.

72. Oertel YC, Oertel JE. Thyroid cytology and histology. Baillieres Best Pract Res Clin Endocrinol Metab. 2000;14:541–57.

73. Szporn AH, Yuan S, Wu M, Burstein DE. Cellular swirls in fine needle aspirates of papillary thyroid carcinoma: a new diagnostic criterion. Mod Pathol. 2006;19:1470–3.

74. Albores-Saavedra J, Wu J. The many faces and mimics of papillary thyroid carcinoma. Endocr Pathol. 2006;17:1–18.

75. Das DK. Intranuclear cytoplasmic inclusions in fine-needle aspiration smears of papillary thyroid carcinoma: a study of its morphological forms, association with nuclear grooves, and mode of formation. Diagn Cytopathol. 2005;32:264–8.

76. Tielens ET, Sherman SI, Hruban RH, Ladenson PW. Follicular variant of papillary thyroid carcinoma. A clinicopathologic study. Cancer. 1994;73:424–31.

77. Baloch ZW, Gupta PK, Yu GH, Sack MJ, LiVolsi VA. Follicular variant of papillary carcinoma. Cytologic and histologic correlation. Am J Clin Pathol. 1999;111:216–22.

78. El Hag IA, Kollur SM. Benign follicular thyroid lesions versus follicular variant of papillary carcinoma: differentiation by architectural pattern. Cytopathology. 2004;15:200–5.

79. Gallagher J, Oertel YC, Oertel JE. Follicular variant of papillary carcinoma of the thyroid: fine-needle aspirates with histologic correlation. Diagn Cytopathol. 1997;16:207–13.

80. Renshaw AA, Gould EW. Why there is the tendency to "overdiagnose" the follicular variant of papillary thyroid carcinoma. Am J Clin Pathol. 2002;117:19–21.

81. Filie AC, Chiesa A, Bryant BR, Merino MJ, Sobel ME, Abati A. The Tall cell variant of papillary carcinoma of the thyroid: cytologic features and loss of heterozygosity of metastatic and/or recurrent neoplasms and primary neoplasms. Cancer. 1999;87:238–42.

82. Ostrowski ML, Merino MJ. Tall cell variant of papillary thyroid carcinoma: a reassessment and immunohistochemical study with comparison to the usual type of papillary carcinoma of the thyroid. Am J Surg Pathol. 1996;20:964–74.

83. Gamboa-Dominguez A, Candanedo-Gonzalez F, Uribe-Uribe NO, Angeles-Angeles A. Tall cell variant of papillary thyroid carcinoma. A cytohistologic correlation. Acta Cytol. 1997;41:672–6.

84. Das DK, Mallik MK, Sharma P, Sheikh ZA, Mathew PA, Sheikh M, et al. Papillary thyroid carcinoma and its variants in fine needle aspiration smears.

A cytomorphologic study with special reference to tall cell variant. Acta Cytol. 2004;48:325–36.

85. Ferreiro JA, Hay ID, Lloyd RV. Columnar cell carcinoma of the thyroid: report of three additional cases. Hum Pathol. 1996;27:1156–60.

86. Mizukami Y, Nonomura A, Michigishi T, Noguchi M, Nakamura S, Hashimoto T. Columnar cell carcinoma of the thyroid gland: a case report and review of the literature. Hum Pathol. 1994;25:1098–101.

87. Jayaram G. Cytology of columnar-cell variant of papillary thyroid carcinoma. Diagn Cytopathol. 2000;22:227–9.

88. Wenig BM, Thompson LD, Adair CF, Shmookler B, Heffess CS. Thyroid papillary carcinoma of columnar cell type: a clinicopathologic study of 16 cases. Cancer. 1998;82:740–53.

89. Fujimoto Y, Obara T, Ito Y, Kodama T, Aiba M, Yamaguchi K. Diffuse sclerosing variant of papillary carcinoma of the thyroid. Clinical importance, surgical treatment, and follow-up study. Cancer. 1990;66: 2306–12.

90. Triggiani V, Ciampolillo A, Maiorano E. Papillary thyroid carcinoma, diffuse sclerosing variant, with abundant psammoma bodies. Acta Cytol. 2003;47: 1141–3.

91. Caplan RH, Wester S, Kisken AW. Diffuse sclerosing variant of papillary thyroid carcinoma: case report and review of the literature. Endocr Pract. 1997;3:287–92.

92. Berho M, Suster S. The oncocytic variant of papillary carcinoma of the thyroid: a clinicopathologic study of 15 cases. Hum Pathol. 1997;28:47–53.

93. Beckner ME, Heffess CS, Oertel JE. Oxyphilic papillary thyroid carcinomas. Am J Clin Pathol. 1995;103:280–7.

94. Khanum O, Wang S, Hameed A. Fine needle aspiration cytology of a papillary oncocytic neoplasm of the thyroid gland. Acta Cytol. 1999;43:976–8.

95. Akslen LA, LiVolsi VA. Prognostic significance of histologic grading compared with subclassification of papillary thyroid carcinoma. Cancer. 2000;88: 1902–8.

96. Johnson TL, Lloyd RV, Thompson NW, Beierwaltes WH, Sisson JC. Prognostic implications of the tall cell variant of papillary thyroid carcinoma. Am J Surg Pathol. 1988;12:22–7.

97. van den Brekel MW, Hekkenberg RJ, Asa SL, Tomlinson G, Rosen IB, Freeman JL. Prognostic features in tall cell papillary carcinoma and insular thyroid carcinoma. Laryngoscope. 1997;107:254–9.

98. Herrera MF, Hay ID, Wu PS, Goellner JR, Ryan JJ, Ebersold JR, et al. Hurthle cell (oxyphilic) papillary thyroid carcinoma: a variant with more aggressive biologic behavior. World J Surg. 1992;16:669–74. discussion 774–665.

99. Imamura Y, Kasahara Y, Fukuda M. Multiple brain metastases from a diffuse sclerosing variant of papillary carcinoma of the thyroid. Endocr Pathol. 2000;11:97–108.

100. Gupta S, Sodhani P, Jain S, Kumar N. Morphologic spectrum of papillary carcinoma of the thyroid: role of cytology in identifying the variants. Acta Cytol. 2004;48:795–800.

101. Nair M, Kapila K, Karak AK, Verma K. Papillary carcinoma of the thyroid and its variants: a cytohistological correlation. Diagn Cytopathol. 2001;24: 167–73.

102. Baloch ZW, LiVolsi VA. Cytologic and architectural mimics of papillary thyroid carcinoma Diagnostic challenges in fine-needle aspiration and surgical pathology specimens. Am J Clin Pathol. 2006; 125(Suppl):S135–44.

103. Fletcher JR. Medullary (solid) carcinoma of the thyroid gland. A review of 249 cases. Arch Surg. 1970;100:257–62.

104. Williams ED. A review of 17 cases of carcinoma of the thyroid and phaeochromocytoma. J Clin Pathol. 1965;18:288–92.

105. Williams ED. The origin and associations of medullary carcinoma of the thyroid. Monogr Neoplast Dis Var Sites. 1970;6:130–40.

106. Williams CR, Brewer DB. Medullary carcinoma of the thyroid. Br J Surg. 1969;56:437–43.

107. Collins BT, Cramer HM, Tabatowski K, Hearn S, Raminhos A, Lampe H. Fine needle aspiration of medullary carcinoma of the thyroid. Cytomorphology, immunocytochemistry and electron microscopy. Acta Cytol. 1995;39:920–30.

108. Papaparaskeva K, Nagel H, Droese M. Cytologic diagnosis of medullary carcinoma of the thyroid gland. Diagn Cytopathol. 2000;22:351–8.

109. Bose S, Kapila K, Verma K. Medullary carcinoma of the thyroid: a cytological, immunocytochemical, and ultrastructural study. Diagn Cytopathol. 1992;8: 28–32.

110. Forrest CH, Frost FA, de Boer WB, Spagnolo DV, Whitaker D, Sterrett BF. Medullary carcinoma of the thyroid: accuracy of diagnosis of fine-needle aspiration cytology. Cancer. 1998;84:295–302.

111. McIver B, Hay ID, Giuffrida DF, Dvorak CE, Grant CS, Thompson GB, et al. Anaplastic thyroid carcinoma: a 50-year experience at a single institution. Surgery. 2001;130:1028–34.

112. Us-Krasovec M, Golouh R, Auersperg M, Besic N, Ruparcic-Oblak L. Anaplastic thyroid carcinoma in fine needle aspirates. Acta Cytol. 1996;40:953–8.

113. Bauman ME, Tao LC. Cytopathology of papillary carcinoma of the thyroid with anaplastic transformation. A case report. Acta Cytol. 1995;39:525–9.

114. Shvero J, Gal R, Avidor I, Hadar T, Kessler E. Anaplastic thyroid carcinoma. A clinical, histologic, and immunohistochemical study. Cancer. 1988;62:319–25.

115. Sclabas GM, Staerkel GA, Shapiro SE, Fornage BD, Sherman SI, Vassillopoulou-Sellin R, et al. Fine-needle aspiration of the thyroid and correlation with histopathology in a contemporary series of 240 patients. Am J Surg. 2003;186:702–9. discussion 709–710.

116. Adeniran AJ, Zhu Z, Gandhi M, Steward DL, Fidler JP, Giordano TJ, et al. Correlation between genetic alterations and microscopic features, clinical manifestations, and prognostic characteristics of thyroid papillary carcinomas. Am J Surg Pathol. 2006;30: 216–22.

117. Xing M. BRAF mutation in papillary thyroid cancer: pathogenic role, molecular bases, and clinical implications. Endocr Rev. 2007;28:742–62.

118. Kimura ET, Nikiforova MN, Zhu Z, Knauf JA, Nikiforov YE, Fagin JA. High prevalence of BRAF mutations in thyroid cancer: genetic evidence for constitutive activation of the RET/PTC-RAS-BRAF signaling pathway in papillary thyroid carcinoma. Cancer Res. 2003;63:1454–7.

119. Nikiforova MN, Lynch RA, Biddinger PW, Alexander EK, Dorn 2nd GW, Tallini G, et al. RAS point mutations and PAX8-PPAR gamma rearrangement in thyroid tumors: evidence for distinct molecular pathways in thyroid follicular carcinoma. J Clin Endocrinol Metab. 2003;88:2318–26.

120. Pizzolanti G, Russo L, Richiusa P, Bronte V, Nuara RB, Rodolico V, et al. Fine-needle aspiration molecular analysis for the diagnosis of papillary thyroid carcinoma through BRAF V600E mutation and RET/PTC rearrangement. Thyroid. 2007;17:1109–15.

121. Sapio MR, Posca D, Raggioli A, Guerra A, Marotta V, Deandrea M, et al. Detection of RET/PTC, TRK and BRAF mutations in preoperative diagnosis of thyroid nodules with indeterminate cytological findings. Clin Endocrinol (Oxf). 2007;66:678–83.

122. Sapio MR, Posca D, Troncone G, Pettinato G, Palombini L, Rossi G, et al. Detection of BRAF mutation in thyroid papillary carcinomas by mutant allele-specific PCR amplification (MASA). Eur J Endocrinol. 2006;154:341–8.

123. Nikiforov YE, Steward DL, Robinson-Smith TM, Haugen BR, Klopper JP, Zhu Z, et al. Molecular testing for mutations in improving the fine-needle aspiration diagnosis of thyroid nodules. J Clin Endocrinol Metab. 2009;94:2092–8.

124. Nikiforova MN, Tseng GC, Steward D, Diorio D, Nikiforov YE. MicroRNA expression profiling of thyroid tumors: biological significance and diagnostic utility. J Clin Endocrinol Metab. 2008;93: 1600–8.

125. Calin GA, Croce CM. MicroRNA signatures in human cancers. Nat Rev Cancer. 2006;6:857–66.

126. Weber F, Teresi RE, Broelsch CE, Frilling A, Eng C. A limited set of human MicroRNA is deregulated in follicular thyroid carcinoma. J Clin Endocrinol Metab. 2006;91:3584–91.

127. Pallante P, Visone R, Ferracin M, Ferraro A, Berlingieri MT, Troncone G, et al. MicroRNA deregulation in human thyroid papillary carcinomas. Endocr Relat Cancer. 2006;13:497–508.

Staging Systems for Differentiated Thyroid Carcinomas

6

Ronnie Meiyi Wong and Glenn D. Braunstein

Introduction

A multitude of retrospective studies have identified prognostic factors for the mortality and recurrence rates of thyroid carcinoma. Using a combination of these factors, many medical institutions have developed their own systems for the staging of thyroid carcinoma and the system used depends on physician or medical center preference. The stage of cancer generally refers to the extent, or invasion of disease, and how far the cancer has metastasized. The goal of each staging system is to provide a more precise depiction of the tumor, to aid the physician in the selection of the best course of treatment for the patient, and to assist in the prediction of disease-specific mortality. Depending on which system is utilized, major prognostic factors can include histologic variant, tumor grade, patient age, tumor size, lymph node involvement, invasion of adjacent structures surrounding the neck, or distant metastasis to other organs.

Most staging systems described in this chapter incorporate these prognostic factors while some may also include gender or extent of thyroidectomy performed as contributing features. Some systems restrict their staging and applicability to the relatively low risk and long-term survivability of the well-differentiated papillary (PTC) and

follicular thyroid carcinomas (FTCs). Other staging systems include the higher risk, less differentiated thyroid carcinomas, namely medullary (MTC) and the more fatal anaplastic thyroid carcinomas (ATCs).

In general, the majority of all thyroid cancers are well-differentiated PTC and FTC which have a more favorable mortality outcome and recurrence rate when compared to patients with MTC and ATC. However, a worse prognosis is usually observed with any type of thyroid cancer that has aggressively invaded through the thyroid capsule or metastasized to distant organs. While distant metastasis is relatively rare among well-differentiated thyroid carcinoma (WDTC), the lungs and bones are the most common sites of spread and can dramatically increase mortality rates [1–3]. As a result, thyroid cancer encompasses a wide spectrum of disease resulting in staging, mortality, and recurrence rates that can vary considerably depending on the system used. Thus, staging of thyroid cancer should factor in these differing prognostic factors so physicians can avoid over-treating low-risk patients as well as under-treating high-risk patients who need more aggressive treatments.

This chapter introduces the major staging systems for thyroid carcinomas as well as their corresponding survival and mortality rates. These systems are then applied to data from the Thyroid Cancer Center at Cedars-Sinai Medical Center (CSMC) based in Los Angeles, California. This analysis is done in order to compare each staging system's accuracy with predicting survival within this patient population. This database was established

R.M. Wong • G.D. Braunstein (✉)
Divison of Endocrinology, Diabetes, and Metabolism,
Department of Medicine, Cedars-Sinai Medical Center,
8700 Beverly Blvd, Los Angeles, CA 90048, USA
e-mail: braunstein@cshs.org

G.D. Braunstein (ed.), *Thyroid Cancer*, Endocrine Updates 30,
DOI 10.1007/978-1-4614-0875-8_6, © Springer Science+Business Media, LLC 2012

in 2007 and includes many variables such as patient demographics, tumor type, size, and various treatment modalities of thyroid carcinoma patients. It currently has approximately 1000 differentiated thyroid carcinoma patients and is a retrospective chart review of patients from primary surgeons and select endocrinologists at CSMC.

Common staging Systems

AGES System

Developed in 1987 by Mayo Clinic physicians for PTC, AGES is defined as *a*ge, histologic *g*rade, *e*xtrathyroidal extent, and tumor *s*ize. It is difficult to apply to most patients because tumor grade is rarely reported on pathology reports [4, 5]. Additionally, determining tumor grade requires additional time, expense, and expertise which are not always readily available or possible at all medical centers [4–6]. Table 6.1 shows how to compute the AGES score and its corresponding 25-year cause-specific mortality rate among the Mayo Clinic's 860 PTC patients [5, 7, 8]. This system was later expanded and Mayo Clinic physicians introduced the MACIS staging system in 1993 which eliminated grade and included surgery type.

AMES System

The AMES binary system was developed in 1985 at the Lahey Clinic and refers to a patient's *a*ge, *m*etas-

tases, *e*xtent of tumor, and tumor *s*ize [4, 9]. Size was found to be a very important factor in this system as 50% of older patients with tumors ≥5 cm died of their disease [9]. Cady and Rossi found that their 20-year survival rate among the low-risk group was 98% versus 54% in their high-risk group [9, 10]. As Table 6.2 shows, differentiated thyroid cancer (DTC) patients are either Pstaged as low or high risk [8–11]. Figures 6.1 and 6.2 show overall survival of DTC patients at CSMC using this system.

Clinical Class System/University of Chicago System

Developed in 1990 at the University of Chicago, the Clinical Class system incorporates intra- and extrathyroidal tumors, nodal tissue involvement, and distant metastasis. It is applicable to DTC and divides patients into four different classes: class I includes patients with disease limited to the thyroid (T1/T2); class II patients have lymph node involvement (N1); class III patients have extrathyroidal invasion or incompletely resected lymph nodes; and class IV includes patients with distant metastasis (M1) [11, 12]. A 20-year disease-specific mortality in each class was 1, 3, 14, and 70% respectively [11]. Figures 6.3 and 6.4 show overall survival of DTC patients at CSMC.

Table 6.1 AGES system

+0.05 × Age if ≥ 40 years old, +0 if <40 years
+1 if Grade 2 (poorly differentiated FTC), +3 if grade 3 or 4 (poorly differentiated PTC or tumors with anaplastic components)
+1 if Extrathyroidal invasion present
+3 if Distant metastasis is present
+0.2 × tumor size in cm
= AGES Score

Total score	Risk group	25-year mortality rate(%)
<4	1	2
4–4.9	2	24
5–5.9	3	49
≥6	4	93

Created using data from Hay [7]

Table 6.2 AMES system

Low-risk group

A. All younger patients without distant metastases (men <41, women <51)

B. All older patients with:
   1. Intrathyroidal PTC or FTC with minor tumor capsular involvement and
   2. Primary cancers <5 cm and
   3. No distant metastases

High-risk group

A. All patients with distant metastases

B. All older patients with:
   1. Extrathyroidal PTC or FTC with major tumor capsular involvement and
   2. Primary cancers ≥5 cm regardless of extent of disease

Reproduced with permission from Cady and Rossi [9] Copyright 1998 Elsevier

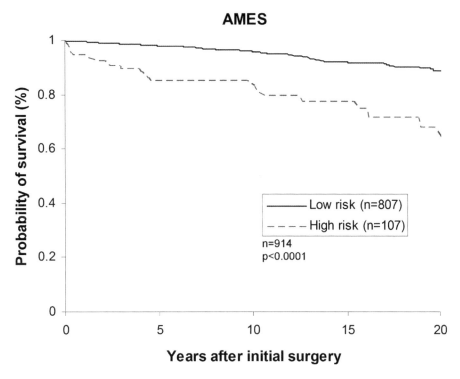

Fig. 6.1 Overall survival of 914 PTC patients using the AMES system

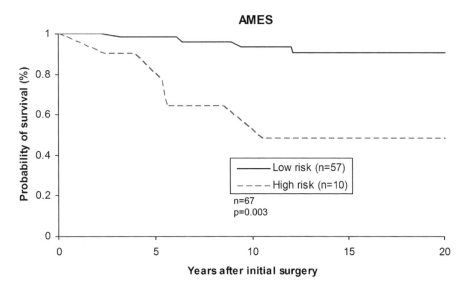

Fig. 6.2 Overall survival of 67 FTC patients using the AMES system

DAMES System

Developed at the Karolinska Hospital and Institute, the DAMES staging system's prognostic factors include *D*NA ploidy, *a*ge, *m*etastasis, *e*xtent, and *s*ize of tumor. Similar to the AGES system, the DAMES system is rarely used because determining DNA ploidy requires complex flow and image cytophotometry which is expensive and time consuming [5, 13]. Using both types of cytophotometry to analyze DNA, a histogram is created to show how many chromosomes are in

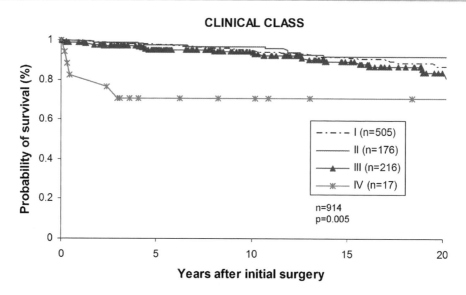

Fig. 6.3 Overall survival of 914 PTC patients using the Clinical Class system

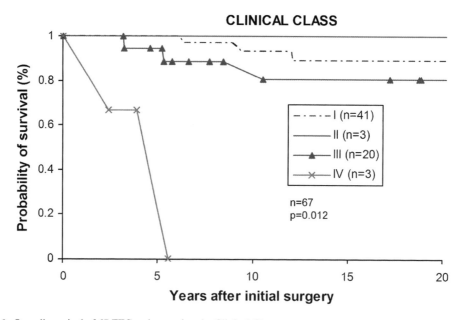

Fig. 6.4 Overall survival of 67 FTC patients using the Clinical Class system

the cell. An aneuploid tumor has DNA that is outside a specified region and is considered a more aggressive tumor than a euploid tumor [13].

The DAMES system divides PTC patients among three risk groups. The low-risk group includes patients in the AMES low-risk category with euploid tumors. The intermediate risk group includes those in the AMES high-risk group with euploid tumors. The high-risk group includes patients in the AMES high-risk group with aneuploid tumors, which carries a worse prognosis [13, 14]. The DAMES high-risk group follows a similar biological pattern as that of ATC [13]. No patients in their study were AMES low risk with aneuploid tumors [13]. The death rates for the 73 patients in the low-, intermediate-, and high-risk groups were 2% at 8.4 years, 4.5% at 10 years, and 100% at 2 years, respectively [13].

EORTC System

Developed in 1979, the European Organization for Research on the Treatment of Cancer (EORTC) system is among the oldest thyroid cancer staging systems. EORTC is a scoring system based on multivariate analysis from 23 different European hospitals. It is applicable to all histologic types of thyroid carcinoma and assigns a numeric score to significant variables such as patient age, gender, thyroid cancer type, extrathyroidal invasion, and distant metastases [8, 15]. Table 6.3 shows how each risk group is computed as well as its five-year disease-specific survival rate [15]. Figures 6.5 and 6.6 show overall survival of thyroid carcinoma patients at CSMC.

MACIS System

Developed in 1993 from physicians at the Mayo clinic and adapted from the AGES staging system, MACIS is an acronym for *m*etastases, *a*ge, *c*ompleteness of resection, *i*nvasion, and tumor *s*ize [4, 5, 11, 15–17]. Through multifactorial analysis of these variables, they developed a scoring system for papillary thyroid cancer where each characteristic is assigned a numeric score. Survival rates are determined based on this total weighted score divided between four risk groups. Table 6.4 shows how MACIS is

Table 6.3 EORTC System

+Age at diagnosis
+12 if patient is male
+10 if MTC or if principal cell type is poorly differentiated FTC
+45 if ATC
+10 if extrathyroidal (T3)
+15 if one distant metastasis is present
±15 if multiple distant metastases is present
= EORTC Score

Total score	Risk group	5-year survival rate(%)
<50	I	95
50–65	II	80
66–83	III	51
84–108	IV	33
≥109	V	5

Reproduced with permission from D'Avanzo et al. [8]

computed and how each score corresponds to a 20-year disease-specific survival rate [5, 8, 16, 17]. Figure 6.7 shows overall survival of PTC patients at CSMC.

Memorial Sloan Kettering System

The Memorial Sloan Kettering staging system was developed in 1994 and through their data on 1,038 differentiated thyroid cancer patients, researchers found that age, tumor size, histology type and subtype, extrathyroidal extension, and distant metastasis were significant factors in their staging of thyroid cancer [16, 18–21]. Nodal tissue involvement was not found to be a significant factor in this system. High grade, as shown in Table 6.5, is defined as FTC tumors with extracapsular invasion and Hurthle cell or tall cell variant [22]. Patients were classified as either low, intermediate, or high risk based on these criteria. Table 6.5 shows how each risk group is defined [16, 18–20, 22].

Sloan Kettering found that among the low-, intermediate-, and high-risk groups, 20-year disease-free survival rates were 99%, 85%, and 57% respectively [19, 20]. Figures 6.8 and 6.9 show overall survival of DTC patients at CSMC.

Noguchi Thyroid Clinic System

The Noguchi Thyroid Clinic system was developed in 1994 for PTC and includes three risk groups. Its prognostic factors include age, lymph node involvement, and gender [14, 23]. Although poorly differentiated PTC has a worse prognosis when compared to well differentiated PTC, this was not included in their initial analysis. Additionally, researchers excluded patients who had primary tumors of <10 mm, those aged >80, and patients with distant metastases [23]. As a result, the remaining patients were categorized into three risk groups as shown in greater detail in Table 6.6 [23]. Ten-year survival rates among males in the excellent-, intermediate-, and poor-risk groups were 98%, 90%, and 74% respectively.

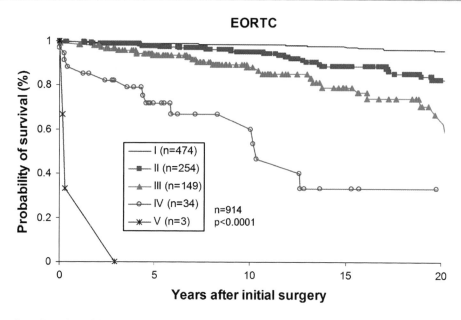

Fig. 6.5 Overall survival of 914 PTC patients using the EORTC system

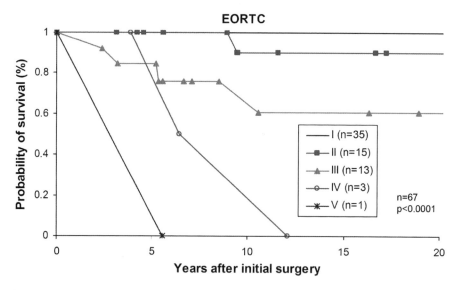

Fig. 6.6 Overall survival of 67 FTC patients using the EORTC system

Among female patients, 10-year survival rates in each group were 99%, 96%, and 89% respectively [23]. Figure 6.10 shows overall survival of PTC patients for both genders at CSMC. The survival curve for FTC was excluded due to the low number of FTC patients that fit Noguchi's criteria in the CSMC database.

NTCTCS System

In 1986, the National Thyroid Cancer Treatment Cooperative Study (NTCTCS) compiled data from 14 different medical centers and 1,600 patients [4, 11]. The goal was to establish a widely accepted staging system and to determine the effectiveness of each center's treatment modalities [24]. Researchers used these data and developed their four-stage classification system for differentiated thyroid carcinomas. Each stage is detailed in Table 6.7 and includes differentiated thyroid cancers as well as MTC [24]. The NTCTCS concluded that age at diagnosis, tumor type, tumor size, extrathyroidal invasion, nodal, and distant metastases are contributing factors. Their research found that five-year disease-specific survival rates for PTC stages I–IV were 100%, 100%, 93.8% and 78.5% respectively [24]. Additionally, five-year disease-specific survival rates for FTC nonoxyphilic stages I–IV were 100%, 100%, 81.9%, and 37.1% respectively [24]. Figures 6.11 and 6.12 show overall survival among DTC patients at CSMC.

Table 6.4 MACIS system

+3 if distant metastasis present
+3.1 if patient ≤39 years of age at surgery or 0.08 x age ≥40
+1 if tumor incompletely resected
+1 if local invasion present
+0.3 × tumor size (cm)

Total score	Stage	20-year survival rate(%)
<6	I	99
6–6.99	II	89
7–7.99	III	56
>8	IV	24%

Created using data from Hay et al. [5]

Ohio State System

Although not as widely used as the others, the Ohio State Scoring system was developed in 1994 and includes tumor size, lymph node involvement, multifocality, distant metastasis, and extrathyroidal invasion as prognostic factors in stage and mortality [11, 14, 15, 25]. This is one of the few staging systems that incorporates multifocality as a prognostic factor. Table 6.8 shows how differentiated thyroid cancer patients are categorized and their 30-year disease-specific mortality rates [4, 11]. Figures 6.13 and 6.14 show overall survival for DTC patients at CSMC.

SAG System

Developed in 1993 for well-differentiated thyroid carcinomas at the University of Bergen (Norway), the SAG system is another prognostic scoring system for PTC that is divided into three risk groups. SAG stands for *sex*, *age*, and *grade* [26, 27]. Grade is based on vascular invasion, marked nuclear atypia, and tumor necrosis [26, 27]. Vascular invasion is usually associated with FTC but can also be found in some PTC cases. Nuclear atypia, as defined by Akslen [26], includes tumor cell nuclei with considerable pleomorphism and

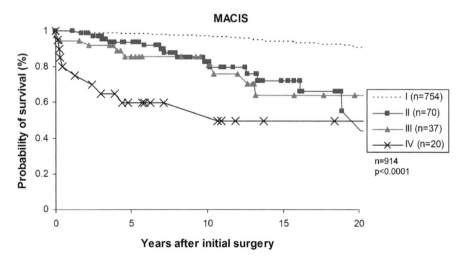

Fig. 6.7 Overall survival of 914 PTC patients using the MACIS system

Table 6.5 Memorial Sloan Kettering system

	Low risk	Intermediate risk		High risk	
Age	<45	<45	>45	>45	
Tumor size	<4 cm	>4 cm	<4 cm	>4 cm	
Histology	PTC	FTC and/or high grade[a]	PTC	FTC and/or high grade	
Extrathyroidal extension	(T1/T2)	(T3/T4)	(T1/T2)	(T3/T4)	
Distant metastasis	M0	M1	M0	M1	

Reproduced with permission from Shaha et al. [19]. Copyright 1994 Elsevier
[a]High grade defined as tumors with extracapsular invasion, Hurthle cell, or tall cell variant

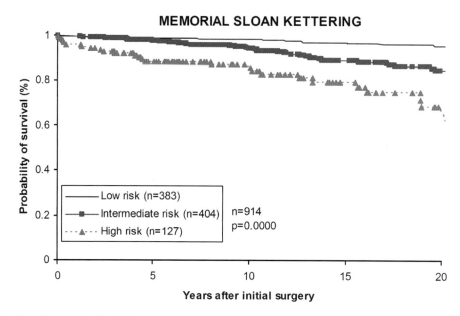

Fig. 6.8 Overall survival of 914 PTC patients using the MSK system

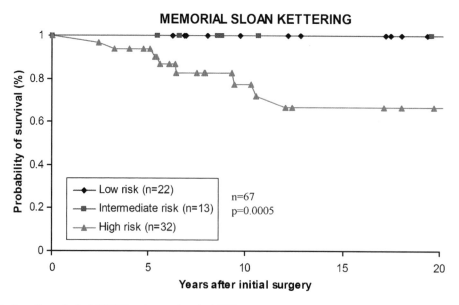

Fig. 6.9 Overall survival of 67 FTC patients using the MSK system

Table 6.6   Noguchi thyroid clinic

	Excellent				Intermediate[a]				Poor	
Age	<45	≤60	<50	50–55	>60	45–55	56–65	50–55	>55	
Gender	M	M	F	F	M	M	F	F	M	All other F
Lymph node	N0, N1	N0	N0, N1	N0	N0	N1	N0	N1	N1	

[a]Also includes females >65 and with tumor size <30 mm

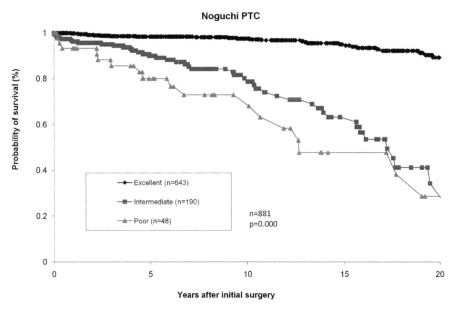

Fig. 6.10   Overall survival of 881 PTC patients using the Noguchi system

hyperchromasia in at least one high-power field. However, this may also be associated with DNA aneuploidy as in the DAMES staging system and, as a result, may not be a practicable system for some medical centers. Additionally, tumor necrosis is defined as the absence or presence of necrotic areas within the tumor [26]. Vascular invasion, marked nuclear atypia and tumor necrosis, is also referred to as the VAN score, with grade 1 (low grade) meaning that none of these are present and grade 2 (high grade) meaning that any one of these features are present [26]. Table 6.9 shows how patients are scored and its corresponding 15-year mortality rate [26].

TNM System

First developed in 1940 and updated multiple times with the latest revision published in 2010 (7th edition), the TNM staging system is one of the oldest cancer staging systems in existence. It is a joint classification effort between the Union Internationale Contre le Cancer (UICC) and the American Joint Commission on Cancer (AJCC). This system can be applied to as many as 23 different human organs and it is one of the more universally accepted staging systems for thyroid cancer. TNM stands for tumor size (T), lymph node involvement (N), and presence of distant metastasis (M) [4, 27–31]. Tumor size refers to the largest nodule found and lymph node involvement can either be found in the central (level VI) or lateral compartments of the neck and can change a patient's stage from III to IV depending on age and thyroid cancer type.

There are very minor changes in the 7th edition from the 6th edition which was published in 2002. The changes are as follows: T1 has further divided intrathyroidal tumors into T1a (≤1 cm) and T1b (>1–2 cm), solitary tumors are now classified as *s* (instead of a) and multifocal as *m* (instead of b), and

Table 6.7 NTCTCS system

	Tumor type			
	Papillary Carcinoma		Follicular Carcinoma	
	Age <45 years	Age ≥45 years	Age <45 years	Age ≥45 years
Primary tumor size (cm)				
<1	I	I	I	II
1–4	I	II	I	III
>4	II	III	II	III
Primary tumor description				
Microscopic multifocal	I	II	I	III
Macroscopic multifocal or macroscopic tumor capsule invasion	I	II	II	III
Microscopic extraglandular invasion	I	II	I	III
Macroscopic extraglandular invasion	II	III	II	III
Poor differentiation	NA	NA	III	III
Metastases				
Cervical lymph node metastases	I	III	I	III
Extracervical lymph node metastases	III	IV	III	IV
	Medullary Carcinoma			
C-cell hyperplasia	I			
Tumor size< 1 cm	II			
Tumor size≥ 1 cm or positive cervical lymph nodes	III			
Extraglandular invasion or extracervical metastases	IV			

All anaplastic carcinomas are Stage IV
NA Not applicable
Copyright 1998 Wiley. Used with permission from Sherman et al. [24]

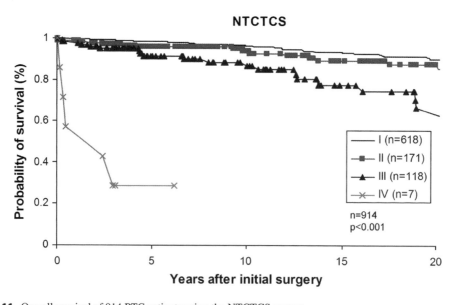

Fig. 6.11 Overall survival of 914 PTC patients using the NTCTCS system

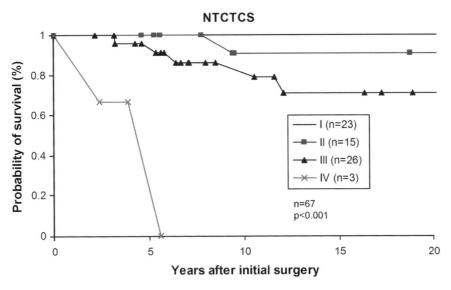

Fig. 6.12 Overall survival of 67 FTC patients using the NTCTS system

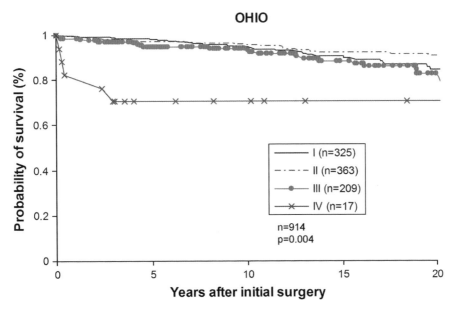

Fig. 6.13 Overall survival of 914 PTC patients using the OHIO State Scoring system

Table 6.8 Ohio State system

Stage	Criteria	30-Year Disease Specific Mortality
I	Tumors ≤1.49 cm, no lymph node or distant metastasis	0%
II	Tumors 1.5 to 4.49 cm or lymph node involvement or >3 intrathyroidal multifocal tumors (any size)	6%
III	Tumors ≥4.5 cm or extrathyroidal extension	14%
IV	Distant metastasis present	65%

Reproduced with permission from Sherman [11]

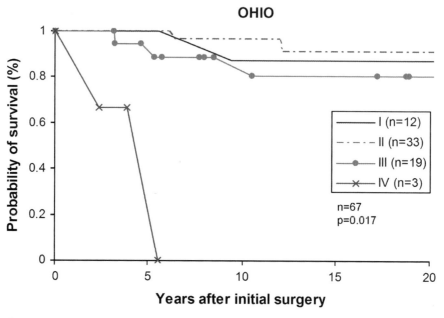

Fig. 6.14 Overall survival of 67 FTC patients using the OHIO State Scoring system

Table 6.9 SAG system

+1 if male
+1 if aged ≥70 years
+1 if vascular invasion, marked nuclear atypia, or
tumor necrosis is present
= SAG score

Total score	Risk group	15-year mortality rate (%)
0	I	1.7
1	II	12
2-3	III	61

Copyright 1993 Wiley. Used with permission from Akslen [26]

the original terms "resectable" and "unresectable" anaplastic carcinomas are replaced with "moderately advanced" and "very advanced." However, these editions differ from the 5th edition in that tumor size was originally T1 for intrathyroidal tumors ≤1 cm, T2 for intrathyroidal tumors 1 cm to ≤4 cm, and T3 for intrathyroidal tumors >4 cm. T4 included any tumor size with extrathyroidal extension [30, 31]. Additionally, the Mx(distant metastasis cannot be assessed) classfication was eliminated. All anaplastic thyroid carcinomas were also originally categorized as stage IV but updated in the 7th edition to include stages IVA for intrathyroidal

tumors and IVB for extrathyroidal tumors, and IVC (all ATC patients with distant metastases) [30, 31]. Additionally among differentiated TC patients over the age of 45, the 6th and 7th edition groups these patients >45 with minimal extrathyroidal extension as stage III and further divides type of extrathyroidal invasion as stage IVA or IVB [30, 31]. All patients in this age group with distant metastases are classified as stage IVC [30, 31].

The TNM staging is applicable to all four types of thyroid cancer but the specific type of thyroid cancer plays an important role in determining stage. For example, PTC and FTC are classified in a range of stages from I to IV while ATC is categorized into stage IV only. Age of patient is an important feature in this system as a patient with PTC distant metastasis can either be given a stage II if under age 45 or a stage IVC if aged 45 and older. The thyroid is the only organ that uses age in the AJCC staging system with a division of patients below or above the age of 45 [30, 31]. As a result, younger patients less than 45 years of age with WDTC cannot be given a stage of III or IV, despite having distant metastases. Additional information on the TNM staging system is found in Tables 6.10 and 6.11.

Table 6.10 TNM system, 7th edition

Tumor size (T)

All categories may be subdivided: (s) solitary tumor and (m) multifocal tumor (the largest determines the classification)

TX	Primary tumor cannot be assessed
T0	No evidence of primary tumor
T1	Intrathyroidal tumor ≤2 cm
T1a	Intrathyroidal tumor ≤1 cm
T1b	Intrathyroidal tumor >1 cm but not more than 2 cm
T2	Intrathyroidal tumor >2 cm but not more than 4 cm
T3	Intrathyroidal tumor >4 cm or tumor of any size with minimal
	Extrathyroidal extension (i.e., sternothyroid muscle or perithyroid soft tissues)
T4a	Moderately advanced disease
	Any size tumor with extension or invasion to subcutaneous soft tissues, larynx, trachea, esophagus, or recurrent laryngeal nerve
T4b	Very advanced disease tumor invading prevertebral fascia, encasing mediastinal vessels or carotid artery

All anaplastic thyroid cancers are considered T4

T4a	Intrathyroidal anaplastic carcinoma
T4b	Extrathyroidal anaplastic carcinoma

Lymph nodes (N)

NX	Regional lymph nodes cannot be assessed
N0	No regional lymph node metastasis
N1	Regional lymph node metastasis
N1a	Metastasis to Level VI (pretracheal, paratracheal, and prelaryngeal/Delphian lymph nodes)
N1b	Metastasis to unilateral, bilateral, or contralateral cervical (Levels I, II, III, IV or V) or superior mediastinal lymph nodes (Level VII)

Distant metastasis (M)

M0	No distant metastasis
M1	Any distant metastasis

Table 6.10 reproduced with permission from AJCC Cancer Staging Manual [31]

Table 6.11 TNM system, 7th edition

	PTC/FTC <45 years of age	PTC/FTC ≥45 years	MTC Any age	ATC Any age
Stage I	Any T, any N, M0	T1, N0, M0	T1, N0, M0	N/A
Stage II	Any T, any N, M1	T2, N0, M0	T2-3, N0, M0	N/A
Stage III	N/A	T3, N0, M0 T1–T3, N1A, M0	T1–T3, N1A, M0	N/A
Stage IVA	N/A	T1–T3, N1B, M0 T4a, N0–N1, M0	T4a, any N, M0 T1–T3, N1B, M0	T4a, any N, M0
Stage IVB	N/A	T4b, any N, M0	T4b, any N, M0	T4b, any N, M0
Stage IVC	N/A	Any T, any N, M1	Any T, any N, M1	Any T, any N, M1

Table 6.11 reproduced with permission from [31]

Figures 6.15–6.18 show overall survival of DTC patients at CSMC using the TNM staging system for both the 7th and 5th editions.

Data from the AJCC Cancer Staging Manual (7th edition) show five-year disease-specific survival rates for stages I to IV for PTC is 100%, 100%, 93%, and 51%; FTC is 100%, 100%, 71%, and 50%; MTC is 100%, 98%, 81%, and 28%, respectively; and ATC stage IV is approximately 7% [29].

Four classifications can further be used to describe the TNM grouping. Clinical classification (c) is used before surgery has occurred and can take

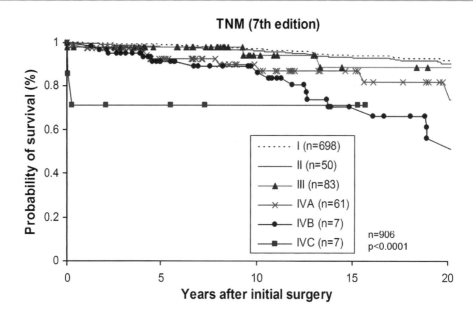

Fig. 6.15 Overall survival of 906 PTC patients using the TNM 7th System edition

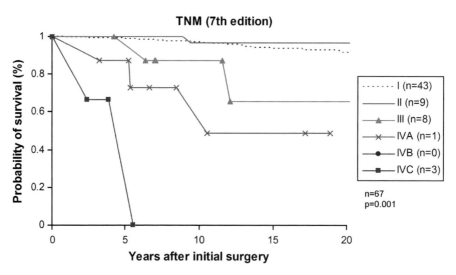

Fig. 6.16 Overall survival of 67 FTC patients using the TNM 7th System edition

place during a physical examination or imaging procedure. This aids in the selection of treatment and surgery. Pathologic classification (p) uses anatomic information from the initial surgery and pathologic report. Retreatment classification (r) is for purposes of further treatment of a recurring cancer. Finally, autopsy classification (a) occurs during a postmortem examination where a cancer was incidentally found [30, 31]. These classifications are placed before the TNM grouping to provide further information to physicians. For example, under the TNM 7th edition, a multifocal PTC patient with no metastasis under age 45 who has undergone surgery would be grouped as pT1mN0M0, stage 1.

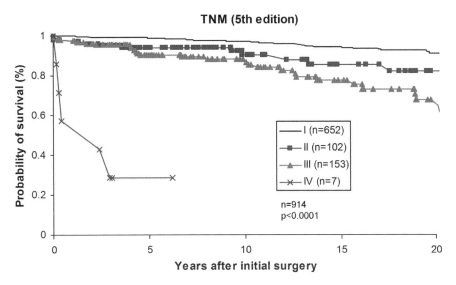

Fig. 6.17 Overall survival of 914 PTC patients using the TNM 5th System edition

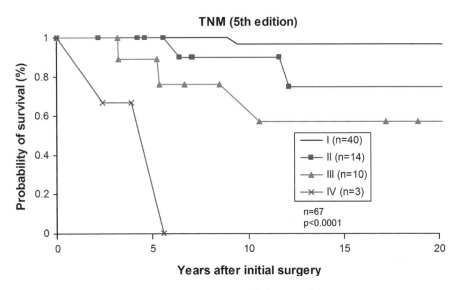

Fig. 6.18 Overall survival of 67 FTC patients using the TNM 5th System edition

UAB-MDACC System

The University of Alabama (Birmingham) and M.D. Anderson Cancer Center (Houston) developed this staging system for well-differentiated thyroid cancers in 1999. Using multivariate analysis, the UAB-MDACC system includes only patient age and distant metastasis as prognostic factors [14, 15, 32]. These two factors are used to define low-, intermediate-, and high-risk patients. Table 6.12 shows how each risk group is defined.

Passler et al's research found that their low-, intermediate-, and high-risk patients had a 5-year disease-specific survival rate of 99.4, 87.8, and 54.4%, respectively [15]. Figures 6.19 and 6.20 show overall survival for DTC patients at CSMC using this classification.

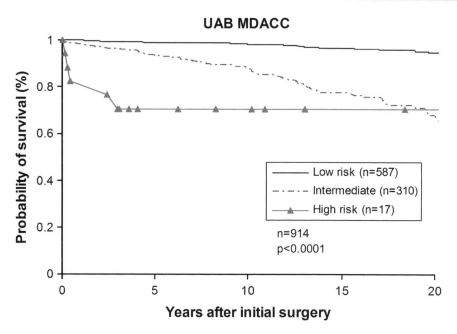

Fig. 6.19 Overall survival of 914 PTC patients using the UAB-MDACC system

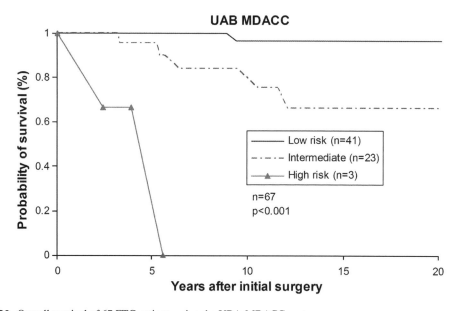

Fig. 6.20 Overall survival of 67 FTC patients using the UBA-MDACC system

University of Munster System

Developed in 1995, the University of Munster system includes differentiated thyroid cancer patients and defines tumor invasion (T4) or distant metastases (M1) as high risk. All other patients are considered low risk [14, 15, 33]. University of Munster data found that the 5-year survival rate among the high-risk group was 83% and among the low risk group was 97% [33]. Figures 6.21 and 6.22 show overall survival of DTC patients at CSMC.

Table 6.12 UAB-MDACC system

	Low risk	Intermediate risk	High risk
Age	<50	≥50	Any age
Distant metastasis	Not present	Not present	Present

Created using data from Beenken et al. [32]

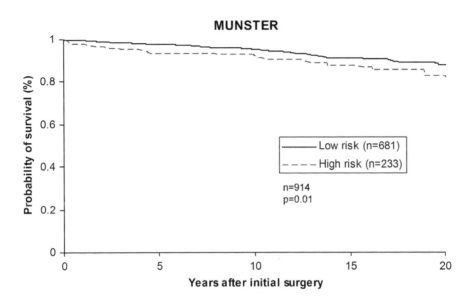

Fig. 6.21 Overall survival of 914 PTC patients using the University of Munster system

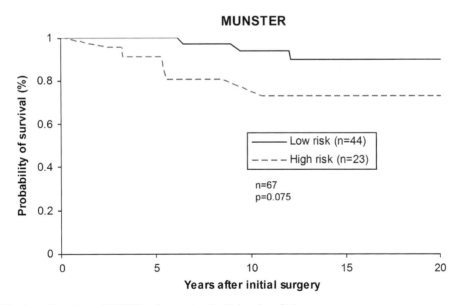

Fig. 6.22 Overall survival of 67 FTC patients using the University of Munster system

Virgen de la Arrixaca University Hospital at Murcia (Spain) System

Between the years 1970 and 1995, approximately 200 patients were treated at the Virgen de la Arrixaca University Hospital for PTC. Using multivariate analysis, they developed a scoring system specifically for PTC, and determined age, tumor size, extrathyroidal spread, and histologic variant of PTC were prognostic factors [14, 34]. Longer survival rates occurred in those patients younger than 50 years of age, having tumor sizes less than 4 cm, tumors with intrathyroidal spread

only and among those with histological variants that did not include solid, tall-cell or poorly differentiated variants of PTC [34]. Table 6.13 shows how each low-, intermediate-, and high-risk group's scores are calculated as well as their 10-year tumor-related survival rate [14, 34]. Figure 6.23 shows overall survival of PTC patients at CSMC using this system.

Comparison of Staging Systems Using Csmc Data

Table 6.14 shows overall 5-, 10-, 15-, and 20-year survival for each staging system that is applicable to the CSMC cohort with all having significant p values of <0.05 with the exception of Munster FTC, Noguchi FTC (both genders) and the Virgen de la Arrixaca University Hospital Systems.

The systems AGES, DAMES, and SAG were not included in these analyses because not all of their prognostic factors were available in the CSMC data set. Overall survival is also included using the Kaplan–Meier method for this population. The relative importance of each staging system to CSMC's data was determined using the proportion of variation explained (PVE).

Table 6.13 Virgen de la Arrixaca University at Murcia system

3× age (1 if <50, 2 if ≥50)
+2× size of tumor (1 if 1–4 cm, 2 if >4 cm)
+6× spread (1 if intrathyroidal, 2 if extrathyroidal)
+2× histologic variant (1 if well-differentiated, follicular variant or diffuse
sclerosis, 2 if solid or tall cell, 3 if poorly differentiated PTC)
= Virgen de la Arrixaca University at Murcia Score

Total score	Risk group	10-year survival rate(%)
<18	Low	100
18–22	Medium	77
>22	High	39

Reproduced with permission from Sebastian et al. [34]

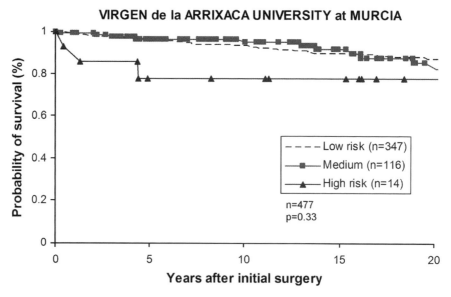

Fig. 6.23 Overall survival of 477 PTC patients using the Virgen de la Arrixaca University system

Table 6.14 Overall survival of PTC and FTC in each staging system

| Staging System | No. of pts | No. of deaths | Overall survival | | | | p value |
			5-yr	10-yr	15-yr	20-yr	(log rank)
EORTC – PTC							
I	474	17	0.99	0.98	0.98	0.96	<0.0001
II	254	25	0.98	0.95	0.89	0.83	
III	149	27	0.94	0.88	0.79	0.67	
IV	34	15	0.72	0.67	0.33	0.00	
V	3	3	0.00	0.00	0.00	0.00	
EORTC – FTC							
I	35	0	1.00	1.00	1.00	1.00	<0.0001
II	15	1	1.00	0.90	0.90	0.90	
III	13	4	0.85	0.76	0.61	0.61	
IV	3	2	1.00	0.50	0.00	0.00	
V	1	1	1.00	0.00	0.00	0.00	
Clinical class – PTC							
I	505	46	0.98	0.94	0.91	0.87	0.0050
II	176	10	0.98	0.97	0.91	0.91	
III	216	26	0.95	0.94	0.89	0.84	
IV	17	5	0.71	0.71	0.71	0.71	
Clinical class – FTC							
I	41	3	1.00	0.93	0.89	0.89	0.0120
II	3	0	1.00	1.00	1.00	1.00	
III	20	3	0.95	0.89	0.81	0.81	
IV	3	2	0.67	0.00	0.00	0.00	
MACIS – PTC							
I	754	48	0.98	0.97	0.94	0.91	<0.0001
II	70	16	0.94	0.83	0.72	0.55	
III	37	9	0.86	0.86	0.64	0.64	
IV	20	9	0.60	0.60	0.50	0.50	
NTCTCS – PTC							
I	618	42	0.98	0.96	0.93	0.90	<0.0001
II	171	19	0.96	0.94	0.89	0.87	
III	118	21	0.91	0.88	0.77	0.66	
IV	7	5	0.29	0.00	0.00	0.00	
NTCTCS – FTC							
I	23	0	1.00	1.00	1.00	1.00	<0.0001
II	15	1	1.00	0.91	0.91	0.91	
III	26	5	0.96	0.86	0.71	0.71	
IV	3	2	0.67	0.00	0.00	0.00	
OHIO – PTC							
I	325	30	0.98	0.95	0.91	0.85	0.0040
II	363	26	0.97	0.96	0.92	0.91	
III	209	26	0.95	0.94	0.88	0.83	
IV	17	5	0.71	0.71	0.71	0.71	
OHIO – FTC							
I	12	1	1.00	0.88	0.88	0.88	0.0170
II	33	2	1.00	0.96	0.91	0.91	
III	19	3	0.94	0.89	0.80	0.80	
IV	3	2	0.67	0.00	0.00	0.00	

(continued)

Table 6.14 (continued)

| Staging System | No. of pts | No. of deaths | Overall survival | | | | p value |
			5-yr	10-yr	15-yr	20-yr	(log rank)
MSK – PTC							
Low risk	383	13	0.99	0.98	0.97	0.96	0.0001
Intermediate risk	404	40	0.98	0.94	0.89	0.84	
High risk	127	27	0.88	0.87	0.79	0.69	
MSK – FTC							
Low risk	22	0	1.00	1.00	1.00	1.00	0.0001
Intermediate risk	13	0	1.00	1.00	1.00	1.00	
High risk	32	8	0.94	0.78	0.64	0.64	
UAB MDACC – PTC							
Low risk	587	24	0.99	0.98	0.97	0.95	0.0001
Intermediate risk	310	58	0.93	0.88	0.77	0.68	
High risk	17	5	0.71	0.71	0.71	0.71	
UAB MDACC – FTC							
Low risk	41	1	1.00	0.97	0.97	0.97	0.0001
Intermediate risk	23	5	0.95	0.84	0.66	0.66	
High risk	3	2	0.67	0.00	0.00	0.00	
Munster – PTC							
Low risk	681	56	0.98	0.95	0.91	0.88	0.0100
High risk	233	31	0.93	0.93	0.88	0.83	
Munster – FTC							
Low risk	44	3	1.00	0.94	0.90	0.90	0.0750
High risk	23	5	0.91	0.80	0.73	0.73	
AMES – PTC							
Low risk	807	62	0.98	0.96	0.92	0.89	0.0001
High risk	107	25	0.85	0.85	0.77	0.68	
AMES – FTC							
Low risk	57	4	0.98	0.93	0.90	0.90	0.0030
High risk	10	4	0.90	0.64	0.48	0.48	
Noguchi – PTC							
Excellent	643	32	0.98	0.98	0.95	0.89	0.0001
Intermediate	190	45	0.90	0.80	0.63	0.34	
High risk	48	17	0.80	0.73	0.48	0.29	
Virgen de la Arrixaca – PTC							
Low risk	347	36	0.96	0.93	0.90	0.87	0.3300
Medium risk	116	12	0.96	0.96	0.92	0.85	
High risk	14	3	0.78	0.78	0.78	0.78	
TNM 7th ed – PTC							
I	698	48	0.98	0.96	0.93	0.90	0.0001
II	50	3	0.98	0.94	0.89	0.89	
III	83	10	0.92	0.90	0.87	0.82	
IVA	61	17	0.91	0.89	0.70	0.56	
IVB	7	2	0.71	0.71	0.71	0.00	
IVC	7	5	0.29	0.00	0.00	0.00	
TNM 7th ed – FTC							
I	43	1	1.00	0.97	0.97	0.97	0.0010
II	9	2	1.00	0.88	0.66	0.66	
III	8	3	0.88	0.73	0.49	0.00	

(continued)

Table 6.14 (continued)

| Staging System | No. of pts | No. of deaths | Overall survival | | | | p value |
			5-yr	10-yr	15-yr	20-yr	(log rank)
IVA	1	0	1.00	1.00	1.00	1.00	
IVB	0	0	0.00	0.00	0.00	0.00	
IVC	3	2	0.67	0.00	0.00	0.00	
TNM 5th ed – PTC							
I	652	40	0.99	0.97	0.94	0.91	0.0001
II	102	13	0.94	0.90	0.85	0.82	
III	153	29	0.90	0.88	0.78	0.68	
IV	7	5	0.29	0.00	0.00	0.00	
TNM 5th ed – FTC							
I	40	1	1.00	0.97	0.97	0.97	0.0001
II	14	2	1.00	0.90	0.75	0.75	
III	10	3	0.89	0.76	0.57	0.57	
IV	3	2	0.67	0.00	0.00	0.00	

Table 6.15 PVE of all applicable staging systems for PTC and FTC

| PTC | | | FTC | | |
Staging system	PVE (%)	Ranking	Staging system	PVE (%)	Ranking
EORTC	13.1	1	EORTC	30.9	1
Noguchi	11.5	2	UAB MDACC	28.7	2
UAB MDACC	9.4	3	NTCTCS	27.6	3
MACIS	8.7	4	MSK	24.5	4
TNM 7th ed	7.1	5	TNM 7th ed	20.2	5
MSK	7.0	6	TNM 5th ed	17.8	6
TNM 5th ed	6.9	7	Ohio	15.1	7
NTCTCS	5.5	8	Clinical class	13.7	8
AMES	3.7	9	AMES	6.8	9
Clinical class	1.7	10			
Ohio	1.5	11			
Munster	0.3	12			

The PVE was calculated to determine which system was the best method for our data set using SAS 9.2. PVE is a widely accepted and common measurement tool that has been used in many comparison studies to predict survival [8, 14, 15, 27, 35, 36]. Its advantages include the ability to directly compare qualitative variables as well as show which system has the best prognostic information [35, 36]. The mathematical formula is: $PVE = 1 - \exp(-G^2/n)$, with G standing for the maximum likelihood ratio [36].

As shown in Table 6.15, the greater the PVE value, with a range from 0 to 100, the stronger the association between each system on sur-

vival rates and the better the predictability of that system. As a result, PVE for CSMC data for PTC concluded that the EORTC, Noguchi and UAB-MDACC systems were best suited for predicting survival in this patient population. CSMC's papillary thyroid carcinoma's PVE rankings are not consistent with the Lang [14], Brierly [27], or Passler [15] studies. The Lang et al. study found that the MACIS (PVE = 18.7), TNM 6th edition (PVE = 17.9), and EORTC (PVE = 16.6) systems were most applicable to their PTC patient population [14]. The Brierly et al. study found that the TNM (PVE = 23.3), AGES (PVE = 23.1), and MACIS

(PVE = 20.6) systems were most applicable to their patient population [27]. The Passler et al. study found that the MACIS (PVE = 15), EORTC (PVE = 12.87), and the TNM 5th edition (PVE = 10.22) systems were most applicable to their patient population [15].

Additionally, among CSMC's follicular thyroid carcinoma population, the EORTC, UAB-MDACC, and NTCTCS system's PVE values were most applicable to predicting survival in this specific subtype of thyroid carcinoma. This was not consistent with the Passler [15] or Lang [35, 36] studies. The Passler et al. study found that the EORTC (PVE = 17), TNM 5th edition (PVE = 16.6), and Clinical Class (PVE = 15.8) systems were most applicable to their FTC patient population [14], whereas the Lang et al. study found that the TNM 6th edition (PVE = 22.4) and the Clinical Class (PVE = 21.2) systems were most applicable to their patient population [36].

CSMC data may differ from other studies because of differing sample sizes and data collection methods. Additionally, many studies report cause-specific survival while our data report all-cause survival only. However, all studies report relatively low PVE values which show that these staging systems have a less than perfect survival predictability [14, 15, 27]. In conclusion, it remains unclear as to which staging system is most applicable in predicting survival in patients with DTC [14].

Conclusion

Currently, the TNM staging system is the most universally accepted system in the staging of thyroid carcinomas. It is also the most available, easily applicable, and has the least amount of areas of discrepancy when compared to the other staging systems. However, due to the extent of surgical resection, surgeon expertise, pathologic skills in reading specimens, and differing treatment modalities among endocrinologists at various institutions, it is difficult to accept a universal staging system that is applicable to DTC patients across all medical institutions. Therefore, any new staging system that is introduced should be compared to the TNM

system, validated across various data sets, and then proven to be applicable among all thyroid carcinoma patients in any medical institution.

References

1. Shaha AR, Shah JP, Loree TR. Differentiated thyroid cancer presenting initially with distant metastasis. Am J Surg. 1997;174(5):474–6.
2. Shaha AR, Ferlito A, Rinaldo A. Distant metastases from thyroid and parathyroid cancer. ORL J Otorhinolaryngol Relat Spec. 2001;63(4):243–9.
3. Shoup M, Stojadinovic A, Nissan A, et al. Prognostic indicators of outcomes in patients with distant metastases from differentiated thyroid carcinoma. J Am Coll Surg. 2003;197(2):191–7.
4. Wartofsky L, Van Norstrand D. Staging of thyroid cancer. In: Wartofsky L, Van Nostrand D, editors. Thyroid cancer, a comprehensive guide to clinical management. 2nd ed. Totowa, NJ: Humana Press; 2006. p. 87–95.
5. Hay ID, Bergstralh EJ, Goellner JR, Ebersold JR, Grant CS. Predicting outcome in papillary thyroid carcinoma: development of a reliable prognostic scoring system in a cohort of 1779 patients surgically treated at one institution during 1940 through 1989. Surgery. 1993;114(6):1050–8.
6. Sugitani I, Nobukatsu K, Fujimoto Y, Yanagisawa K. A novel classification system for patients with PTC: addition of the new variables of large (3 cm or great) nodal metastases and reclassification during the follow-up period. Surgery. 2004;135(2):139–48.
7. Hay ID, Grant CS, Taylor WF, McConahey WM. Ipsilateral lobectomy versus bilateral lobar resection in papillary thyroid carcinoma: a retrospective analysis of surgical outcome using a novel prognostic scoring system. Surgery. 1987;102(6):1088–95.
8. D'Avanzo A, Ituarte P, Treseler P, et al. Prognostic scoring systems in patients with follicular thyroid cancer: a comparison of different staging systems in predicting the patient outcome. Thyroid. 2004;14(6):453–8.
9. Cady B, Rossi R. An expanded view of risk-group definition in differentiated thyroid carcinoma. Surgery. 1998;104(6):947–53.
10. Haigh PI, Urbach DR, Rotstein LE. AMES prognostic index and extent of thyroidectomy for well-differentiated thyroid cancer in the US. Surgery. 2004;136(3):609–16.
11. Sherman SI. Toward a standard clinicopathologic staging approach for differentiated thyroid carcinoma. Semin Surg Oncol. 1999;16:12–5.
12. DeGroot LJ, Kaplan EL, McCormick M, Straus FH. Natural history, treatment, and course of papillary thyroid carcinoma. J Clin Endocrinol Metab. 1990;71(2):414–24.

13. Pasieka JL, Zedenius J, Auer G, et al. Addition of nuclear DNA content to the AMES risk-group classification for papillary thyroid cancer. Surgery. 1992;112(6):1154–60.

14. Lang BH, Lo CY, Chan WF, Lam KY, Wan KT. Staging systems for papillary thyroid carcinoma, a review and comparison. Ann Surg. 2007;245(3):366–78.

15. Passler C, Prager G, Scheuba C, Kaserer K, Zettinig G, Niederle B. Application of staging systems for differentiated thyroid carcinoma in an endemic goiter region with iodine substitution. Ann Surg. 2003; 237(2):227–34.

16. Shaha AR, Shah JP, Loree R. Patterns of failure in differentiated carcinoma of the thyroid based on risk groups. Head Neck. 1998;20(1):26–30.

17. Leite KRM, de Araujo VC, Meirelles MIR, Lopes Costa AL, Camara-Lopes LH. No relationship between proliferative activity and the MACIS prognostic scoring system in papillary thyroid carcinoma. Head Neck. 1999;21(7):602–5.

18. Shaha AR, Shah JP, Loree R. Risk group stratification and prognostic factors in papillary carcinoma of thyroid. Ann Surg Oncol. 1996;3(6):534–8.

19. Shaha AR, Loree TR, Shah JP. Intermediate-risk group for differentiated carcinoma of thyroid. Surgery. 1994;116(6):1036–41.

20. Shaha AR. Implications of prognostic factors and risk groups in the management of differentiated thyroid cancer. Laryngoscope. 2004;114(3):393–402.

21. Shah JP, Loree TR, Dharker D, Strong EW, Begg C. Prognostic factors in differentiated carcinoma of the thyroid gland. Am J Surg. 1992;164(6): 658–61.

22. Kuriakose MA, Hicks WL, Loree TR, Yee H. Risk group-based management of differentiated thyroid carcinoma. J R Coll Surg Edinb. 2001;46(4): 216–23.

23. Noguchi S, Murakami N, Kawamoto H. Classification of papillary cancer of the thyroid based on prognosis. World J Surg. 1994;18(4):552–8.

24. Sherman SI, Brierley JD, Sperling M, et al. Prospective multicenter study of thyroid carcinoma treatment, initial analysis of staging and outcome. Cancer. 1998;83(5):1012–21.

25. Mazzaferri EL, Jhiang SM. Long-term impact of initial surgical and medical therapy on papillary and follicular thyroid cancer. Am J Med. 1994;97(5):418–28.

26. Akslen LA. Prognostic importance of histologic grading in papillary thyroid carcinoma. Cancer. 1993; 72(9):2680–5.

27. Brierley JD, Panzarella T, Tsang RW, Gospodarowicz MK, O'Sullivan S. A comparison of different staging systems predictability of patient outcome, thyroid carcinoma as an example. Cancer. 1997;79(12):2414–23.

28. Shaha AR. TNM classification of thyroid carcinoma. World J Surg. 2007;31(5):879–87.

29. American Cancer Society: Learn about cancer website. How is thyroid cancer staged? http://www. cancer.org/cancer/Thyroid cancer/Detailed Guide/ thyroid-cancer survival rates. Accessed 9 Dec 2010.

30. Comparison guide: Cancer staging manual fifth versus sixth edition. http://www.springer.com/cda/content/ document/cda_downloaddocument/cancer_staging_ comparison_guide.pdf?SGWID=0-0-45-148294-0. Accessed 26 Aug 2007

31. Edge SE, Byrd DR, Carducci MA, Compton CA, editors. AJCC cancer staging manual. 7th ed. New York, NY: Springer; 2009.

32. Beenken S, Roye D, Weiss H, Sellers M, Urist M, Diethelm A, et al. Extent of surgery for intermediate-risk well-differentiated thyroid cancer. Am J Surg. 2000; 179(1):51–6.

33. Lerch H, Schober O, Kuwert T, Hans-Bernard S. Survival of differentiated thyroid carcinoma studied in 500 patients. J Clin Oncol. 1997;15(5): 2067–75.

34. Sebastian SO, Gonzalez JM, Paricio P, et al. Papillary thyroid carcinoma, prognostic index for survival including the histological variety. Arch Surg. 2000;135(3):272–7.

35. Schemper M. The relative importance of prognostic factors in studies of survival. Stat Med. 1993; 12(24):2377–82.

36. Lang BH, Lo CY, Chan WF, Lam KY, Wan KY. Staging systems for follicular thyroid carcinoma: application to 171 consecutive patients treated in a tertiary referral center. Endocr Relat Cancer. 2007; 14(1):29–42.

Papillary Thyroid Carcinoma

7

Wendy Sacks and Glenn D. Braunstein

Introduction

Papillary thyroid carcinoma (PTC) is the most common type of thyroid cancer, comprising 80% of all thyroid carcinomas [1, 2]. From 1973 to 2002, the incidence of all thyroid cancers increased 2.4-fold, and the increase was virtually entirely due to an increase in papillary carcinomas (Fig 7.1). Over this 30-year period, the incidence of PTC increased more by 5 per 100,000, a 2.9-fold increase [3]. Despite the increasing incidence of PTC, the mortality from thyroid cancer has remained stable over the years (Fig 7.2) [3].

Many thyroid cancers are found as nonpalpable, incidentally discovered nodules. In fact, papillary thyroid microcarcinoma (PTMC), defined by the World Health Organization as thyroid cancer less than or equal to 1 cm, accounts for 49% of the increase in PTC noted by Davies et al. [3]. Furthermore, 87% of the increase in PTC is due to cancers less than or equal to 2 cm in size [3]. One explanation for the increased incidence of PTC is an increase in diagnostic scrutiny due to advances in ultrasonography and fine needle aspiration (FNA) biopsy; however, since the increase occurs across all tumor sizes, other factors may also play a role [4–7].

PTC is more common in women than men (3:1), but men have twice the risk of dying from PTC than women [8]. PTC tends to occur in younger patients in their third or fourth decades of life, the median age at diagnosis is 48 years old [9], and while mortality rates are low among those under age 40, mortality rates rise incrementally over the age of 40 [10–12].

Predisposing factors for thyroid cancer include a family history of thyroid cancer [13] as well as exposure to ionizing radiation in childhood or adolescence. Hereditary nonmedullary thyroid cancer occurs as a minor component of other familial cancer syndromes such as familial adenomatous polyposis, Gardner's syndrome, Cowden's disease, Carney's complex, Werner's syndrome, and papillary renal neoplasia or it can occur as a primary feature, termed familial non-medullary thyroid cancer (FNMTC). FNMTC accounts for 3.2–6.2% of all thyroid cancer and PTC is the most common histologic subtype [14]. Several studies have shown that FNMTC has a slightly more aggressive behavior than sporadic cancers namely, higher rates of multi-centric tumors, local invasion, lymph node metastases, and recurrence [15–17]. Disease-free survival is lower than that in patients with sporadic disease, and disease-specific survival is lower for FNMTC if more than three individuals are involved in the patient's family [15, 16, 18, 19]. While FNTC has an autosomal-dominant pattern of inheritance with incomplete penetrance, the genetic basis for FNMTC is poorly understood. Unlike in familial medullary thyroid

W. Sacks (✉) • G.D. Braunstein
Division of Endocrinology, Diabetes, and Metabolism, Department of Medicine, Cedars-Sinai Medical Center, Los Angeles, CA 90048, USA
e-mail: sacksw@cshs.org

G.D. Braunstein (ed.), *Thyroid Cancer*, Endocrine Updates 30, DOI 10.1007/978-1-4614-0875-8_7, © Springer Science+Business Media, LLC 2012

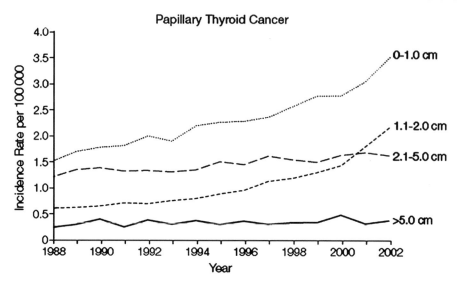

Fig. 7.1 Increasing incidence of papillary thyroid carcinoma < 2 cm [3]

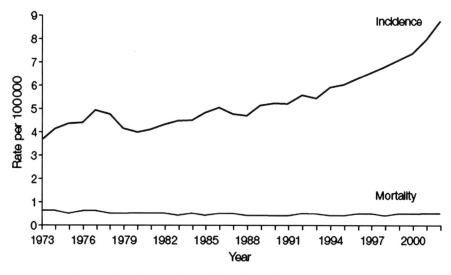

Fig. 7.2 Increasing incidence of thyroid cancer in the United States [3]

cancer, genes conferring the predisposition for thyroid cancer have not been identified. Early screening is recommended for those who have one or more first-degree relatives with nonmedullary thyroid carcinoma [14, 19, 20].

In the past, ionizing radiation was used to treat conditions such as acne, birthmarks, suspected thymic enlargement ringworm, and enlarged tonsils. This exposure as well as exposure to Chernobyl radioactivity [21–23] in childhood

increase the risk of malignancy in a thyroid nodule from 5–10% up to 30–50% [24] and radiation-related cancers have been observed more than 40 years after initial exposure [25, 26]. Radiation effects on the thyroid are discussed in depth later in this chapter.

While the majority of patients with thyroid cancer can be cured, the biological behavior of PTC varies widely from clinically insignificant papillary microcarcinomas to locally invasive tumors that may progress to distant metastases and eventually lead to death. Clinically, it is not possible to predict which tumors will behave more aggressively; however, various staging systems (see Chap. 6) provide parameters which can be used to determine a patient's prognosis. In addition, factors unaccounted for in staging systems must also be considered such as histologic variants of PTC, including columnar or tall-cell, insular, and sclerosing which are staged like common forms of PTC; however, they have a more aggressive phenotype [27]. Management of PTC outlined in this chapter will emphasize a risk-stratified approach in which a patient's risk for cancer recurrence and mortality is assessed prior to treatment in order to minimize unnecessary therapies and to avoid treatment complications and side effects.

Diagnosis and Management Approach

Most patients are found to have a thyroid nodule on a physical exam done by their physician or by self-palpation; however, many thyroid nodules are also found by imaging studies done for other reasons. Five percent of nodules over 1 cm in size are found by palpation [28], whereas one or more nodules are seen on neck ultrasound in over 50% of the population [29]. Current practice management for thyroid nodules typically includes an FNA biopsy to identify the 5–7% of thyroid nodules that are malignant (see Chaps. 3 and 5).

Management Approach to PTC

The traditional paradigm for treatment of PTC has shifted slightly over the years toward a risk-stratified approach. An evaluation of a patient's individual risk for recurrence and mortality determines the management approach which entails the extent of initial surgery, postoperative treatment with radioactive iodine (RAI), and the degree of TSH suppression. In general, those patients at low risk for recurrence and mortality have smaller tumors (1–4 cm), no local or regional

invasion, or distant metastases, while those at high risk have larger tumors (>4 cm), local and regional invasion, and/or distant metastases. Moderate-risk patients have microscopic invasion of tumor into the perithyroidal soft tissues, cervical lymph node metastases, and aggressive tumor histology or vascular invasion [30]. Accurate staging of PTC based on clinico-pathologic features after initial resection of the cancer is also important to assess risk. Two staging systems for thyroid cancer – AJCC/UICC tumor, node, metastasis (TNM) and MACIS (metastases, age, completeness of resection, invasion and tumor size) scoring system – have demonstrated consistent and similar survival and recurrence results [31, 32]; however, the AJCC/UICC TNM staging system is used for cancer registries and is recommended for all patients with thyroid carcinomas, particularly PTC [30].

Once the diagnosis of thyroid cancer has been established, thyroidectomy is the next recommended therapy. For PTC under 1 cm in size or if PTMC is found incidentally when surgery is performed for reasons other than thyroid cancer, a hemithyroidectomy may be sufficient (see section on microcarcinomas). However, for patients with tumors greater than 1 cm in size, lobectomy is associated with a 15% higher recurrence rate ($P=0.04$) and 31% higher risk of cancer death ($P=0.04$) and, therefore, subtotal or total thyroidectomy is the treatment of choice [33]. In addition, nodal metastases, particularly in the central compartment (level VI), are a hallmark of PTC and correlate with persistence and recurrence of PTC [34, 35]. Therefore, central compartment lymph node dissection (CLND) is also advocated as part of the initial surgery for PTC [36, 37].

Preoperative Ultrasound

Studies demonstrate lymph node metastases to be present in 38–90% of patients at the time of initial surgery [10, 38, 39]. The pattern of drainage of PTC to nodal metastases is initially to the central compartment (level VI) lymph nodes followed by ipsilateral spread to lateral lymph nodes (levels II, III, IV, V) [40, 41]. High-resolution ultrasonography performed prior to surgery has a sensitivity ranging from 36.7 to 83.5% [42–44] and specificity of 89.3 to 97.7% for identifying lymph node metastases [42]. Macroscopic (≥1 cm) lymph nodes are oftentimes not palpable prior to surgery or intraoperatively; therefore, current guidelines recommend performing a high-resolution ultrasound (US) to assess both the thyroid gland and lymph nodes prior to surgery [30]. One study reports that preoperative US detected unappreciated abnormal lymph nodes in 20% of patients, altered the surgical procedure 39% of the time, and decreased cervical recurrence to 6% [42]. However, preoperative US is unreliable in identifying the central compartment lymph nodes, because this compartment is obscured by the thyroid gland. Furthermore, level VI lymph node metastases are oftentimes microscopic and not found by intraoperative palpation. Thus, a complete resection of PTC should include a dissection of the central compartment lymph nodes in most cases.

Surgery

One of the primary goals of surgery for thyroid carcinoma is to completely remove the tumor in its entirety, including extrathyroidal spread and any involved lymph nodes. There has been some controversy over the years regarding the optimal surgery for treatment of PTC. Some studies have not demonstrated a benefit of total thyroidectomy verses lobectomy [45, 46]. In a large population-based study, Haigh et al. used the SEER database to assess the optimal extent of surgery for survival of low-risk and high-risk PTC patients. They did not find a significant difference in 5- and 10-year survival between less than total versus near-total thyroidectomy in either the low-risk (95% and 89%) or high-risk groups (84–73%). Since the median follow-up in their study was 7.5 years, longer follow-up may have been needed to see a survival difference [46]. The authors also acknowledge that for higher-risk patients, more aggressive surgery has been shown to decrease recurrence [46]. A review from the Mayo Clinic in 1987 of

1500 patients demonstrated no difference in recurrence or survival after 25 years of follow-up for low-risk patients with tumors between 1 and 4 cm in size whether thyroidectomy or lobectomy was performed ($P = 0.15$) [47].

Since that time, the Mayo Clinic and others have demonstrated improved disease-free survival and cause-specific survival in patients who have undergone total thyroidectomy versus lobectomy [34, 48–50]. Specifically, of 1,685 low-risk patients from the Mayo Clinic, 14% had local recurrence after lobectomy versus only 2% after total thyroidectomy [34]. The effects of adjuvant therapies such as RAI remnant ablation are not accounted for in these studies and may confound the data. Jonklaas et al. published outcome data of almost 3,000 patients with differentiated thyroid cancer, 78% of which had PTC [51]. Their analysis demonstrated improved overall survival for AJCC/TNM5 stage II patients (age <45 years: tumor >4 cm and macroscopic extraglandular invasion; age >45 tumor size 1–4 cm, microscopic multifocal or macroscopic multifocal with capsule invasion, or microscopic extraglandular invasion) considered low-risk as well as for high-risk patients (AJCC/TNM5 stages III and IV) who underwent total thyroidectomy. For those AJCC/TNM5 stage I patients, overall survival was not affected by extent of surgery [51]. Despite the conflicting conclusions, the current recommendation for surgical management of PTC is for a total thyroidectomy for all tumors greater than 1 cm in size. Additional benefits of total thyroidectomy are that it allows for complete resection of multicentric tumors which occur in 36–44% of PTC cases, simplifies radioiodine therapy, and facilitates monitoring for recurrence using RAI scans and thyroglobulin levels [30].

Complete surgical resection means removal of involved lymph nodes. As mentioned above, central compartment lymph node metastases are seen up to 90% of the time while lateral compartment nodes are less common. Prophylactic CLND is controversial and there are currently no prospective, randomized controlled trials that provide data to explain the impact of CLND on recurrence or disease-specific mortality in PTC.

In 2007, White et al. performed an evidence-based analysis of the literature evaluating the need for CLND and while the studies are retrospective, they found that total thyroidectomy plus CLND decreases recurrence of PTC, improves disease-specific survival, reduces levels of serum thyroglobulin, and increases rates of athyroglobulinemia [52]. While still controversial, performing a CLND at the time of initial surgery is currently recommended for PTC. Although CLND increases the risk for surgical complications, including recurrent laryngeal nerve injury and hypocalcemia, in the hands of an experienced thyroid surgeon these risks are minimized [52, 53]. Furthermore, reoperation for recurrence in the central neck is associated with more complications [52]. However, this again can be minimized by an experienced surgeon [54–56]. Prophylactic lateral neck dissection is not recommended. Ito et al. demonstrated that a modified lateral neck dissection did not improve lymph node recurrence-free survival in patients without preoperatively detectable metastatic nodes ($P = 0.4$) [57].

Radioactive Iodine (RAI)

Following surgery for PTC, most physicians employ the use of RAI for remnant ablation of residual thyroid tissue or as adjuvant therapy for treatment of residual thyroid cancer and to permit accurate staging of PTC [58, 59]. In addition, ablation of remnant thyroid tissue improves the value of serum thyroglobulin as a tumor marker [60, 61] and increases the specificity of subsequent I-131 scans to detect thyroid cancer recurrences [62]. In the past, RAI treatment was recommended for almost all patients with PTC other than the very low risk PTMC patients because in addition to ease of follow-up, RAI was thought to decrease PTC recurrence and improve survival rates [48, 63–71]. However, more recent reviews of the literature suggest that RAI treatment may not improve disease-free survival or mortality for low and moderate risk patients [72–83]. There are many deficiencies in

the literature that make it difficult to compare study outcomes, including (1) a lack of prospective, randomized controlled trials [84]; (2) a lack of consistency in categorizing patients as low risk or high risk; (3) pooling of histologic subtypes that behave differently; (4) ethnic and geographic differences in total incidence and incidence of different histological types of PTC which are not accounted for in analyses; (5) recurrence and death from thyroid cancer can be seen many years after the initial diagnosis; therefore, outcome data are dependent on duration of the studies which is highly variable; and 6) methods for detecting recurrence of disease have improved over time which make it difficult to compare older studies with more recent ones. For these reasons, an individualized approach should be taken when deciding whether to treat with I-131 RAI. This decision should be based upon an individual's risk for recurrence and death. The 2009 updated American Thyroid Association guidelines for management of DTC recommended postoperative radioiodine ablation for American Joint Committee on Cancer (AJCC/TNM, Sixth Edition) stage III/IV disease, stage II disease in patients younger than age 45 years (and select patients 45 years or older), and select cases of stage I disease, especially those with multifocal disease, nodal metastases, extrathyroidal or vascular invasion, and/or more aggressive histologies [30].

For maximum radioiodine uptake after thyroidectomy, concentrations of thyroid hormone should drop sufficiently to allow the endogenous thyroid stimulating hormone (TSH) to rise to above 25–30 mU/L [85, 86] or if using recombinant human TSH (rhTSH), levels between 51 and 82 mU/L result in maximal thyrocyte stimulation [87]. Withdrawal of thyroxine for 4 weeks results in the desired elevations of TSH; however, to prevent hypothyroidism in patients for that length of time, liothyronine can be used up to 2 weeks prior to treatment [88–90]. RhTSH (Thyrogen ©) can be used rather than thyroid hormone withdrawal for remnant ablation in those patients who are unable to tolerate the side effects of hypothyroidism or in those patients whose TSH levels do not elevate appropriately with withdrawal. In fact, many physicians start patients on thyroxine suppression in the hospital after thyroidectomy and use rhTSH in preparation for RAI treatment. A prospective randomized study by Pacini and colleagues compared RAI ablation with a dosage of 30 mCI in patients who received rhTSH versus withdrawal of thyroid hormone and found that both methods are equally effective [91]. Furthermore, studies have shown a decreased amount of radiation exposure after rhTSH likely due to increased renal radioiodine clearance when one is not hypothyroid [92]. Also needed for optimization of RAI uptake for ablation is adherence to a low-iodine diet for 10–14 days prior to treatment (<50 μg/day of dietary iodine) as well as avoidance of other potential contaminants such as iodinated contrast used for CT scans [93, 94]. The Thyroid Cancer Survivor's website is an excellent resource for patients to learn how to choose foods low in iodine (www.thyca.org). Serum thyroglobulin (Tg) levels at the time of ablation are also useful in predicting clinical recurrence; a negative Tg has an excellent negative predictive value for residual disease, while the risk of persistent disease increases with higher stimulated Tg levels [95, 96].

Pretherapy RAI scans with small doses of I-131 or I-123 may be useful when the amount of remnant tissue is unknown or if the results would alter the decision of whether to treat and with what dose to treat. Experts do not recommend standard use of pretherapy radioiodine scans because of the potential for "stunning" of thyroid tissue by introduction of a pretreatment dose of radioiodine which may compromise the uptake and effectiveness of the treatment dose [30, 97–101]. Stunning is further discussed in Chap. 13. Post-therapy scans performed 2–10 days after I-131 treatment are more sensitive for exposing areas of metastatic disease involvement when compared with low-dose diagnostic scans [97, 102, 103] because the sensitivity relates directly to the amount of radioiodine given [62, 104]. Evidence of metastases on post-treatment scans enables the physician to determine the intensity of need for future monitoring and treatments [104].

Thyroid Hormone Suppression Therapy (THST)

Standard treatment for PTC is surgery and I-131 RAI ablation followed by thyroid hormone suppression therapy (THST). Because data have shown that TSH stimulates normal and neoplastic thyroid cell proliferation, radioiodine uptake, and thyroglobulin (Tg) production [96, 105–109], in theory, suppression with L-thyroxine should reduce the ability of TSH to stimulate growth of thyroid cancer cells [110, 111]. Thyroid hormone replacement to produce a TSH of 0.4 mU/L is necessary to suppress thyroglobulin [112]; yet there is no consensus as to the level of TSH below the lower limit of the normal range (<0.1 or 0.1–0.4 mU/L) that is optimal for initial and long-term treatment of PTC. The degree of TSH suppression required should be based on a patient's individual risk for cancer recurrence and death, but the adverse effects seen on the bones and cardiovascular system [111, 113] must also factor into the decision. A patient's risk for adverse effects such as osteoporosis and heart arrhythmias must be weighed against the benefits of thyroxine suppression for improving disease-free survival and mortality from PTC.

Studies have shown regression of tumor recurrences and fewer cancer-related deaths with THST. Mazzaferri and Kloos demonstrated a 25% decrease in locoregional and distant recurrences over a 40-year follow-up period in their cohort of PTC patients treated with THST after surgery (P<0.0002) [48]. Patients who were treated with total thyroidectomy plus RAI and THST had even lower rates of recurrence (P<0.02) compared to surgery alone or surgery plus THST [48]. Pujol et al. demonstrated improved disease-free survival for those patients treated with THST independent of the initial disease stage [114]. They also showed that independent of initial disease stage, patients with a greater degree of suppression (<0.1 mU/L) had a better disease-free survival than those who were not suppressed (TSH ≥1.0 mU/L) [114]. Not all studies confirm these results and the debate continues over which patients benefit from THST and to what extent the TSH needs to be suppressed.

A review of THST by Biondi and colleagues in 2005 showed no clear benefit except in patients with persistent or recurrent disease [111]. An analysis of a cohort of 2936 patients from the National Thyroid Cancer Treatment Cooperative Study Group (NTCTCSG) revealed a significant improvement in overall survival in TNM5 stage II, III, and IV patients who maintained subnormal or undetectable TSH levels ($P=0.0003$, $P=0.016$, $P=0.016$, respectively) [51, 115]. Low-risk (stage I) patients did not demonstrate improved overall survival with THST [51]. Limitations to this study include short duration of follow-up, different management styles among the study centers that make up the NTCTCSG, and relatively few TSH values for each patient [51]. A Dutch study of 366 patients with differentiated thyroid carcinoma all treated with surgery and I-131 RAI ablation showed that TSH levels of 2 mU/L were associated with increased cancer-specific death and recurrence, while there was no difference in death or recurrence for those patients with TSH between 0.1 and 0.4 mU/L. In addition, a TSH level >4.5 mU/L was an independent predictor of death [116].

These studies suggest that a lower TSH is important for high-risk patients to prevent recurrence and cancer-specific death and that low-risk patients do not require such an aggressive TSH suppression [51, 116]. In addition, most recurrences occur within the first 5–10 years after initial treatment for PTC so it would follow that one would treat more aggressively during this time period. The ATA guidelines reflect these factors in their recommendations [30]. For high-risk and moderate-risk thyroid cancer patients, the initial TSH goal is <0.1 mU/L and, if disease-free at follow-up, TSH 0.1–0.5 mU/L for 5–10 years [30]. Low-risk thyroid cancer patients need less suppression with an initial TSH goal of 0.1–0.5 mU/L and 0.3–2 mU/L if disease-free at follow-up. Biondi and Cooper propose an algorithm for early and long-term THST that not only takes into account a patient's risk of recurrence and death from thyroid cancer, but also assesses a patient's comorbidities such as age, osteoporosis, and cardiovascular disease to determine the optimal level of TSH suppression [117] (see Tables 7.1 and 7.2).

Monitoring

There is a great deal of variability among physicians managing the follow-up care of thyroid cancer patients, but as with other areas of thyroid cancer management, it is important to individualize care based on a patient's survival and recurrence risks. Long-term monitoring of papillary thyroid cancer must take into account the patient's risk for recurrent disease which occurs up to 35% of the time within the first decade after diagnosis [48]. While recurrence rates are fairly high, overall survival for NTCTCSG stage I patients is 98% and stage II is 87% over 14 years [51]. Overall survival decreases for stage III and IV patients (70% and 20%, respectively) over the 14-year follow-up period [51]. Patients at higher risk for recurrence and death from PTC include male patients, patients over the age of 60, presence of extrathyroidal or distant metastases, and tumor features such as poor histological subtypes and larger size. High-risk patients may require more intense surveillance necessitating scans and

Table 7.1 Suggested initial thyrotropin targets in thyroid cancer patients according to risk assessment

		Risk of cancer recurrence and progression		
		High	Intermediate	Low
Risk from T$_4$ therapy	*High*	<0.1 mU/L[a]	<0.1 mU/L[a]	0.5–1 mU/L
	Intermediate	<0.1 mU/L[b]	<0.1 mU/L[b]	0.5–1 mU/L
	Low	<0.1 mU/L	<0.1 mU/L	0.1–0.5 mU/L

[a]With high risk from L-T4: consider cardiovascular drugs, calcium, vitamin D, and antiresorptive drugs
[b]With intermediate risk from L-T4 and high or intermediate risk of tumor progression: consider β-adrenergic blocking drugs, calcium, and vitamin D
L-T4 levothyroxine
From Biondi and Cooper [117]

Table 7.2 Suggested thyrotropin targets in thyroid cancer patients according to risk assessment during follow-up

| | | Risk of cancer recurrence and progression | | |
		High	Intermediate	Low
Risk from T_4 therapy	*High*	<0.1 mU/L persistent or metastatic disease; 0.1–0.5 mU/L if disease free for 5–10 years[a]	0.5–1 mU/L if disease free for 5–10 years, then 1–2m U/L	1–2 mU/L
	Intermediate	<0.1 mU/L persistent or metastatic disease[b]; 0.1–0.5 mU/L if disease free for 5–10 years	0.1–0.5 mU/L if disease free for 5–10 years, then 1–2 mU/L	1–2 mU/L
	Low	<0.1 mU/L persistent or metastatic disease[c]; 0.1–0.5 mU/L if disease free for 5–10 years	0.1–0.5 mU/L if disease free for 5–10 years, then 0.3–2 mU/L	0.3–2 mU/L

[a]With high risk from L-T4 with persistent/metastatic disease: TSH suppression should be adapted to the clinical situation
[b]With intermediate risk from L-T4 with persistent/metastatic disease: consider cardiovascular drugs, calcium, and vitamin D
[c]With low risk from L-T4 with persistent/metastatic disease: periodic cardiovascular and BMD assessment
From Biondi and Cooper [117]

thyroglobulin levels every 6 months, while low-risk patients may only need to be seen every year or every other year. Monitoring studies include US of the neck as well as other imaging modalities such as MRI, CT, and FDG-PET scans when indicated, radioiodine whole body scanning, and serum thyroglobulin levels. After surgery and RAI treatment, serum thyroglobulin (Tg) measurements should be undetectable and therefore Tg can be used as a tumor marker to monitor for the presence of recurrent or residual thyroid cancer [60, 61, 118]. Thyroglobulin levels reach their nadir approximately 3 months after surgery and RAI ablation [119]. An elevated Tg provides evidence that residual thyroid tissue or cancer still persists with a sensitivity of 85–95% during thyroid hormone withdrawal [120, 121] and 98–99% with rhTSH stimulation [118, 122]. Sensitivity of Tg for detecting disease falls to 50% with poorly differentiated thyroid cancer or when TSH is suppressed [120, 121]. One problem with serum thyroglobulin is assay variability which is likely due to differences in specificity for Tg isoforms and persists despite attempts at standardization [123–127]. In addition, assay method variability makes serial monitoring of Tg difficult if different laboratories are used. Therefore, it is prudent to use the same lab when testing Tg and if a patient has to switch doctors or get blood tests done in a

different lab, a new baseline should be established [123]. Lastly, a problem for 25% of thyroid cancer patients is the presence of thyroglobulin antibodies which interferes with Tg measurements usually causing a falsely low Tg concentration [128–130]. Even though the Tg is not a useful marker when antibodies are present, following the trend in thyroglobulin antibodies can be helpful when monitoring for recurrence of disease. Persistence of thyroglobulin antibodies can be thought of as an indirect measure of recurrent or residual thyroid cancer [127].

Monitoring thyroglobulin levels in the very low-risk patients who have not had total thyroidectomy or RAI remnant ablation is not very helpful. In a study of 80 patients with PTMC who had less than total thyroidectomy and no radioiodine ablation, the most sensitive test for identifying recurrence of disease was ultrasound of the neck [131]. The high sensitivity of US in detecting recurrences has been confirmed in additional studies [132, 133]. In addition, rhTSH-stimulated Tg levels correlated to the amount of thyroid remnant in the neck (based on WBS uptake) and not to thyroid cancer recurrence [131]. Long-term follow-up for this group of patients can be limited to neck US [131], although a rising level of serum Tg in the face of adequate TSH suppression may be indicative of tumor growth.

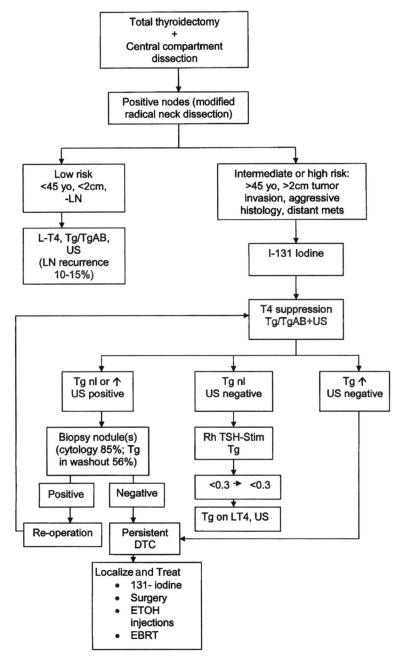

Fig. 7.3 Management algorithm for follow-up of papillary thyroid carcinoma. ETOH ethanol; EBRT external beam irradiation therapy

Low-risk patients who have undergone total thyroidectomy and RAI remnant ablation should be followed between 6 months and 1 year with serum Tg on thyroxine suppression and neck US (Fig 7.3). If the Tg is undetectable (<0.1 ng/mL), a TSH-stimulated Tg should be performed [134, 135]. Because TSH-stimulated Tg levels are highly sensitive but not specific, the false positive rate for detecting recurrence is high [136, 137]. Therefore, in certain circumstances, such as when a low-risk patient has a suppressed Tg <0.1 ng/mL, one may consider following Tg and US while on suppression rather than doing an unnecessary stimulation test [135]. For low-risk patients who have had remnant ablation, a negative rhTSH-stimulated Tg, and a negative neck US, future monitoring entails only annual clinical exam and TSH-suppressed Tg measurement [30]. A diagnostic WBS is not required during follow-up for low-risk patients, but may be valuable in the follow-up of intermediate or high-risk patients or in low-risk patients with Tg antibodies [30].

High risk patients should be followed with thyroglobulin levels and cervical US followed by a TSH-stimulated diagnostic whole body 131-I scan if the Tg is elevated, but US shows no evidence of thyroid bed or cervical nodal disease (Fig 7.3). If there is evidence of recurrence or persistent PTC on US, a FNA biopsy for cytology and Tg in the needle washings followed by an en bloc resection of the involved LN compartment is indicated. Explanations for an elevated Tg with a negative whole body scan (WBS) include: poor compliance with thyroid hormone withdrawal; contamination with stable iodine; lack of uptake by noniodine avid disease; human anti-mouse antibody (HAMA) interference with the Tg assay; or a false positive Tg.

Elevated levels of Tg without Tg antibodies are most likely an indicator for local recurrence or metastases. A TSH-stimulated Tg greater than 2.0ng/mL occurs in approximately 20% of patients and is sensitive for identifying patients with persistent tumor [121, 135, 138]. Ultrasonography and radioiodine scans are recommended for localization of disease but RAI scans are only 50–69% sensitive for detecting thyroid malignancies [139–141]. Other imaging modalities such as CT scans, MRI, bone scintigraphy, and FDG PET scans are used to localize the source of Tg production. The approximately 40% of lesions that are no longer iodine avid may be metastases with dedifferentiation which portends a worse prognosis [139, 140, 142, 143]. 18F-FDG PET studies can be used to localize iodine-refractory recurrent or metastatic thyroid cancer with a sensitivity of 50–78% and specificity of 90–100% [141, 144, 145]. Because PET scans usually show activity of dedifferentiated tumors, PET positive lesions are associated with

a worse prognosis. TSH stimulation prior to FDG PET improves its sensitivity for localizing small lesions, but only changed management 6% of the time in one study [146]. The 2009 thyroid cancer guidelines list the following uses for 18-FDG PET scanning:

• Initial staging and follow-up of high-risk patients with poorly differentiated thyroid cancers unlikely to concentrate RAI in order to identify sites of disease that may be missed with RAI scanning on conventional imaging
• Initial staging and follow-up of invasive or metastatic Hurthle cell carcinoma
• A prognostic tool for identifying which patients with known distant metastases are at highest risk for disease-specific mortality
• A selection tool to identify those patients unlikely to respond to additional RAI therapy
• A measurement of post-treatment response following external beam irradiation, surgical resection, embolization, or systemic therapy [30]

The combination of PET and CT improves diagnostic assessment by providing more accurate information particularly for miliary lung metastases which are often missed by FDG-PET alone, while CT has a 100% sensitivity for lung metastases [147].

Treatment of persistent or metastatic papillary thyroid cancer relies first on localizing the disease and then determining which of the possible therapeutic options – surgery, high dose RAI, external beam radiation therapy (EBRT), and targeted chemotherapies – will best serve the patient (Fig. 7.3). These decisions should be carefully coordinated by members of a multispecialty team while also making sure to include the patient's goals and wishes. Surgery for nodal and extranodal metastases can improve survival in some patients [148] and, when possible, should be considered to alleviate symptoms of bulky disease. Approximately 80% of patients with regional nodal metastatases respond to empiric doses of I-131 RAI treatment and it works best for those patients without bulky disease. Additionally, RAI treatment for iodine-avid pulmonary metastases may extend 5-year survival (60% treated vs. 30% untreated) [149, 150]. Treatment of metastases with RAI should be repeated every 6–12 months until the disease is ablated or until there is no longer iodine uptake. However, complete remission is not common and one must consider the increased risk for second primary malignancies with cumulative doses of I-131 above 800–1,000 mCi [151]. When surgery is not feasible for gross residual disease or metastases, treatment with EBRT for local disease and/or targeted chemotherapy for widespread metastases may improve survival. Chow and colleagues demonstrated greater local regional control rate at a 5-year follow-up (67 vs. 38%, $P = 0.001$) in patients with gross residual disease who received EBRT after initial surgery for PTC [152]. Several phase II studies have shown that drugs such as Sorafenib that target the Ras-Braf-MAP kinase pathways can result in a partial response in anywhere from 13–21% of patients and stability of disease in up to 60% of patients with metastatic disease [153–155].

Papillary Microcarcinoma (PTMC)

As mentioned above, PTMC incidence is increasing. The frequency of PTMC at autopsy appears to be relatively high, the incidence ranging from 2% up to 36% in one review of 20 studies from various countries [156]. This 18-fold difference brings up the problem of ascertainment bias due to differences in sectioning technique and geographic regions. Interestingly, autopsy studies show that the sex distribution is nearly equal as opposed to the marked female predominance of clinical cancers, and prevalence of PTMC is higher in adults compared to young people [156]. In addition, several surgical series of patients treated for benign thyroid disease have reported the incidental coexistence of occult PTMC with a prevalence ranging from 1.3 to 21.6% [156].

Not all microcarcinomas remain clinically occult and a subset of patients with PTMC has a presentation that is clinically similar to conventional papillary thyroid carcinoma. Many studies have examined the clinicopathologic features and treatments that may affect disease-free and cause-specific survival. Similar to PTC, lymph node metastases are present in 40–60% of patients with papillary microcarcinomas [157, 158]. A retro-

spective study of 243 patients with PTMC from Italy found a correlation between the size of the tumor and presence of metastatic disease or recurrence at the time of initial diagnosis. Locoregional and distant metastases as well as recurrence of disease were more common in patients with PTMC larger than or equal to 8 mm [157]. In addition, the threshold size for LN metastases was approximately 5 mm and that for extrathyroidal growth 10 mm [159]. Those patients with PTMC presenting with LN metastases had significantly worse disease-free survival than those who presented without LN metastases [157, 158, 160–162]; however, the clinical significance of this for cause-specific survival is not clear. Some studies have reported higher mortality rates in those patients with lymph node metastases [163, 164]; however, other studies note no difference in survival whether lymph nodes are involved or not [157, 165]. Pacini et al. demonstrated that multifocal PTMC is common in both low- and high-risk patients but they did not find predictors of multifocality [166].

The Mayo Clinic published one of the largest series of PTMCs over a 60-year period [167]. Out of the 900 patients with PTMC, 23% had multifocal disease, 30% had lymph node metastases, 2% had extrathyroidal spread, and 0.3% had distant metastatic spread. The 40-year cause-specific mortality was excellent at 0.7%, while recurrence rates ranged between 5 and 8% at 40 years. Twenty-year recurrence rates were higher for multifocal tumors (11% vs 4%) and for those patients who had lymph node involvement at the time of diagnosis (16% vs 0.8%) [167].

Traditionally, the management of PTMC echoes that of larger papillary carcinomas; however, some studies suggest that a less aggressive approach may be acceptable (see Fig 7.4). Bilimoria et al. found that for patients with tumors less than 1 cm in size, there is no significant difference in rates of recurrence or survival if the patient had a lobectomy or a total thyroidectomy ($P = 0.24$ and $P = 0.83$, respectively) [33]. In a prior Mayo Clinic review of a smaller series of PTMC patients, an increased extent of initial surgery was associated with lower recurrence rates, but in their larger series, recurrence rates

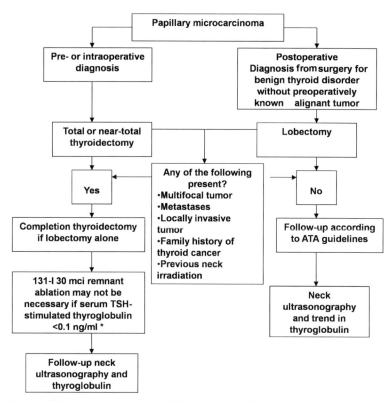

Fig. 7.4 Management algorithm for papillary thyroid microcarcinoma. Adapted from Mazzaferri [168]

did not differ statistically between patients treated with unilateral lobectomy or bilateral resection, as long as complete tumor resection was achieved ($P=0.54$) [10]. Perhaps, even monitoring alone without surgery is feasible in this population of low-risk thyroid cancer patients. Ito et al. studied the natural course of PTMC by offering patients either surgical resection or observation [169]. Approximately 70% opted for immediate surgery and 30% chose observation. After 5 years of follow-up, 60–71% of the tumors were unchanged and 6–16% decreased in size. Fifteen to 29% of the tumors increased in size and lateral lymph node metastases developed in only 1.2% of patients. Ultimately, however, 34% of the patients in the observation group subsequently chose to undergo surgery for primarily emotional reasons [169]. The American Thyroid Association (ATA) rec-

ommends a near-total or total thyroidectomy for PTMC; however, if the diagnosis is made postoperatively, completion thyroidectomy is not required [30]. In summary, predictors of recurrence of PTMC include multifocal and bilateral disease, palpable lateral lymph nodes at presentation, and extent of initial surgery.

Postoperative management of PTMC using RAI for remnant ablation (RAI) is somewhat controversial. In the past, patients with PTMC were treated similarly to patients with larger cancers. However, more recent data such as that from the Mayo Clinic suggest that survival and recurrence are unaffected by whether or not patients received remnant ablation. Hay et al. showed that RAI remnant ablation does not result in an improved tumor recurrence rate at any site at 20 years, even for those patients with multifocal disease [167]. Therefore, current ATA guidelines recommend against RAI ablation for single or multifocal microcarcinomas as long as there is no evidence of extracapsular invasion, incomplete tumor resection, or distant metastases [30].

Special Circumstances

Pregnancy

Thyroid nodules found during pregnancy should be evaluated as if the patient were not pregnant other than performing a radionucleotide scan which is contraindicated. It is unclear whether nodules are more likely to be malignant in pregnant women than in nonpregnant women [170], because there are no population-based studies looking at this question. Ninety percent of thyroid cancers diagnosed during pregnancy are PTC [171]. PTC does not appear to be more aggressive when found during pregnancy. In a study of 61 pregnant women found to have thyroid cancer, there were no significant differences in physical or tumor pathological features, treatment or outcome when compared to women who were not pregnant [172, 173]. Favorable outcomes occurred in those women for whom surgery was delayed until after delivery even if there was lymph node involvement [172]. A larger study of 129 women diagnosed with thyroid cancer during pregnancy found no difference in mortality when compared to 466 women whose thyroid cancer was diagnosed in the postpartum period. In addition, the frequency of locoregional and distant metastases did not differ when compared to 2,270 nonpregnant age-matched controls [171]. They also found that thyroidectomy was not associated with maternal or neonatal complications when performed during pregnancy [171]. Current recommendations suggest that nodules with cytology favoring PTC discovered during pregnancy should be monitored for growth until midgestation (weeks 24 through 26). If there is growth, surgery is recommended during the second trimester to decrease the risk for miscarriage [174]. If the tumor is stable in size or found midgestation, one may wait until after delivery to perform surgery [30, 175, 176]. In women suspected

of having cancer or if FNA suggests the nodule is suspicious for thyroid cancer, one should consider thyroid hormone suppression with a goal TSH of 0.1–1.0 [177].

Tuttle et al. reported the first study that looked retrospectively at women with thyroid cancer who became pregnant after the thyroid cancer had already been treated. If the thyroid cancer was well controlled with a low or undetectable Tg level and no evidence of disease on ultrasound, neither recurrence nor progression of disease was seen at 5 years after the pregnancy. However, women with prepregnancy elevations in Tg or US evidence of disease demonstrated increases in Tg and new evidence of disease on US within 5 years of the postpartum period [178]. Women with clinical evidence of persistent or recurrent thyroid cancer who desire pregnancy should be counseled for the possibility of an increased risk for worsening of disease during or after gestation.

Thyroid Cancer in Children

Two percent of all thyroid cancer cases are diagnosed in patients under age 20 [179]. Thyroid cancers are the third most common solid tumor, and the most common endocrine malignancy in children. From 2003 to 2007, incidence rates of thyroid cancer in the United States for males and females under age 14 and adolescents ages 15–19 were 6 and 19 per 1,000,000, respectively [180]. In addition, in the late adolescent years, the incidence of differentiated thyroid cancer increases and the female to male ratio mimics that of adults (3:1) [180].

Pediatric thyroid cancer typically presents with a solitary thyroid nodule and while the majority of all thyroid nodules are benign, the risk for malignancy in children is greater than that in adults, 20% versus 5% respectively [181, 182]. Factors that increase the risk for malignancy in this age group include age less than 10 years, a family history of thyroid cancer, and a history of ionizing radiation to the head or neck and iodine deficiency [183–187]. The method for diagnosing thyroid cancer in this population is by use of ultrasound for nodules over 0.5 cm and fine-needle aspiration biopsy [187].

Children and adolescents often present with more extensive spread of thyroid cancer than adults. Lymph node involvement is seen in 40–80% of children [187–191] and the frequency of distant metastases at initial presentation is higher in children than in adults with an incidence of 20–30% [188, 191]. Despite the advanced nature of the thyroid cancer in this young age group, there is a favorable prognosis with 20-year survival rates of 90–99% [192].

Surgical management for children with thyroid cancer is not specifically addressed in the most recent ATA guidelines [30]. Since 40% of PTC in children is multifocal and since some authors have found higher rates of recurrence with lobectomy alone, total thyroidectomy is recommended in this age group [187, 192–194]. As with adults, lymph node disease is often present at initial presentation and controversy exists over whether or not to do prophylactic central compartment neck dissection (CLND). Some studies have shown improved rates of lymph node-free survival after CLND in children [195]; however, there is a risk of increased morbidity with more extensive surgery. Experts recommend that CLND be performed in children if lymph nodes are detected on intraoperative palpation or by preoperative ultrasound [187].

Postoperative management of thyroid cancer in children and adolescents includes I-131 RAI adjuvant therapy for the majority of cases. This recommendation is based on retrospective studies that demonstrate decreased recurrence rates and improved survival with RAI treatment [195, 196]. Similar to adults, children are treated 4–6 weeks post-thyroidectomy and need to maintain a low-iodine diet. Unlike adults, this younger age group can achieve an optimal TSH (>30 mU/L) after 2 weeks of thyroid hormone withdrawal. Pretreatment scans are typically performed in children to determine the amount of thyroid bed uptake and if there is evidence of a large remnant, surgery is recommended [182, 193]. There is no consensus on dosing of RAI for children. Some recommend 30mCi and others recommend 80 mCi, reserving larger doses of 150 mCi for those patients with distant metasta-ses (194.181). Long-term follow-up of these young patients is important since recurrences of thyroid cancer have been shown to occur up to 40 years after the initial diagnosis.

Ionizing Radiation

It is well known that external ionizing radiation to the head or neck in childhood or adolescence confers an increased risk for thyroid cancer [197–199]. Approximately 80% of tumors found after childhood exposure to external irradiation to the thyroid are benign and 20% are malignant. Radiation-related thyroid carcinomas are often preceded by or arise simultaneously with benign thyroid adenomas, and hypothyroidism frequently occurs after high-dose radiation to the neck. In 1986, radionuclides including I-131 were released into the environment after the Chernobyl accident and recent reports document over 1,500 cases of thyroid cancer out of 2 million children exposed to radiation from the Chernobyl fallout [200, 201]. For those exposed to radiation under age 15 for reasons including treatment for tinea capitis, enlarged tonsils or enlarged thymus, and atomic bomb survivors, Ron, et al. showed in a pooled analysis of almost 60,000 subjects that the risk for developing thyroid cancer was linear relative to the total amount of exposure. There was an average excess relative risk of 7.7 per Gy, while the excess absolute risk was 4.4 per 10^4 person years per Gy [197]. In one study of over 10,000 children who received radiation treatment for tinea capitis, an estimated exposure of 9 cGy to the thyroid resulted in a fourfold increased risk for malignancy as an adult [202] and the risk increased for those exposed at younger ages and for females [197]. Since this population of patients has an increased risk for thyroid cancer, screening with US and FNA biopsy is warranted.

Conclusion

Papillary thyroid cancer has been increasing in incidence over the last four decades and therefore physicians are seeing more and more patients with the disease. While the majority of

PTC cases have a low risk for recurrence and death from the disease, there are still those low-risk patients who inexplicably develop multiple recurrences, distant metastatic disease, and ultimately die from PTC. Controversy exists over the initial management of such low-risk patients and physicians are faced with difficult decisions in the management of papillary thyroid cancer. Topics such as the extent of surgery, whether or not to perform a prophylactic lymph node dissection, whether or not to treat with RAI, and the degree of thyroxine suppression continue to be debated among thyroidologists. On the other hand, the management for high-risk patients (AJCC/TNM stage II (under 45 years), III and IV disease) is quite well-accepted because studies demonstrate higher rates of recurrence and disease-specific death in this group. Because of the discrepancies and deficiencies in the thyroid cancer literature, a risk assessment needs to be done for each case to provide an individualized approach to treatment and monitoring of thyroid cancer patients.

References

1. Ain KB. Papillary thyroid carcinoma: etiology, assessment, and therapy. Endocrinol Metab Clin North Am. 1995;24:711–60.
2. Schlumberger MJ. Papillary and follicular thyroid carcinoma. N Engl J Med. 1998;338:297–306.
3. Davies L, Welch HG. Increasing incidence of thyroid cancer in the United States, 1973–2002. JAMA. 2006;295:2164–7.
4. Frasca F, Nucera C, Pellegriti G, et al. BRAF V600) mutation and the biology of papillary thyroid cancer. Endocr Relat Cancer. 2008;15:191–205.
5. Pettersson B, Coleman MP, Ron E, et al. Iodine supplementation in Sweden and regional trends in thyroid cancer incidence by histopathologic type. Int J Cancer. 1996;65:13–9.
6. Chen AY, Jemal A, Ward EM. Increasing incidence of differentiated thyroid cancer in the United States, 1988–2005. Cancer. 2009;115:3801–7.
7. Enewold I, Khu K, Ron E, et al. Rising thyroid cancer incidence in the United States by demographic and tumor characteristics, 1980–2005. Cancer Epidemiol Biomarkers Prev. 2009;18:784–91.
8. Altekruse SF, Kosary CL, Krapcho M, et al. SEER cancer statistics review, 1975–2007, National Cancer Institute. Bethesda, MD, http://seer.cancer.gov/csr/1975_2007/, based on November 2009 SEER data submission, posted to the SEER web site, 2010.
9. Horner MJ, Ries LAG, Krapcho M, et al. SEER Cancer statistics review, 1975–2006, National Cancer Institute. Bethesda, MD, http://seer.cancer.gov/csr/1975_2006/, based on November 2008 SEER data submission, posted to the SEER web site, 2009.
10. Hay ID. Papillary thyroid carcinoma. Endocrinol Metab Clin North Am. 1990;19:545–76.
11. Ries LAG, Eisner MP, Kosary CL. SEER cancer statistic review, 1973–1997. Bethesda, MD: National Cancer Institute; 2000.
12. Mazzaferri EL, Jhiang SM. Long-term impact of initial surgical and medical therapy on papillary and follicular thyroid cancer. Am J Med. 1994;97:418–28.
13. Hemminki K, Eng C, Chen B. Familial risks for non-medullary thyroid cancer. J Clin Endocrinol Metab. 2005;90:5747–53.
14. Vriens MR, Insoo S, Moses W, et al. Clinical features and genetic predisposition to hereditary nonmedullary thyroid cancer. Thyroid. 2009;19(12):1343–9.
15. Alsanea O, Wada N, Ain K, et al. Is familial non-medullary thyroid carcinoma more aggressive than sporadic thyroid cancer? A multicenter series. Surgery. 2000;128:1043–50.
16. Uchino S, Noguchi S, Kawamoto H, et al. Familial non-medullary thyroid carcinoma characterized by multifocality and a high recurrence rate in a large study population. World J Surg. 2002;26:897–902.
17. Lupoli G, Vitale G, Caraglia M, et al. Familial papillary thyroid microcarcinoma: a new clinical entity. Lancet. 1999;353:637–9.
18. Triponez F, Wong M, Sturgeon C, et al. Does familial non-medullary thyroid cancer adversely affect survival? World J Surg. 2006;30:787–93.
19. Sippel RS, Caron NR, Clark OH. An evidence-based approach to familial non-medullary thyroid cancer: screening, clinical management, and follow-up. World J Surg. 2007;31:924–33.
20. Pal T, Vogl FD, Chappuis PO, et al. Increased risk for non-medullary thyroid cancer in the first degree relatives of prevalent cases of non-medullary thyroid cancer: a hospital-based study. J Clin Endocrinol Metab. 2001;86:5307–12.
21. Schneider AB, Ron E, Lubin J. Dose-response relationships for radiation-induced thyroid cancer and thyroid nodules: evidence for the prolonged effects of radiation on the thyroid. J Clin Endocrinol Metab. 1993;77:362–9.
22. Shibaba Y, Yamashita S, Masyakin VB, et al. 15 years after Chernobyl: new evidence of thyroid cancer. Lancet. 2001;358:1965–6.
23. Hegedus L. Clinical practice. The thyroid nodule. N Engl J Med. 2004;351:1764–71.
24. Robbins J, Merino MJ, Boice JD, et al. Thyroid cancer: a lethal endocrine neoplasm. Ann Intern Med. 1991;115:133–47.
25. Ron E, Lubin JH, Shore RE, et al. Thyroid cancer after exposure to external radiation: a pooled analysis of seven studies. Radiat Res. 1995;141(3):259–77.
26. Shore RE, Xue X-N. Comparative thyroid cancer risk of childhood and adult radiation exposure and estimation of lifetime risk. In: Thomas D, Karaoglou A,

Williams ED, editors. Radiation and thyroid cancer. Singapore: World Scientific Publishing; 1999. p. 491–8.

27. Burman KD, Ringel MD, Wartofsky L. Unusual types of thyroid neoplasms. Endocrinol Metab Clin North Am. 1996;25:49–68.

28. Mazzaferri EL. Management of a solitary thyroid nodule. N Engl J Med. 1993;328:553–9.

29. Ezzat S, Sarti DA, Cain DR, Braunstein GD. Thyroid incidentalomas: prevalence by palpation and ultrasound. Arch Intern Med. 1994;154:1838–940.

30. Cooper DS, Doherty MD, Haugen BR, et al. Revised American thyroid association management guidelines for patients with thyroid nodules and differentiated thyroid cancer. Thyroid. 2009;19(11):1167–214.

31. Lang BH, Lo CY, Chan WF, et al. Staging systems for papillary thyroid carcinoma: a review and comparison. Ann Surg. 2007;245:366–78.

32. Pacini F, Schlumberger M, Harmer C, et al. Postsurgical use of radioiodine (131I) in patients with papillary and follicular thyroid cancer and the issue of remnant ablation: a consensus report. Eur J Endocrinol. 2005;153:651–9.

33. Bilimoria KY, Bentrem DJ, Ko CY, et al. Extent of surgery affects survival for papillary thyroid cancer. Ann Surg. 2007;246(3):375–84.

34. Hay ID, Grant CS, Bergstralh EJ, et al. Unilateral total lobectomy: is it sufficient surgical treatment for patients with AMES low-risk papillary thyroid carcinoma? Surgery. 1998;124(6):958–64. discussion 964–6.

35. Mazzaferri EL, Jhiang SM. Differentiated thyroid cancer long-term impact of intial therapy. Trans Am Clin Climatol Assoc. 1995;106:151–70.

36. Tzvetov G, Hirsch D, Shraga-Slutsky I, et al. Welldifferentiated thyroid carcinoma: comparison of microscopic and macroscopic disease. Thyroid. 2009; 19:487–94.

37. Pereira JA, Jimeno J, Miquel J, et al. Nodal yield, morbidity, and recurrence after central neck dissection for papillary thyroid carcinoma. Surgery. 2005;138(6):1095–101.

38. Noguchi S, Noguchi A, Murakami N. Papillary carcinoma of the thyroid. I. Developing pattern of metastasis. Cancer. 1970;26:1053–60.

39. Gimm O, Rath FW, Dralle H. Pattern of lymph node metastases in papillary thyroid carcinoma. Br J Surg. 1998;85:252–4.

40. Dralle H, Machens H. Lymph node dissection in thyroid cancer. In: Gubbard JGH, Inabnet WB, Chung-Yau L, editors. Endocrine surgery, principles and practice. New York: Springer; 2009. p. 173–93.

41. Machens A, Hinze R, Thomusch O, et al. Pattern of nodal metastasis for primary and reoperative thyroid cancer. World J Surg. 2002;26:22–8.

42. Kouvaraki MA, Shapiro SE, Fornage BD, et al. Role of preoperative ultrasonography in the surgical management of patients with thyroid cancer. Surgery. 2003;134:946–54.

43. Shimamoto K, Satake H, Sawaki A, et al. Preoperative staging of thyroid papillary carcinoma with ultrasonography. Eur J Radiol. 1998;29:4–10.

44. Stulak JM, Grant CS, Farley DR, et al. Value of preoperative ultrasonography in the surgical management of initial and reoperative papillary thyroid cancer. Arch Surg. 2006;141:489496.

45. Wanebo H, Coburn M, Teates D, et al. Total thyroidectomy does not enhance disease control or survival even in high-risk patients with differentiated thyroid cancer. Ann Surg. 1998;227:912–21.

46. Haigh PI, Urbach DR, Rotstein LE. Extent of thyroidectomy is not a major determinant of survival in lowor high-risk papillary thyroid cancer. Ann Surg Oncol. 2005;12(1):81–9.

47. Hay ID, Grant CS, Taylor WF, et al. Ipsilateral lobectomy versus bilateral lobar resection in papillary thyroid carcinoma: a retrospective analysis of surgical outcome using a novel prognostic scoring system. Surgery. 1987;102:1088–95.

48. Mazzaferri EL, Kloos RT. Current approaches to primary therapy for papillary and follicular thyroid cancer. J Clin Endocrinol Metab. 2001;86(4):1447–63.

49. DeGroot LJ, Kaplan EL, Straus FH, et al. Does the method of management of papillary thyroid carcinoma make a difference in outcome? World J Surg. 1994;18:123–30.

50. Hay I, McConahey WM, Goellner JR. Managing patients with carcinoma: insights gained from the Mayo Clinics's experience of treating 2,512 consecutive patients doing 1940 though 2000. Trans Am Clin Climatol Assoc. 2002;113:241–60.

51. Jonklass J, Sarlis NJ, Litofsky D, et al. Outcomes of patients with differentiated thyroid carcinoma following initial therapy. Thyroid. 2006;16(12):1229–42.

52. White ML, Gauger PG, Doherty GM. Central lymph node dissection in differentiated thyroid cancer. World J Surg. 2007;31:895–904.

53. Bhattacharyya N, Fried MP. Assessment of the morbidity and complications of total thyroidectomy. Arch Otolaryngol Head Neck Surg. 2002;128(4): 389–92.

54. Schuff KG, Weber SM, Givi B, et al. Efficacy of nodal dissection for treatment of persistent/recurrent papillary thyroid cancer. Laryngoscope. 2008;118: 768–75.

55. Kim MK, Mandel SH, Baloch Z, et al. Morbidity following central compartment reoperation for recurrent or persistent thyroid cancer. Arch Otolaryngol Head Neck Surg. 2004;130:12141–1216.

56. Alvarado R, Sywak MS, Delbridge L, Sidhu SB. Central lymph node dissection as a secondary procedure for papillary thyroid cancer: is there added morbidity? Surgery. 2009;145:514–8.

57. Ito Y, Tomoda C, Uruno T, et al. Preoperative ultrasonographic examination for lymph node metastasis: usefulness when designing lymph node dissection for papillary microcarcinoma of the thyroid. World J Surg. 2004;28:498–501.

58. Brierley JD, Panzarella T, Tsang RW, et al. A comparison of different staging systems predictability of patient outcome. Thyroid carcinoma as an example. Cancer. 1997;79:2414–23.

59. Hay ID, Thompson GB, Grant CS, et al. Papillary thyroid carcinoma managed at the Mayo Clinic during six decades (1940–1999): temporal trends in initial

therapy and long-term outcome in 2444 consecutively treated patients. World J Surg. 2001;26:879–85.

60. Okosieme OE, Parkes AB, Premawardhana LD, et al. Thyroglobulin: current aspects of its role in autoimmune thyroid disease and thyroid cancer. Minerva Med. 2003;94:319–30.

61. Schlumberger M, Pacini F, Wiersinga WM, et al. Follow-up and management of differentiated thyroid carcinoma: a European perspective in clinical practice. Eur J Endocrinol. 2004;151:539–48.

62. Sherman S. Thyroid carcinoma. Lancet. 2003;361: 501–11.

63. Lo CY, Chan WF, Lam KY, et al. Optimizing the treatment of AMES high-risk papillary thyroid carcinoma. World J Surg. 2004;28:1103–9.

64. Cunningham MP, Duda RB, Recant W, et al. 1990 Survival discriminants for differentiated thyroid cancer. Am J Surg. 1990;160:344–7.

65. Shoup M, Stojadinovic A, Nissan A, et al. Prognostic indicators of outcomes in patients with distant metastases from differentiated thyroid carcinoma. J Am Coll Surg. 2003;197:191–7.

66. Samaan NA, Schultz PN, Haynie TP, et al. Pulmonary metastasis of differentiated thyroid carcinoma: treatment results in 101 patients. J Clin Endocrinol Metab. 1985;60:376–80.

67. Tseng LM, Lee CH, Wang HC, et al. The surgical treatment and prognostic factors of well-differentiated thyroid cancers in Chinese patients: a 20-year experience. Zhonghua Yi Xue Za Zhi (Taipei). 1996;58:121–31.

68. Varma VM, Beierwaltes WH, Nofal MM, et al. Treatment of thyroid cancer. Death rates after surgery and after surgery followed by sodium iodide I-131. JAMA. 1970;214:1437–42.

69. Mihailovic J, Stefanovic L, Malesevic M. Differentiated thyroid carcinoma with distant metastases: probability of survival and its predicting factors. Cancer Biother Radiopharm. 2007;22:250–5.

70. Massin JP, Savoie JC, Garnier H, et al. Pulmonary metastases in differentiated thyroid carcinoma. Study of 58 cases with implications for the primary tumor treatment. Cancer. 1984;53:982–92.

71. Wong JB, Kaplan MM, Meyer KB, et al. Ablative radioactive iodine therapy for apparently localized thyroid carcinoma. A decision analytic perspective. Endocrinol Metab Clin North Am. 1990;19:741–60.

72. Zidan J, Kassem S, Kuten A. Follicular carcinoma of the thyroid gland: prognostic factors, treatment, and survival. Am J Clin Oncol. 2000;23:1–5.

73. Sanders LE, Silverman M. Follicular and Hurthle cell carcinoma: predicting outcome and directing therapy. Surgery. 1998;124:967–74.

74. Segal K, Shpitzer T, Hazan A, et al. Invasive well-differentiated thyroid carcinoma: effect of treatment modalities on outcome. Otolaryngol Head Neck Surg. 2006;134:819–22.

75. Pelizzo MR, Toniato A, Boschin IM, et al. Locally advanced differentiated thyroid carcinoma: a 35-year mono-institutional experience in 280 patients. Nucl Med Commun. 2005;26:965–8.

76. Coburn M, Teates D, Wanebo HJ. Recurrent thyroid cancer. Role of surgery versus radioactive iodine (I131). Ann Surg. 1994;219:587–93.

77. Davis NL, Gordon M, Germann E, et al. Efficacy of 131I ablation following thyroidectomy in patients with invasive follicular thyroid cancer. Am J Surg. 1992;163:472–5.

78. Cross S, Wei JP, Kim S, et al. Selective surgery and adjuvant therapy based on risk classifications of well-differentiated thyroid cancer. J Surg Oncol. 2006;94:678–82.

79. Kim S, Wei JP, Braveman JM, et al. Predicting outcome and directing therapy for papillary thyroid carcinoma. Arch Surg. 2004;139:390–4.

80. Pelizzo MR, Boschin IM, Toniato A, et al. Papillary thyroid microcarcinoma (PTMC): prognostic factors, management and outcome in 403 patients. Eur J Surg Oncol. 2006;32:1144–8.

81. Loh KC, Greenspan FS, Gee L, et al. Pathological tumor-node metastasis (pTNM) staging for papillary and follicular thyroid carcinomas: a retrospective analysis of 700 patients. J Clin Endocrinol Metab. 1997;82:3553–62.

82. DeGroot LJ, Kaplan EL, McCormick M, et al. Natural history, treatment, and course of papillary thyroid carcinoma. J Clin Endocrinol Metab. 1990;71:414–24.

83. Podnos YD, Smith DD, Wagman LD, et al. Survival in patients with papillary thyroid cancer is not affected by the use of radioactive isotope. J Surg Oncol. 2007;96:3–7.

84. Mazzaferri E. A randomized trial of remnant ablation–in search of an impossible dream? J Clin Endocrinol Metab. 2004;89:3662–4.

85. Schlumberger M, Tubiana M, De Vathaire F, et al. Long-term results of treatment of 283 patients with lung and bone metastases from differentiated thyroid carcinoma. J Clin Endocrinol Metab. 1986;63:960–7.

86. Edmonds CJ, Hayes S, Kermode JC, et al. Measurement of serum TSH and thyroid hormones in the management of treatment of thyroid carcinoma with radioiodine. Br J Radiol. 1977;50:799–807.

87. Torres MS, Ramirez L, Simkin PH, et al. Effect of various doses of recombinant human thyrotropin on the thyroid radioactive iodine uptake and serum levels of thyroid hormones and thyroglobulin in normal subjects. J Clin Endocrinol Metab. 2001;86:1660–4.

88. Sanchez R, Espinosa-de-los-Monteros AL, Mendoza V, et al. Adequate thyroid stimulating hormone levels after levothyroxine discontinuation in the follow-up of patients with well-differentiated thyroid carcinoma. Arch Med Res. 2002;33:478–81.

89. Grigsby PW, Siegel BA, Bekker S, et al. Preparation of patients with thyroid cancer for 131I scintigraphy or therapy by 1–3 weeks of thyroxine discontinuation. J Nucl Med. 2004;45:567–70.

90. Serhal DI, Nasrallah MP, Arafah BM. Rapid rise in serum thyrotropin concentrations after thyroidectomy or withdrawal of suppressive thyroxine therapy in preparation for radioactive iodine administration to patients with differentiate thyroid cancer. J Clin Endocrinol Metab. 2004;89:3285–9.

91. Pacini F, Molinaro E, Castagna MG, et al. Ablation of thyroid residues with 30 mCi (131)I: a comparison in thyroid cancer patients prepared with recombinant human TSH or thyroid hormone withdrawal. J Clin Endocrinol Metab. 2002;87:4063–8.

92. Pilli T, Brianzoni E, Capoccetti F, et al. A comparison of 1850 (50mCi) and 3700 MBQ (100mCi) 131-iodine administered doses for recombinant thyrotropin-stimulated postoperative thyroid remnant ablation in differentiated thyroid cancer. J Clin Endocrinol Metab. 2007;92:3542–6.

93. Maxon HR, Thomas SR, Boehringer A, et al. Low iodine diet in I-131 ablation of thyroid remnants. Clin Nucl Med. 1983;8:123–6.

94. Pluijmen MJ, Eustatia-Rutten C, Goslings BM, et al. Effects of low-iodide diet on postsurgical radioiodide ablation therapy in patients with differentiated thyroid carcinoma. Clin Endocrinol. 2003;58: 428–35.

95. Kim TY, Kim WB, Kim ES, et al. Serum thyroglobulin levels at the time of 131-I remnant ablation just after thyroidectomy are useful for early prediction of clinical recurrence in low-risk patients with differentiated thyroid carcinoma. J Clin Endocrinol Metab. 2005;90:1440–5.

96. Heemstra KA, Liu YY, Stokkel M, et al. Serum thyroglobulin concentrations predict disease-free remission and death in differentiated thyroid carcinoma. Clin Endocrinol. 2007;66:58–64.

97. Sherman SI, Tielens ET, Sostre S, et al. Clinical utility of posttreatment radioiodine scans in the management of patients with thyroid carcinoma. J Clin Endocrinol Metab. 1994;78:629–34.

98. Muratet JP, Giraud P, Daver A, et al. Predicting the efficacy of first iodine-131 treatment in differentiated thyroid carcinoma. J Nucl Med. 1997;38:1362–8.

99. Leger AF, Pellan M, Dagousset F, et al. A case of stunning of lung and bone metastases of papillary thyroid cancer after a therapeutic dose (3.7Gbq) of 131I and review of the literature: implications for sequential treatments. Br J Radiol. 2005;78:428–32.

100. Morris LF, Waxman AD, Braunstein GD. The nonimpact of thyroid stunning: remnant ablation rates in 131I-scanned and nonscanned individuals. J Clin Endocrinol Metab. 2001;86:3507–11.

101. Silberstein EB. Comparison of outcomes after (123) I versus (131)I pre-ablation imaging before radioiodine ablation in differentiated thyroid carcinoma. J Nucl Med. 2007;48:1043–6.

102. Fatourechi V, Hay ID, Mullan BP, et al. Are posttherapy radioiodine scans informative and do they influence subsequent therapy of patients with differentiated thyroid cancer? Thyroid. 2000;10:573–7.

103. Waxman A, Ramanna L, Chapman NB, et al. The significance of I-131 scan dose in patients with thyroid cancer: determination of ablation. J Nucl Med. 1981; 22:861–5.

104. Reynolds J. Percent 131I uptake and post-therapy 131I scans: their role in the management of thyroid cancer. Thyroid. 1997;7:281–4.

105. Brabant G. Thyrotropin suppressive therapy in thyroid carcinoma: what are the targets? J Clin Endocrinol Metab. 2008;93:1167–9.

106. Potter E, Horn R, Scheumann GF, et al. Western blot analysis of thyrotropin receptor expression in human thyroid tumors and correlation with TSH-binding. Biochem Biophys Res Commun. 1994;205:361–7.

107. Spencer CA, LoPresti JS, Fatemi S, et al. Detection of residual and recurrent differentiated thyroid carcinoma by serum thyroglobulin measurement. Thyroid. 1999;9:435–41.

108. Pacini F, Lari R, Mazzeo S, et al. Diagnostic value of a single serum thyroglobulin determination on and off thyroid suppressive therapy in the follow-up of patients with differentiated thyroid cancer. Clin Endocrinol. 1985;23:45–411.

109. Ichikawa YE, Saito Y, Abe MH, et al. Presence of TSH receptor in thyroid neoplasms. J Clin Endocrinol Metab. 1976;42:395–8.

110. Hoelting T, Tzelman S, Siperstein AE, et al. Biphasic effects of thyrotropin on invasion and growth of papillary and follicular thyroid cancer in vitro. Thyroid. 1995;5:35–40.

111. Biondi B, Filetti S, Schlumberger M. Thyroid-hormone suppression therapy and thyroid cancer: a reassessment. Nat Clin Pract Endocrinol Metab. 2005;1:32–8.

112. Burmeister LA, Goumaz MO, Mariash CN, et al. Levothyroxine dose requirements for thyrotropin suppression in the treatment of differentiated thyroid cancer. J Clin Endocrinol Metab. 1992;75:344–50.

113. Flynn RW, Bonellie SR, Jung RT, et al. Serum thyroid-stimulating hormone concentration and morbidity from cardiovascular disease and fractures in patients on long-term thyroxine therapy. J Clin Endocrinol Metab. 2010;95(1):186–93.

114. Pujol P, Daures JP, Nsakala N, et al. Degree of thyrotropin suppression as a prognostic determinant in differentiated thyroid cancer. J Clin Endocrinol Metab. 1996;81:4318–23.

115. Cooper DS, Specker B, Ho M, et al. Thyrotropin suppression and disease progression in patients with differentiated thyroid cancer: results from the National Thyroid Cancer Treatment Cooperative Registry. Thyroid. 1998;8:737–44.

116. Hovens GC, Stokkel MP, Kievit J, et al. Associations of serum thyrotropin concentrations with recurrence and death in differentiated thyroid cancer. J Clin Endocrinol Metab. 2007;92:2610–5.

117. Biondi B, Cooper DS. Benefits of thyrotropin suppression versus the risks of adverse effects in differentiated thyroid cancer. Thyroid. 2010;20(2): 135–46.

118. Castagna D, Brilli L, Pilli T, et al. Limited value of repeat recombinant human thyrotropin (rhTSH)-stimulated thyroglobulin testing in differentiated thyroid carcinoma patients with previous negative rhTSH-stimulated thyroglobulin and undetectable basal serum thyroglobulin levels. J Clin Endocrinol Metab. 2008;93:76–81.

119. LoPresti J, Atkinson E, Maceri D, et al. The reference pattern of serum thyroglobulin (Tg) decline, measured by sensitive assay, can be used as a staging parameter for non-RAI treated low-risk papillary thyroid cancer (PTC) patients. Amer Thyroid Associan West Palm Beach, FL 2009; Abstract# 151.

120. Mueller-Gaertner HW, Schneider C. Clinical evaluation of tumor characteristics predisposing serum thyroglobulin to be undetectable in patients with differentiated thyroid cancer. Cancer. 1988;61:976–81.

121. Haugen BR, Pacini F, Reiners C, et al. A comparison of recombinant human thyrotropin and thyroid hormone withdrawal for the detection of thyroid remnant or cancer. J Clin Endocrinol Metab. 1999; 84:3877–85.

122. Kloos RT. Mazzaferri El. A single recombinant human thyrotrophin-stimulated serum thyroglobulin measurement predicts differentiated thyroid carcinoma metastases three to five years later. J Clin Endocrinol Metab. 2005;90:5047–57.

123. Spencer CA, Bergoglio LM, Kazarosyan M, et al. Clinical impact of thyroglobulin (Tg) and Tg autoantibody method differences on the management of patients with differentiated thyroid carcinomas. J Clin Endocrinol Metab. 2005;90(10):5566–75.

124. Ferrari L, Biancolini D, Seregni E, et al. Critical aspects of immunoradiometric thyroglobulin assays. Tumori. 2003;89:537–9.

125. Schulz R, Bethauser H, Stempka L, et al. Evidence for immunological differences between circulating and tissue-derived thyroglobulin in men. Eur J Clin Invest. 1989;19:459–63.

126. Feldt-Rasmussen U, Profilis C, Colinet E, et al. Human thyroglobulin reference material (CRM 457). II. Physicochemical characterization and certification. Ann Biol Clin. 1996;54:343–8.

127. Spencer CA, Takeuchi M, Kazarosyan M, et al. Serum thyroglobulin autoantibodies: prevalence, influence on serum thyroglobulin measurement, and prognostic significance in patients with differentiated thyroid carcinoma. J Clin Endocrinol Metab. 1998;83(4):1121–7.

128. Mariotti S, Barbesino G, Caturegli P, et al. Assay of thyroglobulin in serum with thyroglobulin autoantibodies: an unobtainable goal? J Clin Endocrinol Metab. 1995;80:468–72.

129. Hollowell JG, Staehling NW, Flanders WD, et al. Serum TSH, T(4), and thyroid antibodies in the United States population (1988 to 1994): National Health and Nutrition Examination Survey (NHANES III). J Clin Endocrinol Metab. 2002;87:489–99.

130. Spencer CA, LoPresti JS, Fatemi S, et al. Detection of residual and recurrent differentiated thyroid carcinoma by serum thyroglobulin measurement. Thyroid. 1999;9:435–41.

131. Torlontano M, Crocetti U, Augello G, et al. Comparative evaluation of recombinant human thyrotropin-stimulated thyroglobulin levels, 131I whole-body scintigraphy, and neck ultrasonography in the follow-up of patients with papillary thyroid microcarcinoma who have not undergone radioiodine therapy. J Clin Endocrinol Metab. 2006;91:60–3.

132. Pacini F, Molinaro E, Castagna MG, et al. Recombinant human thyrotropin-stimulated serum thyroglobulin combined with neck ultrasonography has the highest sensitivity in monitoring differentiated thyroid carcinoma. J Clin Endocrinol Metab. 2003;88:3668–73.

133. Kouvaraki MA, Shapiro SE, Fornage BD, et al. Role of preoperative ultrasonography in the surgical management of patients with thyroid cancer. Surgery. 2003;134:946–54.

134. Schlumberger M, Berg G, Cohen O, et al. Follow-up of low-risk patients with differentiated thyroid carcinoma: a European perspective. Eur J Endocrinol. 2004;150:105–12.

135. Mazzaferri EL, Robbins RJ, Spencer CA, et al. A consensus report of the role of serum thyroglobulin as a monitoring method for low-risk patients with papillary thyroid carcinoma. J Clin Endocrinol Metab. 2003;88(4):1433–41.

136. Smallridge RC, Meek SE, Morgan MA, et al. Monitoring thyroglobulin in a sensitive immunoassay has comparable sensitivity to recombinant human TSH-stimulated thyroglobulin in follow-up of thyroid cancer patients. J Clin Endocrinol Metab. 2007;92:82–7.

137. Iervasi A, Iervasi G, Ferdeghini M, et al. Clinical relevance of highly sensitive Tg assay in monitoring patients treated for differentiated thyroid cancer. Clin Endocrinol. 2007;67:434–41.

138. Haugen BR, Ridgway EC, McLaughlin BA, McDermott MT. Clinical comparison of whole-body radioiodine scan and serum thyroglobulin after stimulation with recombinant human thyrotropin. Thyroid. 2002;12:37–43.

139. Iwata M, Kasagi K, Misaki T, et al. Comparison of whole-body 18F-FDG PET, 99mTc-MIBI SPECT, and post-therapeutic 131I-Na scintigraphy in the detection of metastatic thyroid cancer. Eur J Nucl Med Mol Imaging. 2004;31:491–8.

140. Grunwald F, Kalicke T, Feine U, et al. Fluorine-18 fluorodeoxyglucose positron emission tomography and iodine-131 whole-body scintigraphy in the follow-up of differentiated thyroid cancer. Eur J Nucl Med. 1997;24:1342–8.

141. Deitlein M, Scheidhaver K, Voth E, et al. Fleorine-18 fluorodeoxyglucose positron emission tomography and iodine1-131 whole-body scintigraphy in the follow-up of differentiated thyroid cancer. Eur J Nucl Med. 1997;23:1342–8.

142. Schonberger J, Ruschoff J, Grimm D, et al. Glucose transporter 1 gene expression is related to thyroid neoplasm with an unfavorable prognosis: an immunhistochemical study [abstract]. Thyroid. 2002;12:747–54.

143. Schluter B, Bohuslavizki KH, Beyer W, et al. Impact of FDG PET on patients with differentiated thyroid cancer who present with elevated thyroglobulin and negative 131I scan. J Nucl Med. 2001; 42:71–6.

144. Feine U, Lietzenmayer R, Hanke JP, et al. Fluorine-18 FDG and iodine-131 iodide uptake in thyroid cancer. J Nucl Med. 1996;37:1468–72.

145. Grunwald F, Schomburg A, Bender H, et al. Fluorine-18 fluorodeoxyglucose positron emission tomography in the follow up of differentiated thyroid cancer. Eur J Nucl Med. 1996;23:312–9.

146. Leboulleux S, Schroeder PR, Busaidy NL, et al. Assessment of the incremental value of recombinantthyrotropin stimulation before 2-[18F]-fluoro-2-deoxy-d-glucose positron emission tomography/computed tomography imaging to localize residual differentiated thyroid cancer. J Clin Endocrinol Metab. 2009;94(4):1310–6.

147. Zoller M, Kohlfuerst S, Igere I, et al. Combined PET/CT in the follow-up of differentiated thyroid carcinoma: what is the impact of each modality? Eur J Nucl Med Mol Imaging. 2007;34:487–95.

148. Niederle B, Roka R, Schemper M, et al. Surgical treatment of distant metastases in differentiated thyroid cancer: indication and results. Surgery. 1986;100:1088–97.

149. Maxon HR, Smith HS. Radioiodine-131 in the diagnosis and treatment of metastatic well differentiated thyroid cancer. Endocrinol Metab Clin North Am. 1990;19:685–718.

150. Sisson JC, Giordano TJ, Jamadar DA, et al. 131-I treatment of micronodular pulmonary metastases from papillary thyroid carcinoma. Cancer. 1996; 78:2184–92.

151. Sawka AM, Thabane L, Parlea L, et al. Second primary malignancy risk after radioactive iodine treatment for thyroid cancer: a systematic review and meta-analysis. Thyroid. 2009;10(5):451–7.

152. Chow S-M, Law SCK, Mendenhall WM, et al. Papillary thyroid carcinoma: prognostic factors and the role of radioiodine and external radiotherapy. Int J Radiat Oncol Biol Phys. 2002;52:784–95.

153. Gupta-Abramson V, Troxel AB, Nellore A, et al. Phase II trial of sorafenib in advanced thyroid cancer. J Clin Oncol. 2008;26(29):4714–9.

154. Kloos RT, Ringel MD, Knopp MV, et al. Phase II trial of sorafenib in metastatic thyroid cancer. J Clin Oncol. 2009;27(10):1675–84.

155. Nagaiah G, Fu P, Wasman JK, et al. Phase II trial of sorafenib (bay 43–9006) in patients with advanced anaplastic carcinoma of the thyroid (ATC). Proc Am Soc Clin Oncol. 2009;27(15):6058.

156. Pazaitou-Panayiotou K, Capezzone M, Pacini F. Clinical features and therapeutic implication of papillary thyroid microcarcinoma. Thyroid. 2007; 17(11):1085–92.

157. Reddy RM, Grigsby PW, Moley JF, et al. Lymph node metastases in differentiated thyroid cancer under 2cm. Surgery. 2006;140(6):1050–5.

158. Wada N, Duh QY, Sugino K, et al. Lymph node metastasis from 259 papillary thyroid microcarcinomas: frequency, pattern of occurrence and recurrence, and optimal strategy for neck dissection. Ann Surg. 2003;237:399–407.

159. Roti E, Rossi R, Trasforini G, et al. Clinical and histological characteristics of papillary thyroid microcarcinoma: results of a retrospective study in 243 patients. J Clin Endocrinol Metab. 2006;91: 2171–8.

160. Chow SM, Law SC, Chan JK, et al. Papillary microcarcinoma of the thyroid-prognostic significance of lymph node metastasis and multifocality. Cancer. 2003;98(1):31–40.

161. Baudin E, Travagli JP, Ropers J, et al. Microcarcinoma of the thyroid gland: the Gustave-Roussy Institute experience. Cancer. 1998;83(3):553–9.

162. Pellegriti G, Scollo C, Lumera G, et al. Clinical behavior and outcome of papillary thyroid cancers smaller than 1.5cm in diameter: study of 299 cases. J Clin Endocrinol Metab. 2004;89:3713–20.

163. Sellers M, Beenken S, Blankenship A, et al. Prognostic significance of cervical lymph node metastases in differentiated thyroid cancer. Am J Surg. 1992;164:578–81.

164. Podnos YD, Smith D, Wagman LD, Ellenhorn JD. The implication of lymph node metastasis on survival in patients with well-differentiated thyroid cancer. Am Surg. 2005;71:731–4.

165. Kobayashi T, Asakawa H, Komoike Y, et al. Characteristics and prognostic factors in patients with differentiated thyroid cancer who underwent a total or subtotal thyroidectomy: surgical approach for high-risk patients. Surg Today. 1999;29: 200–3.

166. Pacini F, Elisei R, Capezzone M, et al. Contralateral papillary thyroid cancer is frequent at completion thyroidectomy with no difference in low- and high-risk patients. Thyroid. 2001;11(9):877–81.

167. Hay ID, Hutchinson ME, Gonzalez-Losada T, et al. Papillary thyroid microcarcinoma: a study of 900 cases observed in a 60-year period. Surgery. 2008; 144(6):980–8.

168. Mazzaferri EL. Management of low-risk differentiated thyroid cancer. Endocr Pract. 2007;13(5): 498–512.

169. Ito Y, Uruno T, Nakano K, et al. An observation trial without surgical treatment in patients with papillary microcarcinoma of the thyroid. Thyroid. 2003;13: 381–7.

170. Tan GH, Gharib H, Goellner JR, et al. Management of thyroid nodules in pregnancy. Arch Intern Med. 1996;156:2317–20.

171. Yasmeen S, Cress R, Romano PS, et al. Thyroid cancer in pregnancy. Int J Gynaecol Obstet. 2005; 91(1):15–20.

172. Moosa M, Mazzaferri EL. Outcome of differentiated thyroid cancer diagnosed in pregnant women. J Clin Endocrinol Metab. 1997;82:2862–6.

173. Herzon FS, Morris DM, Segal MN, et al. Coexistent thyroid cancer and pregnancy. Arch Otolaryngol Head Neck Surg. 1994;120:1191–3.

174. Mestman JH, Goodwin TM, Montoro MM. Thyroid disorders of pregnancy. Endocrinol Metab Clin North Am. 1995;24:41–71.

175. Nam KH, Yoon JH, Chang HS, et al. Optimal timing of surgery in well-differentiated thyroid carcinoma detected during pregnancy. J Surg Oncol. 2005;91: 199–203.

176. Vini L, Hyer S, Pratt B, et al. Management of differentiated thyroid cancer diagnosed during pregnancy. Eur J Endocrinol. 1999;140:404–6.

177. Rosen IB, Korman M, Walfish PG. Thyroid nodular disease in pregnancy: current diagnosis and management. Clin Obstet Gynecol. 1997;40:81–9.

178. Leboeuf R, Emerick LE, Martorella AJ, et al. Impact of pregnancy on serum thyroglobulin and detection of recurrent disease shortly after delivery in thyroid cancer survivors. Thyroid. 2007;17(6):543–7.

179. Reis LAG, Melbert D, Krapcho M, et al. Seer cancer statistics review, 1975–2006. Bethesda, MD: National Cancer Institute; 2007.

180. Altekruse SF, Kosary CL, Krapcho M, et al. SEER Cancer Statistics Review, 1975–2007, National Cancer Institute. Bethesda, MD, http://seer.cancer.gov/csr/1975_2007/, based on November 2009 SEER data submission, posted to the SEER web site, 2010.

181. Hung W. Solitary thyroid nodules in 93 children and adolescents, a 35-year experience. Horm Res. 1999; 52:15–8.

182. Gharib H, Papini E. Thyroid nodules: clinical importance, assessment, and treatment. Endocrinol Metab Clin North Am. 2007;36:707–35.

183. Hung W, Sarlis NJ. Current controversies in the management of pediatric patients with well-differentiated nonmedullary thyroid cancer: a review. Thyroid. 2002;12(8):683–702.

184. Maule M, Scelo G, Pastore G, et al. Risk of second malignant neoplasms after childhood leukemia and lymphoma: an international study. J Natl Cancer Inst. 2007;99:790–800.

185. Tucker MA, Jones PH, Boice JD, et al. Therapeutic radiation at a young age is linked to secondary thyroid cancer. The Late Effects Study Group. Cancer Res. 1991;51:2885–8.

186. Dinauer CA, Francis GL. Thyroid Cancer in Children. Endocrinol Metab Clin North Am. 2007; 36:779–806.

187. Dinauer CA, Breuer C, Rivkees SA. Differentiated thyroid cancer in children: diagnosis and management. Curr Opin Oncol. 2008;20:59–65.

188. Welch Dinauer CA, Tuttle RM, Robie DK, et al. Clinical features associated with metastasis and recurrence of differentiated thyroid cancer in children, adolescents, and young adults. Clin Endocrinol. 1998;49:619–28.

189. Reiners C, Demidchik YE. Differentiated thyroid cancer in childhood: pathology, diagnosis, therapy. Pediatr Endocrinol Rev. 2003;1 Suppl 2:230–5.

190. Chaukar DA, Rangarajan V, Nair N, et al. Pediatric thyroid cancer. J Surg Oncol. 2005;92:130–3.

191. Okada T, Sasaki F, Takahashi H, et al. Management of childhood and adolescent thyroid carcinoma: long-term follow-up and clinical characteristics. Eur J Pediatr Surg. 2006;16:8–13.

192. Rachmiel M, Charron A, Gupta A, et al. Evidence-based review of treatment and follow up of pediatric patients with differentiated thyroid carcinoma. J Pediatr Endocrinol Metab. 2006;19:1377–93.

193. Parisi MT, Mankoff D. Differentiated pediatric thyroid cancer: correlates with adult disease, controversies in treatment. Semin Nucl Med. 2007;37: 340–56.

194. Borson-Chazot F, Causeret S, Lifante JC, et al. Predictive factors for recurrence from a series of 74 children and adolescents with differentiated thyroid cancer. World J Surg. 2004;28:1088–92.

195. Handkiewicz-Junak D, Wloch J, Roskosz J, et al. Total thyroidectomy and adjuvant radioiodine treatment independently decrease locoregional recurrence risk in childhood and adolescent differentiated thyroid cancer. J Nucl Med. 2007;48:879–88.

196. Chow SM, Law SCK, Mendenhall WM, et al. Differentiated thyroid carcinoma in childhood and adolescence – clinical course and role of radioiodine. Pediatr Blood Cancer. 2004;42:176–83.

197. Ron E, Lubin JH, Shore RE, et al. Thyroid cancer after exposure to external radiation: a pooled analysis of seven studies. Radiat Res. 1995;141(3): 259–77.

198. Foteini P, Efthimiou E. Thyroid cancer after external or internal ionizing irradiation. Hell J Nucl Med. 2009;12(3):266–70.

199. Shore RE. Issues and epidemiological evidence regarding radiation-induced thyroid cancer. Radiat Res. 1992;131:98–111.

200. Dottorini ME, Vignati A, Mazzucchelli L, et al. Differentiated thyroid carcinoma in children and adolescents: a 37-year experience in 85 patients. J Nucl Med. 1998;39:1531–6.

201. Heidenreich WF, Kenigsberg J, Jacob P, et al. Time trends of thyroid cancer incidence in Belarus after the Chernobyl accident. Radiat Res. 1999;151: 617–25.

202. Ron E, Modan B, Preston D, et al. Thyroid neoplasia following low-dose radiation in childhood. Radiat Res. 1989;120(3):516–31.

Follicular Thyroid Carcinoma

8

Jerome Hershman and Adam Lyko

Introduction

Thyroid cancers are classified into four major histopathologic entities: papillary, follicular, medullary, and anaplastic carcinomas. Papillary and follicular thyroid carcinomas are called differentiated thyroid cancers because the cells resemble normal thyroid cells histologically. In many reports, they are grouped together. This chapter will focus on the evaluation and management of follicular thyroid carcinoma that has a unique pathophysiology which differs from that of papillary thyroid cancer. Follicular thyroid carcinoma is defined pathologically as a malignant tumor of the follicular thyroid cells with histopathological characteristics of capsular and vascular invasion [1]. These features differentiate it from follicular adenoma. The follicular thyroid carcinoma is composed of well-differentiated follicular epithelial cells that lack nuclear features of papillary carcinoma. Two variants of follicular carcinoma include the Hurthle cell cancer and insular carcinoma and will also be discussed here [2].

Hurthle cell carcinoma is a follicular cell tumor that contains greater than 75% oncocytic cells and shows capsular or vascular invasion [3, 4].

Survival of patients with Hurthle cell carcinoma is intermediate between follicular carcinoma and the high-grade anaplastic thyroid cancers [5, 6].

Insular thyroid cancer is a poorly differentiated variant of follicular thyroid cancer with an even more aggressive course than Hurthle cell cancer.

Incidence and Epidemiology

Thyroid cancer makes up 2.5% of all cancers and is the most common malignancy of the endocrine system [2, 7, 8]. Approximately 141,000 new cases of follicular carcinomas occur yearly worldwide and account for 0.5% of all cancer deaths [9]. Follicular thyroid carcinoma is the second most common thyroid carcinoma after papillary thyroid cancer, and comprises approximately 10–15% of all thyroid cancers in iodine-replete regions [10]. In areas of iodine deficiency, the incidence of follicular thyroid cancer is much higher and can reach up to 30–40% of all thyroid cancers [11, 12].

The incidence of follicular thyroid carcinoma in the United States has remained relatively stable over the last 30 years in contrast to the overall thyroid cancer incidence which has risen from 3.6 to 8.7 per 100,000 between 1973 and 2002 while the mortality has remained stable at 0.5 per 100,000 [13]. Although the rise in the overall incidence of thyroid cancer can be explained by the increasing detection of small papillary thyroid cancers as a result of more frequent use of medical imaging [14, 15], recent examinations of

J. Hershman (✉) • A. Lyko
Divisions of Endocrinology, Diabetes and Metabolism,
Greater Los Angeles VA and Cedars–Sinai Medical Center,
Endocrinology 111D, Los Angeles, CA 90073, USA
e-mail: jhershmn@ucla.edu

G.D. Braunstein (ed.), *Thyroid Cancer*, Endocrine Updates 30,
DOI 10.1007/978-1-4614-0875-8_8, © Springer Science+Business Media, LLC 2012

a US database show that there is an increase in the incidence of papillary thyroid carcinoma of all sizes in both sexes and various races [15, 16]. Although there may be a trend for increase of follicular cancers, the number is not sufficient to be statistically significant [15]. Minimally invasive follicular thyroid carcinoma has been reported to comprise less than 2% of all thyroid malignancies [17].

The mean age at diagnosis of follicular thyroid carcinoma is in the 6th decade. Follicular thyroid cancer is more common in women than in men with a ratio of 2:1 [3]. In a national surgical database of 6,764 patients with follicular thyroid carcinoma, the 5-year survival rate was 91% and the 10-year survival rate was 85% [10].

Hurthle cell and insular carcinomas carry a worse prognosis than well-differentiated follicular thyroid cancer. In the national surgical database of 1585 patients with Hurthle cell carcinoma, the 5-year survival rate was 91% and the 10-year survival rate was 76% [10]. In a series of 740 thyroid carcinomas, insular thyroid carcinomas comprised 3% and had a 10-year survival rate of 42% [6].

Pathogenesis

Environmental, genetic, and hormonal factors have been implicated in the pathogenesis of follicular thyroid carcinoma. Environmental factors include iodine deficiency as well as ionizing radiation, although radiation exposure confers a much greater risk for papillary thyroid carcinoma than for follicular carcinoma [2, 18]. Chronic TSH elevation has been linked to malignant transformation of follicular cells in a mouse model of thyroid cancer in which the mice had a homozygous mutation of the thyroid hormone beta receptor and developed thyroid cancers with loss of negative feedback resulting in very high serum TSH levels [19]. A family history of thyroid cancer as well as chronic lymphocytic thyroiditis have also been reported as risk factors for follicular thyroid carcinoma [20].

Follicular thyroid carcinoma is thought by some to develop from follicular adenoma [2].

Mutations of the RAS proto-oncogene have been linked to follicular thyroid carcinoma in up to 80% of follicular tumors [21]. The presence of the RAS mutation does not differentiate follicular carcinoma from follicular adenoma but is thought to be an important step in the transformation of follicular cells into carcinoma [22]. RAS mutations are more common in iodine-deficient areas [20].

Another pathogenic genetic mutation reported in follicular thyroid cancer is the PAX8/PPAR-γ rearrangement first reported by Kroll [23]. PPARγ (peroxisome proliferator-activated receptor gamma) is a member of the steroid thyroid nuclear receptor family, and PAX8 is a transcription factor that is essential for normal thyroid gland development [24]. The translocation of t(2;3)(q13;p25) generates a chimeric gene encoding the DNA-binding domain for the thyroid specific transcription factor PAX8 and domains A–F of PPARγ, resulting in an oncoprotein that contributes to malignant transformation of follicular thyroid cells [20, 24]. The RAS mutation and the PAX8/PPARγ rearrangement are the two best examples of different molecular pathways through which follicular thyroid carcinomas can develop [22].

Hurthle cell adenomas and carcinomas, in contrast to differentiated follicular thyroid carcinoma, have a very low frequency of either RAS mutations or PAX8-PPARγ rearrangement, suggesting that they represent a distinct type of thyroid neoplasm [22].

Follicular thyroid carcinoma and follicular adenoma are associated with Cowden syndrome characterized by mutations in the PTEN gene [2, 20, 25]. Insular thyroid carcinoma has also been reported in Cowden syndrome [26]. Cowden syndrome is an autosomal-dominant syndrome caused by germline mutations of the tumor suppressor gene phosphate and tensin homolog (PTEN) located on chromosome 10 [27]. It is characterized by the formation of benign and malignant hamartomas and is the prototype of the PTEN hamartoma tumor syndrome first described in 1963 [28]. Hypermethylation of the PTEN gene is associated with activation of the PI3K/AKT signaling pathway and is thought to promote the development of follicular and anaplastic thyroid carcinomas and breast cancer [29].

Pathology

Follicular thyroid carcinoma is classified into two types: minimally invasive and widely invasive. Minimally invasive carcinoma is characterized by a follicular patterned lesion surrounded by a capsule with associated tumor capsule invasion with full-thickness capsule penetration but not penetration of tumor into surrounding thyroid parenchyma [11]. Small to medium vessel invasion by tumor can be present in the capsule or just outside the capsule [30]. Widely invasive follicular carcinoma shows evidence of capsule penetration with thyroid parenchyma invasion and gross vascular invasion [1] (Fig. 8.1).

Hurthle cell carcinoma is presently classified as a variant of follicular cell carcinoma [31]. This tumor is characterized by oncocytic cells with abundant eosinophilic cytoplasm, abnormal mitochondria which fill the cytoplasm, scant or no colloid, occasional calcifications, and large eosinophilic nucleoli [3]. Diagnosis of Hurthle cell carcinoma requires 75% or more of the follicular tumor cells to be composed of Hurthle cells accompanied by full-thickness capsular invasion and/or vascular invasion [3, 4]. Hurthle cell carcinomas differ from follicular cell carcinomas in that they tend to take up radioactive iodine less often, are more likely to involve cervical lymph nodes, be multifocal or bilateral, and more often have distant metastases on presenta-

tion [32]. Lymph node metastatases can be present in up to 30% of Hurthle cell carcinoma cases [33]. Although management of Hurthle cell carcinomas is the same as that for follicular thyroid carcinomas, Hurthle cell carcinomas represent a distinct clinical entity [34, 35].

Insular carcinoma is a variant of follicular carcinoma that is much more aggressive. Its cardinal features include a tumor cell population arranged in solid nests of small, uniform carcinoma cells or islands of cells separated by a thin, fibrovascular stroma and clefts. There are small follicles containing thyroglobulin and frequent occurrence of necrotic foci. In a report of 183 patients with poorly differentiated thyroid carcinoma, 85% had follicular features [36]. Insular carcinoma made up 50% of the patients, while the other 50% had a solid, uniform, trabecular, or alveolar pattern. Insular carcinoma has a prognosis that is intermediate between differentiated thyroid cancer and anaplastic thyroid cancer. These patients are more likely to have multifocal and bilateral tumors and lymph node involvement than patients with typical follicular thyroid cancer [37].

Follicular variant of papillary carcinoma is defined as a thyroid malignancy with a predominant or exclusive follicular growth pattern displaying the characteristic nuclear features of papillary thyroid carcinoma such as cytoplasmic invaginations with pseudonuclear inclusions, abundant nuclear grooves, and ground glass nuclei

a

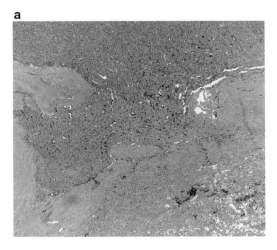

b

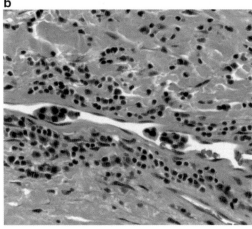

Fig. 8.1 Histopathology of widely invasive follicular thyroid carcinoma with (**a**) capsular invasion and (**b**) vascular invasion

[38]. Follicular variant of papillary carcinoma is classified with papillary thyroid cancer and managed similarly [11]. Older studies may have erroneously considered these cases to be follicular thyroid cancers.

Clinical Features

Approximately 5% of incidentally found thyroid nodules harbor thyroid cancer of which follicular carcinoma is a small minority [39]. Currently, thyroid nodules are most commonly found incidentally, usually as a result of neck imaging studies. Thyroid nodules are very common and present in up to 67% of the general population [40, 41]. The incidence increases with age. A thyroid nodule can be self-diagnosed as a lump in the neck and brought to the attention of the physician, or can be found on routine physical examination. Thyroid nodules are usually asymptomatic. Nodular goiter may cause compressive symptoms including change in voice, dysphagia, cough, pain, or a feeling of pressure in the neck [7]. Clinically, follicular carcinoma presents as a thyroid mass, usually measuring more than 2 cm [1]. Follicular carcinoma most commonly spreads hematogenously, although about 5% of cases may present with metastases to cervical lymph nodes [20]. Approximately 20% of follicular carcinomas present with distant metastatic disease, most commonly to bone and lung [20]. A history of exposure to ionizing radiation, family history of thyroid disease, male sex, and older age increase the risk of thyroid malignancy [7, 42].

Ultrasonography is very helpful in FNA guidance as well as in determination of size and characteristics of thyroid nodules [43]. Ultrasound findings that may indicate a higher risk of malignancy include intrinsic calcification, blurred or ill-defined margin, hypervascularity, or hypoechoic features [44].

Diagnosis

Fine-needle aspiration (FNA) biopsy is the most useful diagnostic test in the evaluation of a thyroid nodule suspected to harbor thyroid cancer [39].

FNA of thyroid nodules has been accepted as a first-line screening test for thyroid carcinoma [42]. It should be performed on nodules >1 cm; however, in patients with symptoms, lymphadenopathy, or history of external radiation to the neck [7], nodules larger than 5 mm should be considered for FNA. Yang et al. report the sensitivity and specificity of FNA for thyroid malignancy of 94 and 98.5% and for thyroid neoplasm of 89.3 and 74%, respectively, in a review of 4,703 thyroid FNA samples [45]. Follicular thyroid carcinoma cannot usually be reliably distinguished from follicular adenoma based on FNA cytology due to the need to show capsular and vascular invasion in follicular carcinoma that is possible only with histopathology but not with cytology [45]. This difficulty results in surgeries for benign disease in approximately 42–77% of thyroid nodules which turn out to be follicular adenoma or hyperplastic colloid nodules on histopathology [46]. In contrast, some cytopathologists believe that the FNA can often differentiate benign from follicular lesions [47]. When the cytologic diagnosis is indeterminate, often called follicular lesion or, recently, follicular lesion of undetermined significance (FLUS), patients are often referred for thyroidectomy, but many endocrinologists use other parameters, such as age, sex, family history, size of nodule, and ultrasound features, to determine whether to refer the patient for surgery or follow the patient with observation alone at intervals of 6–12 months. For example, a nodule over 4 cm in a man of age 50 would be more worrisome, and a nodule of 1.5 cm in a 35-year-old woman would be less likely to be a carcinoma.

Although not used yet in routine clinical practice, genetic, molecular, and immunohistologic markers may allow for distinguishing follicular thyroid cancer from adenoma on FNA cytology [48, 49]. One example is the PAX8-PPARγ rearrangement which is thought to be a strong indicator of follicular carcinoma [22]. Another example is the expression of HBME-1 in follicular carcinomas with RAS mutations [22]. Galectin-3, a β-galactoside-binding protein, has been shown to cause malignant transformation of thyroid cells in vitro and has also been studied as a molecular marker of follicular and papillary carcinoma [50].

Bartolazzi et al. performed immunohistochemical analysis in 465 FNA cytology specimens in a multicenter prospective study [51]. They found a sensitivity of 78% and a specificity of 93% for the diagnosis of cancer, but 22% of cancers were missed by this test. In conjunction with another immunohistochemical marker, HBME-1, galectin-3 has been evaluated in differentiating benign from malignant follicular thyroid carcinoma FNA samples [52]. Molecular markers may be very helpful for evaluating indeterminate FNA results [53–55]. Additionally, microRNA studies have shown two specific microRNAs, 197 and 346, to be significantly overexpressed in follicular thyroid carcinomas [56].

In a series of 1,121 patients undergoing FNA, 103 patients were referred for thyroidectomy due to FNA showing an indeterminate follicular neoplasm of which 21% were confirmed to have a malignancy [57]. Surgery is generally recommended for lesions classified as suspicious or indeterminate; patients with benign FNA results can be followed by repeated ultrasound evaluations at intervals of 1 year [7]. If there is significant growth, the FNA should be repeated. Repeat biopsy is essential for nondiagnostic biopsies [7].

FNA has also been used to detect metastatic disease to lymph nodes. In particular, the detection of thyroglobulin in FNA material from lymph nodes has been found to be an extremely useful and sensitive test for detection of metastatic follicular thyroid carcinoma [58].

Nuclear scintigraphy with radioiodine-^{123}I has also been useful in the evaluation of thyroid nodules because nodules with active uptake are less likely to be malignant [59]. In nodules diagnosed as follicular lesions, radioiodine scans are indicated in the setting of low TSH; if the scan shows that the nodule is "hot," the diagnosis of malignancy is very unlikely.

Measurement of serum TSH level should be performed in all patients with thyroid nodules. A suppressed serum TSH suggests that the nodule may be functional; a radioiodine scan showing that the nodule concentrates radioiodine precludes the need for performing an FNA unless there are definite suggestions of malignancy by a previously performed ultrasound study [60]. Recently, several studies suggest that the height of the serum TSH, even in the normal range, correlates with the diagnosis of malignancy [61–64].

Staging of Follicular Thyroid Cancer

Most staging systems for prognosis of differentiated thyroid cancer included both papillary thyroid cancer and follicular thyroid cancer as a single entity [65]. The much higher proportion of papillary thyroid cancer, more than 80 percent of the cases, probably biased the results. Recently, several studies have applied these staging systems to patients with follicular thyroid cancer to stratify patients into risk groups based on a number of factors. D'Avanzo et al. in San Francisco selected 86 patients with follicular thyroid cancer treated between 1954 and 1998 to compare the results of five staging systems and rate each based on the proportion of explained variance in survival, PVE [66]. Patients with Hurthle cell cancers were excluded. Median follow-up was 11.5 years. All systems were significant predictors of survival. They found that the MACIS system of the Mayo Clinic that scored metastasis, age, completeness of resection, invasion, size was the best predictor (PVE 48%), and the TNM (tumor, node, metastasis) system of the American Joint Committee on Cancer/Union International Centre Cancer, 5th edition, was the worst predictive system (PVE 33%).

Lang et al. in Hong Kong evaluated 14 different staging systems in 171 patients with follicular thyroid cancer who were mainly Chinese [67]. Sixty-one patients had minimally invasive cancer, 26 had angioinvasive cancer, and 84 had widely invasive cancer; 13% had Hurthle cell cancer. Median follow-up was 12 years. PVE was highest for the TNM system (6th edition of the American Joint Committee on Cancer/Union International Centre Cancer) 22.4% (Table 8.1). The clinical class system of the University of Chicago [68] was second with PVE of 21.2%. This system is simple: class 1 is disease limited to the thyroid gland; class 2 is locoregional lymph node involvement; class 3 is extrathyroid tumor invasion; and class 4 is distant metastases. The complex MACIS system was third with a PVE of 20.4%. The recently revised guidelines of the

Table 8.1 Cancer-specific survival of follicular thyroid carcinoma

Staging	Patients	Deaths	5 year (%)	10 year (%)	15 year (%)
TNM	171	20			
I	94	2	97.5	97.5	97.5
II	25	2	96.4	90.8	90.8
III	27	3	95.8	82.4	82.4
IVA	6	1	100.0	80.0	80.0
IVB	1	1	0.00	0.00	0.00
IVC	18	11	60.4	40.3	40.3

From Lang et al. [67] Reproduced with permission

American Thyroid Association recommended that all patients with differentiated thyroid cancer be staged by the TNM, 6th edition [69].

In a tabulation of 13 series that included 623 patients with histologic staging showing minimally invasive follicular thyroid carcinoma, the recurrence rate ranged from 5 to 43% and the death rate ranged from 2 to 43% [66]. In seven series that included 365 patients with widely invasive follicular thyroid carcinoma, the recurrence rate was 65% and the death rate was 53% [66].

Therapy

Surgical Treatment of Follicular Thyroid Carcinoma

For patients with a diagnosis of follicular thyroid cancer based on FNA and imaging characteristics, a complete or near-complete thyroidectomy is the procedure of choice (Fig. 8.2). In patients with widely invasive follicular thyroid cancer, ipsilateral dissection of the central and possibly the lateral cervical compartments is also recommended [70]. In contrast, for patients with minimally invasive follicular thyroid carcinoma, a near-total thyroidectomy or lobectomy is probably sufficient without dissection of lymph nodes.

In many patients with the diagnosis of follicular thyroid neoplasm based on FNA, lobectomy or subtotal thyroidectomy is appropriate. When the final pathologic diagnosis is follicular thyroid cancer, or follicular variant of papillary thyroid cancer, completion thyroidectomy is usually advised, preferably within one week of the original surgery, although it can also be performed

several weeks later after healing has occurred. This scenario occurs in 10–30% of patients with follicular thyroid neoplasms. In order to avoid second operations, some surgeons recommend that the first operation is a total or near-total thyroidectomy, even though the diagnosis of follicular thyroid carcinoma is not likely beforehand. For patients with minimal capsular invasion, thyroid lobectomy provides definitive treatment because these patients usually have an excellent prognosis. For patients with angioinvasion, with or without capsular invasion, complete thyroidectomy is indicated because these patients have a moderate prognosis with 10-year survival of about 75% [66]. Because Hurthle cell carcinomas are more aggressive, complete thyroidectomy with nodal dissection is indicated because these patients are also more likely to have lymph node involvement. However, because most Hurthle cell lesions are adenomas rather than carcinomas, many patients will have lobectomy followed by completion thyroidectomy for Hurthle cell cancers determined by permanent sections. Most surgeons are more likely to employ complete thyroidectomy as the initial surgery for lesions over 4 cm because this increases the possibility of malignancy.

In one series of 65 patients, 32 had an initial lobectomy followed by completion total thyroidectomy in 25 patients after a median duration of 7 weeks following the initial surgery; total thyroidectomy was performed in 15 patients; and subtotal thyroidectomy was performed in 11 patients followed by reoperation in two [71]. Intraoperative frozen section, performed in 39 patients, yielded a correct diagnosis of follicular thyroid cancer in only three patients (8%), whereas

Flow diagram for the management of follicular thyroid lesion and follicular thyroid carcinoma

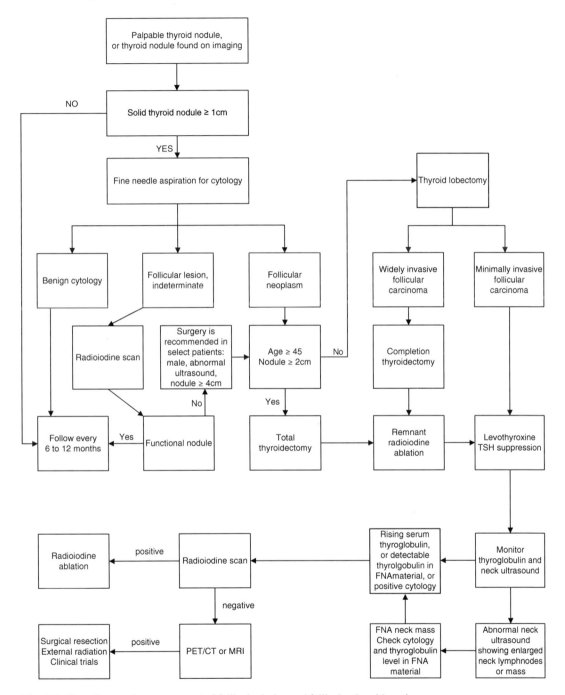

Fig. 8.2 Flow diagram for management of follicular lesion and follicular thyroid carcinoma

it was as high as 50% in a smaller series [72]. Permanent complications of surgery occurred in 3% of patients [71].

In another series of 207 patients with follicular thyroid carcinoma, 113 (54.6%) underwent total thyroidectomy, 16 (7.7%) underwent near-total thyroidectomy, and 56 (27.1%) underwent completion thyroidectomy [70]. Minimally invasive thyroid carcinoma was found in 127 (61.4%) patients and widely invasive cancer was found in 80 (38.6%) of patients [70]. In the minimally invasive group, 12 (9.4%) patients had distant metastases at time of diagnosis compared with 30 (37.5%) patients in the widely invasive group, and six (5.2%) patients in the minimally invasive group developed distant metastases compared to 16 (32%) patients in the widely invasive group during the follow-up period [70]. All patients with minimally invasive follicular carcinoma who developed distant metastases were more than 45 years old [70]. The 10-year cancer-specific survival was 93.5% for the minimally invasive group compared to 53.6% in the widely invasive group. The majority of patients in the widely invasive group (92.5%) were >45 years old.

The principal complications of thyroidectomy include hypoparathyroidism and recurrent laryngeal nerve paralysis. Both occur in approximately 1% of patients when the surgery is performed by experienced neck surgeons and are more likely to occur if patients undergo central lymph node dissection. On the other hand, if patients have central neck recurrences that are treated by second surgeries in the same area, the incidence of these complications is considerably higher.

Radioiodine Therapy

Follicular thyroid carcinoma usually has functional sodium/iodide symporter activity that concentrates iodide in the cancer cells. Radioiodine (^{131}I) has been used as adjunctive therapy in the management of differentiated thyroid carcinoma for more than 50 years. The objective of the treatment with radioiodine is to destroy all functioning thyroid cancer tissue. Radioiodine-131 is given to most patients with follicular thyroid carcinoma after thyroidectomy to ablate residual normal thyroid tissue and to destroy the follicular thyroid cancer cells that may remain after surgery. The treatment is not indicated for patients with minimally invasive follicular cancer, but is worthwhile in those with angioinvasion, even in patients with small tumors, because they are predisposed to distant metastases. Although Hurthle cell cancer is less likely than follicular cancer to take up 131I, there are reports of uptake in Hurthle cell cancer [73]. Details of radioiodine therapy are discussed in Chap. 13.

Radioiodine ablative therapy is usually given 6–12 weeks postoperatively. Patients are prepared for 131I ablative therapy by one of two methods currently. After surgery, they are given replacement triiodothyronine for at least 4 weeks that is then withdrawn for two weeks during which the patient follows a low-iodine diet [74]. The goal of the withdrawal is to elevate the serum TSH above 30 mU/L. The ablative dose of 50–100 mCi (1.9–3.8 GBq) is then given. Triiodothyronine is used because it is cleared from the body much more rapidly than T4. The shorter period of withdrawal minimizes the period of hypothyroidism. The patient can be started on a suppressive dose of levothyroxine 48 hours after the radioiodine therapy. In the second method of ablation, the patient starts levothyroxine therapy after surgery and continues it during the radioiodine therapy. Recombinant human TSH is given to stimulate the uptake of the ^{131}I; patients also follow the low-iodine diet for 10–14 days before receiving the ablative dose. A randomized controlled study showed that preparation with thyroid hormone withdrawal or recombinant human TSH gave similar results of successful ablation [75]. Using recombinant TSH to stimulate uptake spares the patient from two weeks of symptoms of hypothyroidism. Four to seven days after the ablative dose, a scan is performed to determine whether there are areas of uptake outside the thyroid bed that are indicative of metastatic disease.

Radioiodine-131 is also used for treatment of metastatic disease. The efficacy of radioiodine therapy is directly related to tumor uptake and retention. Effective tumor uptake is approximately 0.5 % of the radioiodine dose per gram with a biologic half-life of approximately four days. From the administration of 5.6 gigabecquerel (GBq; equivalent to 150 millicuries) of 131I, a tumor may receive as much as 25,000 cGy or four times the absorbed dose that can be delivered by a course of external radiation therapy. Moreover, this dose will be delivered to every functional metastasis, regardless of its size or location in the body, and tumor tissue will receive several hundred times the radiation exposure received by the rest of the body. The treatment is most effective when imaging studies show disappearance of the metastases, but this is not likely to be achieved if there is a large amount of tumor. For example, patients with excellent survival after treatment for pulmonary metastases have tumors that show up on scans but may not show up on chest X-rays. A negative scan after therapy indicates a better prognosis, while a positive scan bodes a poor prognosis [76].

External Beam Radiation Therapy

External beam radiation therapy is used for patients with gross residual disease after thyroidectomy and for recurrent neck disease that cannot be resected and does not take up radioiodine. The series of patients with differentiated thyroid cancer treated by this modality contain many more patients with papillary thyroid cancer and poorly differentiated tumors than those with follicular thyroid cancer. Schwartz et al. reported the results of a therapy for 131 patients, including 25% with follicular or Hurthle cell cancer over a 10-year period [77]. At 4 years, locoregional relapse-free survival was 79% and disease-specific survival was 73%. Patients with high-risk pathology, distant metastases, and gross residual disease had inferior survival. Terezakis et al. reported a series of 76 patients treated during 17 years; the number with follicular cancer was not stated but four had Hurthle cell cancer. The 4-year overall locoregional control rate for all histologic types was 72% and the 4-year overall survival rate for all patients was 55% [78]. In

these recent series, patients received 60 Gray radiation to the tumor. Intensity-modulated radiotherapy was used to diminish dangerous side effects.

Suppression of TSH

Suppression of thyrotropin is indicated following initial therapy for follicular thyroid carcinoma [79]. Patients at low risk for recurrence of thyroid cancer do not require TSH suppression to the same degree as is required for patients at high risk for recurrence [80]. Cooper et al. conducted a registry study looking at the degree of TSH suppression and progression of disease in 617 cases of papillary thyroid carcinoma and 66 cases of follicular thyroid carcinoma and found a significant benefit in proportion to the degree of TSH suppression in higher stages of differentiated thyroid carcinoma; however, a separate multivariate analysis of follicular tumors could not be done due to the low number of cases [81]. Other studies that analyzed follicular together with papillary thyroid carcinoma cases have concluded that high-risk patients benefit from more aggressive TSH suppression than lower-risk patients [82, 83]. Current ATA guidelines recommend suppression of TSH to <0.1 mU/L in the high-risk patients while keeping TSH in the 0.1–0.5 mU/L range in low-risk patients [69]. Monitoring for adverse effects of thyrotoxicosis and making adjustments based on consideration of the risk/benefit ratio is advisable in all patients on TSH suppressive therapy, especially in the elderly and postmenopausal patients [84]. TSH suppression to a level of 0.1–0.3 mU/L has been reported to minimize the risk of iatrogenic thyrotoxicosis [85].

Follow-Up

Patients with a history of follicular thyroid carcinoma require lifelong follow-up because of the possibility of late recurrence of the cancer. Following initial therapy with surgery followed by radioiodine ablation, patients should be seen at intervals of 4–6 months for 5–10 years and then followed on an annual basis. History should include careful questioning regarding pulmonary symptoms or skeletal pain. Physical examination should focus on neck palpation. Laboratory testing includes measurement of serum TSH and thyroglobulin levels. Ultrasonography is the most sensitive test for evaluation of neck lymph node metastases. It is recommended that patients have a TSH-stimulated serum thyroglobulin measurement (with or without a radioiodine whole-body scan) 1 year after the ablative dose of ^{131}I-iodine. If this is negative, then patients do not have to undergo repeated TSH-stimulated scans or thyroglobulin measurements. Radioiodine uptake scans do not need to be done as long as thyroglobulin levels remain undetectable [69].

Detection of Recurrent Disease

Radioiodine whole-body scans have been used for detection of metastatic disease; however, this modality may not detect metastatic disease in tumors which do not take up iodine. Thyroglobulin levels have become much more sensitive in detecting follicular thyroid cancer recurrence than ^{131}I uptake scans [86]. In patients with significantly elevated serum thyroglobulin levels and negative radioiodine scans, other imaging modalities are used for finding the recurrence. These include magnetic resonance imaging, computed tomography, and positron emission tomography.

Treatment of Metastatic Disease

Most studies that evaluate therapy for metastatic thyroid cancer combine follicular carcinoma with papillary carcinoma [76, 87, 88]. Follicular thyroid carcinoma most commonly spreads via the hematogenous route to the bones and lungs, and less often to the brain, liver, adrenal glands, or soft tissues [89]. In a series of 448 patients with follicular thyroid carcinoma, distant metastases were present in 25% of the cases [90]. Shaha et al. reported that 10.5% of follicular thyroid carcino-

mas and 12.2% of Hurthle cell carcinomas present initially with metastatic disease [91].

Sampson et al. have noted a 3-year survival rate of 62% for follicular thyroid cancer patients with initial metastatic disease at presentation compared to 75% for papillary thyroid cancer [92]. The major factors that determined prognosis were age at presentation, site of metastasis, histology, and iodine avidity.

Distant metastatic disease is the most frequent cause of thyroid cancer-related death [76]. The most common immediate causes of death from metastatic follicular thyroid carcinoma are respiratory insufficiency in 46%, airway obstruction in 15%, and circulatory failure in 15% of the cases [93].

Treatment of metastatic disease must be individualized. Modalities include total thyroidectomy, ^{131}I therapy, external beam radiation, surgical metastasectomy, and chemotherapy. Patients who have not had total thyroidectomy need to undergo total thyroidectomy to improve effectiveness of radioiodine therapy and detection of metastases by radioiodine scans, based on the premise that the normal thyroid will concentrate the radioiodine much more avidly than the metastatic thyroid cancer. When the normal thyroid has been completely removed, the serum thyroglobulin levels can be used reliably for detection of metastatic disease [92].

Although there is no clearly defined upper limit to the dose of ^{131}I that can be given, the risk of developing other cancers, including leukemia, becomes significant at doses greater than 600 mCi [76]. In a study of 312 patients in China with differentiated thyroid cancer, of which 62 had follicular carcinoma, the mean cumulative radiation dose was 2,300 mCi (85 GBq) for the treatment of lung metastases and 2,400 mCi (90 GBq) for bone metastases [88]. When there is no uptake of the radioiodine, there is little benefit from ^{131}I therapy. Many studies have been performed to induce re-expression of the sodium/iodide symporter in tumors and thyroid cell lines that do not express it; however, currently, there is no established protocol that will clearly increase radioiodine uptake in cells that lack expression of the symporter.

Sorafenib, a tyrosine kinase inhibitor, has been shown to have a beneficial effect on tumor progression of metastatic follicular carcinoma not responsive to radioiodine therapy [94]. Recent case reports have shown benefit of combining taxane-based chemotherapy with external beam radiation therapy for treatment of locoregional unresectable disease [95].

Lung Metastases

The lung is the most common site of metastases for follicular thyroid carcinoma [96]. Patients with micronodular lung metastases detected by ^{131}I scan may have a better prognosis than patients with macronodular lung metastases [96]. In a series of 96 cases of lung metastatic disease from differentiated thyroid cancer, 31(32%) were due to follicular thyroid carcinomas [97]. Patients with age less than 45, iodine avidity, and miliary-type spread did better than patients who were older, had tumors that did not take up iodine, or had bulky disease. Histology (papillary vs. follicular) did not seem to influence prognosis in patients with metastatic lung disease.

In another series of 272 patients with follicular thyroid carcinoma, 33.7% developed distant metastases to the lung during follow-up [98]. The mean time period between diagnosis and metastatic recurrence was 3.6 years. The 5- and 10-year survival was 68.5 and 54.0%, respectively [98]. Survival did not differ between patients with lung metastases alone and multiorgan metastases.

Thoracic metastasectomy has been used in patients with pulmonary metastases of thyroid cancer, including follicular thyroid carcinoma. In a report from the Mayo Clinic, eight patients out of 48 with pulmonary thyroid cancer metastases had follicular thyroid cancer [99]. Following pulmonary metastasectomy, the 5-year survival for follicular and Hurthle cell cancers was 37% compared to 64% for papillary carcinoma [99]. Although no randomized controlled trials of the efficacy of pulmonary metastasectomy of follicular thyroid carcinoma have been done, it remains a treatment option for patients who are able to tolerate surgery and have resectable disease or potentially resectable dominant lesions [99].

Bone Metastases

Bone metastases occur in 25% of follicular thyroid carcinomas and 35% of Hurthle cell carcinomas [100, 101]. Bone metastases commonly present with pain, fractures, or spinal cord compression [100].

Surgical resection of metastatic disease probably improves survival [102]. External radiotherapy is recommended for bone metastases, which cannot be readily excised surgically [87]. Chemotherapy with tyrosine kinase inhibitors may be another option for these patients.

Summary

Follicular thyroid carcinoma is a distinct differentiated thyroid cancer with unique pathophysiology and prognosis that differs from papillary thyroid carcinoma. Hurthle cell and insular thyroid carcinomas are more aggressive variants of follicular thyroid carcinoma. Follicular thyroid carcinoma makes up 10–15% of all thyroid cancers in iodine-replete regions, and overall survival rate at 5 years is 91% and at 10 years is 85%. Risk factors include older age, iodine deficiency, family history of thyroid cancer, ionizing radiation, and chronic TSH elevation. Genetic changes implicated in pathophysiology of follicular thyroid carcinoma include mutation of RAS proto-oncogene, PAX8/PPARγ rearrangement, as well as mutation of the tumor suppressor gene called the PTEN. The clinical presentation is frequently an incidental thyroid nodule or neck mass. FNA, frequently with ultrasonographic guidance, is the first step in the evaluation of suspicious thyroid nodules. However, cytology does not reliably differentiate follicular adenomas from carcinomas and this often results in surgery for benign disease. Molecular markers, such as PAX8-PPARγ rearrangement, HBME-1 expression, RAS mutations, galectin-3, and microRNA studies may help improve diagnostic accuracy of fine-needle-aspiration cytology. Diagnosis requires demonstration of vascular or capsular invasion by the tumor. Pathologically, two forms of follicular thyroid carcinoma are recognized: minimally invasive and widely invasive. Spread usually occurs hematogenously; however, 5% of cases present with lymph node metastases. Distant metastases are present in 20% of cases at diagnosis and commonly involve bone and lung. Although multiple staging systems have been proposed for follicular thyroid carcinoma, the American Thyroid Association recommends the use of the TNM system. Management of follicular thyroid carcinoma is initially surgical, followed by radioiodine ablation, and then long-term TSH suppression. Follow-up requires monitoring of serum thyroglobulin levels and whole-body radioiodine scanning for detection of metastatic disease. Loco-regional metastases that do not take up ^{131}I can be treated with external beam radiation or surgical excision. Tyrosine kinase inhibitors as oncologic drugs are now used for treatment of diffusely metastatic disease in clinical trials.

Most studies of differentiated thyroid cancers presently have included both papillary and follicular carcinomas together. The realization that follicular thyroid carcinoma is fundamentally different from papillary thyroid carcinoma should lead future research to focus on the unique aspects of follicular thyroid carcinoma as a distinct clinical entity.

References

1. Baloch ZW, LiVolsi VA. Our approach to follicular-patterned lesions of the thyroid. J Clin Pathol. 2007;60:244–50. doi:10.1136/jcp. 2006.038604.
2. DeLellis RA, Lloyd RV, Heitz PU, Eng C. World Health Organization classification of tumours. pathology and genetics of tumours of endocrine organs. Lyon: IARC Press; 2004.
3. Thompson LDR. Malignant neoplasms of the thyroid gland. In: Thompson LDR, editor. Endocrine pathology. Philadelphiam, PA: Elsevier; 2006. p. 101–8.
4. Tallini G, Carcangiu ML, Rosai J. Oncocytic neoplasms of the thyroid gland. Pathol Int. 1992; 42:305–15.
5. Har-el G, Hadar T, Segal K, Levy R, Sidi J. Hurthle cell carcinoma of the thyroid gland. A tumor of moderate malignancy. Cancer. 1986;57:1613–7.
6. Lam KY, Lo CY, Chen KW, Wan KY. Insular and anaplastic carcinoma of the thyroid. Ann Surg. 2000;231: 329–38.
7. Suliburk J, Delbridge L. Surgical management of well-differentiated thyroid cancer: state of the art. Surg Clinc North Am. 2009;89:1171–91.
8. Jemal A, Siegel R, Ward E, Hao Y, Xu J, Thun MJ. Cancer statistics, 2009. CA Cancer J Clin. 2009; 59:225–49.
9. Parkin DM, Bray F, Ferlay J, Pisani P. Global cancer statistics, 2002. CA Cancer J Clin. 2005;55:74–108.
10. Hundahl SA, Fleming ID, Fremgen AM, Menck HR. A National Cancer Data Base report on 53,856 cases of thyroid carcinoma treated in the U.S., 1985–1995. Cancer. 1998;83:2638–48.
11. Rosai J, Carcangiu ML, Delellis RA. Atlas of tumor pathology. Tumors of the thyroid gland. Washington, DC: Armed Forces Institute of Pathology; 1990.
12. Harach HR, Escalante DA, Day ES. Thyroid cancer and thyroiditis in Salta, Argentina: a 40-yr study in relation to iodine prophylaxis. Endocr Pathol. 2002; 13:175–81.
13. Davies L, Welch HG. Increasing incidence of thyroid cancer in the United States, 1973–2002. JAMA. 2006;295(18):2164–7.
14. Kent WDTMMD, Hall SFMMD, Isotalo PAMD, Houlden RLMD, George RLMD, Groome PAP. Increased incidence of differentiated thyroid carcinoma and detection of subclinical disease. CMAJ. 2007;177:1357–61.
15. Enewold L, Zhu K, Ron E, et al. Rising thyroid cancer incidence in the United States by demographic and tumor characteristics, 1980–2005. Cancer Epidemiol Biomarkers Prev. 2009;18:784–91.
16. Chen AY, Jemal A, Ward EM. Increasing incidence of differentiated thyroid cancer in the United States, 1988–2005. Cancer. 2009;115:3801–7.
17. LiVolsi VA, Asa SL. The demise of follicular carcinoma of the thyroid gland. Thyroid. 1994;4:233–6.
18. Knobel M, Medeiros-Neto G. Relevance of iodine intake as a reputed predisposing factor for thyroid cancer. Arq Bras Endocrinol Metabol. 2007;51:701–12.
19. Guigon CJ, Cheng S-Y. Novel non-genomicsignaling of thyroid hormone receptors in thyroid carcinogenesis. Mol Cell Endocrinol. 2009;308:63–9.
20. Kondo T, Ezzat S, Asa SL. Pathogenetic mechanisms in thyroid follicular-cell neoplasia. Nat Rev Cancer. 2006;6:292–306.
21. Lemoine NR, Mayall ES, Wyllie FS, et al. Activated ras oncogenes in human thyroid cancers. Cancer Res. 1988;48:4459–63.
22. Nikiforova MN, Lynch RA, Biddinger PW, et al. RAS point mutations and PAX8-PPAR{gamma} rearrangement in thyroid tumors: evidence for distinct molecular pathways in thyroid follicular carcinoma. J Clin Endocrinol Metab. 2003;88:2318–26.
23. Kroll TG, Sarraf P, Pecciarini L, et al. PAX8-PPARgamma 1 fusion oncogene in human thyroid carcinoma. Science. 2000;289:1357–60.

24. Eberhardt NL, Grebe SK, McIver B, Reddi HV. The role of the PAX8/PPARgamma fusion oncogene in the pathogenesis of follicular thyroid cancer. Mol Cell Endocrinol. 2010;321:50–6.
25. Sogol PB, Sugawara M, Gordon HE, Shellow WV, Hernandez F, Hershman JM. Cowden's disease: familial goiter and skin hamartomas. A report of three cases. West J Med. 1983;139:324–8.
26. Diggelmann HR, Van Daele DJ, O'Dorisio TM, Hoffman HT. Insular thyroid carcinoma in a patient with Cowden syndrome. Laryngoscope. 2010;120:454–7.
27. Hobert JA, Eng C. PTEN hamartoma tumor syndrome: an overview. Genet Med. 2009;11:687–94.
28. Lloyd 2nd KM, Dennis M. Cowden's disease. A possible new symptom complex with multiple system involvement. Ann Intern Med. 1963;58:136–42.
29. Hou P, Ji M, Xing M. Association of PTEN gene methylation with genetic alterations in the phosphatidylinositol 3-kinase/AKT signaling pathway in thyroid tumors. Cancer. 2008;113:2440–7.
30. Heffess CS, Thompson LD. Minimally invasive thyroid follicular carcinoma. Endocr Pathol. 2001;12(4): 417–22.
31. Mazzaferri EL. Practical management of thyroid cancer: a multidisciplinary approach. London: Springer; 2006.
32. Yutan E, Clark OH. Hurthle cell carcinoma. Curr Treat Options Oncol. 2001;2:331–5.
33. Carcangiu ML, Bianchi S, Savino D, Voynick IM, Rosai J. Follicular Hurthle cell tumors of the thyroid gland. Cancer. 1991;68:1944–53.
34. Grant CS. Operative and postoperative management of the patient with follicular and Hurthle cell carcinoma. Do they differ? Surg Clin North Am. 1995; 75:395–403.
35. Kushchayeva Y, Duh QY, Kebebew E, D'Avanzo A, Clark OH. Comparison of clinical characteristics at diagnosis and during follow-up in 118 patients with Hurthle cell or follicular thyroid cancer. Am J Surg. 2008;195:457–62.
36. Volante M, Landolfi S, Chiusa L, et al. Poorly differentiated carcinomas of the thyroid with trabecular, insular, and solid patterns: a clinicopathologic study of 183 patients. Cancer. 2004;100:950–7.
37. Agha A, Glockzin G, Woenckhaus M, Dietmaier W, Iesalnieks I, Schlitt HJ. Insular carcinomas of the thyroid exhibit poor prognosis and long-term survival in comparison to follicular and papillary T4 carcinomas. Langenbecks Arch Surg. 2007;392:671–7.
38. Suster S. Thyroid tumors with a follicular growth pattern. Arch Pathol Lab Med. 2006;130:984–8.
39. Hegedus L. The thyroid nodule. N Engl J Med. 2004; 351:1764–71.
40. Tan GH, Gharib H. Thyroid incidentalomas: management approaches to nonpalpable nodules discovered incidentally on thyroid imaging. Ann Intern Med. 1997;126:226–31.
41. Ezzat S, Sarti DA, Cain DR, Braunstein GD. Thyroid incidentalomas. Prevalence by palpation and ultrasonography. Arch Intern Med. 1994;154:1838–40.
42. Deveci MS, Deveci G, LiVolsi VA, Baloch ZW. Fine-needle aspiration of follicular lesions of the thyroid. Diagnosis and follow-Up. Cytojournal. 2006;3:9.
43. Sahin M, Sengul A, Berki Z, Tutuncu NB, Guvener ND. Ultrasound-guided fine-needle aspiration biopsy and ultrasonographic features of infracentimetric nodules in patients with nodular goiter: correlation with pathological findings. Endocr Pathol. 2006;17: 67–74.
44. Morris LF, Ragavendra N, Yeh MW. Evidence-based assessment of the role of ultrasonography in the management of benign thyroid nodules. World J Surg. 2008;32:1253–63.
45. Yang J, Schnadig V, Logrono R, Wasserman PG. Fine-needle aspiration of thyroid nodules: a study of 4703 patients with histologic and clinical correlations. Cancer. 2007;111:306–15.
46. Mazzaferri EL. Management of a solitary thyroid nodule. N Engl J Med. 1993;328:553–9.
47. Kini SR. Thyroid cytopathology: an atlas and text. 1st ed. Philadelphia, PA: Lippincott Williams & Wilkins; 2008.
48. Cerutti JM, Latini FR, Nakabashi C, et al. Diagnosis of suspicious thyroid nodules using four protein biomarkers. Clin Cancer Res. 2006;12:3311–8.
49. Rossi ED, Raffaelli M, Minimo C, et al. Immunocytochemical evaluation of thyroid neoplasms on thin-layer smears from fine-needle aspiration biopsies. Cancer. 2005;105:87–95.
50. Kato MA, Fahey TJ. Molecular markers in thyroid cancer diagnostics. Surg Clin North Am. 2009;89: 1139–55.
51. Bartolazzi A, Orlandi F, Saggiorato E, et al. Galectin-3-expression analysis in the surgical selection of follicular thyroid nodules with indeterminate fine-needle aspiration cytology: a prospective multicentre study. Lancet Oncol. 2008;9:543–9.
52. Saggiorato E, De Pompa R, Volante M, et al. Characterization of thyroid 'follicular neoplasms' in fine-needle aspiration cytological specimens using a panel of immunohistochemical markers: a proposal for clinical application. Endocr Relat Cancer. 2005;12: 305–17.
53. Freitas BC, Cerutti JM. Genetic markers differentiating follicular thyroid carcinoma from benign lesions. Mol Cell Endocrinol. 2010;321:77–85.
54. Nikiforov YE, Steward DL, Robinson-Smith TM, et al. Molecular testing for mutations in improving the fine-needle aspiration diagnosis of thyroid nodules. J Clin Endocrinol Metab. 2009;94:2092–8.
55. Cantara S, Capezzone M, Marchisotta S, et al. Impact of proto-oncogene mutation detection in cytological specimens from thyroid nodules improves the diagnostic accuracy of cytology. J Clin Endocrinol Metab. 2010;95:1365–9.
56. Weber F, Teresi RE, Broelsch CE, Frilling A, Eng C. A limited set of human MicroRNA is deregulated in follicular thyroid carcinoma. J Clin Endocrinol Metab. 2006;91:3584–91.

57. Tuttle RM, Lemar H, Burch HB. Clinical features associated with an increased risk of thyroid malignancy in patients with follicular neoplasia by fine-needle aspiration. Thyroid. 1998;8:377–83.

58. Borel AL, Boizel R, Faure P, et al. Significance of low levels of thyroglobulin in fine needle aspirates from cervical lymph nodes of patients with a history of differentiated thyroid cancer. Eur J Endocrinol. 2008;158: 691–8.

59. Wilhelm SM. Utility of I-123 thyroid uptake scan in incidental thyroid nodules: an old test with a new role. Surgery. 2008;144:511–5. discussion 5–7.

60. Gharib H, Papini E. Thyroid nodules: clinical importance, assessment, and treatment. Endocrinol Metab Clin North Am. 2007;36:707–35.

61. Boelaert K, Horacek J, Holder RL, Watkinson JC, Sheppard MC, Franklyn JA. Serum thyrotropin concentration as a novel predictor of malignancy in thyroid nodules investigated by fine-needle aspiration. J Clin Endocrinol Metab. 2006;91:4295–301.

62. Haymart MR, Repplinger DJ, Leverson GE, et al. Higher serum thyroid stimulating hormone level in thyroid nodule patients is associated with greater risks of differentiated thyroid cancer and advanced tumor stage. J Clin Endocrinol Metab. 2008;93:809–14.

63. Jonklaas J, Nsouli-Maktabi H, Soldin SJ. Endogenous thyrotropin and triiodothyronine concentrations in individuals with thyroid cancer. Thyroid. 2008;18:943–52.

64. Polyzos SA, Kita M, Efstathiadou Z, et al. Serum thyrotropin concentration as a biochemical predictor of thyroid malignancy in patients presenting with thyroid nodules. J Cancer Res Clin Oncol. 2008;134:953–60.

65. Dulgeroff AJ, Hershman JM. Medical therapy for differentiated thyroid carcinoma. Endocr Rev. 1994;15: 500–15.

66. D'Avanzo A, Ituarte P, Treseler P, et al. Prognostic scoring systems in patients with follicular thyroid cancer: a comparison of different staging systems in predicting the patient outcome. Thyroid. 2004;14: 453–8.

67. Lang BH-H, Lo C-Y, Chan W-F, Lam K-Y, Wan K-Y. Staging systems for follicular thyroid carcinoma: application to 171 consecutive patients treated in a tertiary referral centre. Endocr Relat Cancer. 2007;14:29–42.

68. DeGroot LJ, Kaplan EL, Shukla MS, Salti G, Straus FH. Morbidity and mortality in follicular thyroid cancer. J Clin Endocrinol Metab. 1995;80:2946–53.

69. Cooper DS, Doherty GM, Haugen BR, et al. Revised American thyroid association management guidelines for patients with thyroid nodules and differentiated thyroid cancer. Thyroid. 2009;19:1167–214.

70. Asari R, Koperek O, Scheuba C, et al. Follicular thyroid carcinoma in an iodine-replete endemic goiter region: a prospectively collected, retrospectively analyzed clinical trial. Ann Surg. 2009;249:1023–31.

71. Emerick GT, Duh Q-Y, Siperstein AE, Burrow GN, Clark OH. Diagnosis, treatment, and outcome of follicular thyroid carcinoma. Cancer. 1993;72:3287–95.

72. Tielens ET, Sherman SI, Hruban RH, Ladenson PW. Follicular variant of papillary thyroid carcinoma. A clinicopathologic study. Cancer. 1994;73:424–31.

73. Caplan RH, Abellera RM, Kisken WA. Hurthle cell tumors of the thyroid gland. A clinicopathologic review and long-term follow-up. JAMA. 1984;251: 3114–7.

74. Goldman JM, Line BR, Aamodt RL, Robbins J. Influence of triiodothyronine withdrawal time on 131I uptake postthyroidectomy for thyroid cancer. J Clin Endocrinol Metab. 1980;50:734–9.

75. Pacini F, Ladenson PW, Schlumberger M, et al. Radioiodine ablation of thyroid remnants after preparation with recombinant human thyrotropin in differentiated thyroid carcinoma: results of an international, randomized, controlled study. J Clin Endocrinol Metab. 2006;91:926–32.

76. Durante C, Haddy N, Baudin E, et al. Long-term outcome of 444 patients with distant metastases from papillary and follicular thyroid carcinoma: benefits and limits of radioiodine therapy. J Clin Endocrinol Metab. 2006;91:2892–9.

77. Schwartz DL, Lobo MJ, Ang KK, et al. Postoperative external beam radiotherapy for differentiated thyroid cancer: outcomes and morbidity with conformal treatment. Int J Radiat Oncol Biol Phys. 2009;74: 1083–91.

78. Terezakis SA, Lee KS, Ghossein RA, et al. Role of external beam radiotherapy in patients with advanced or recurrent nonanaplastic thyroid cancer: Memorial Sloan-Kettering Cancer Center experience. Int J Radiat Oncol Biol Phys. 2009;73:795–801.

79. McGriff NJ, Csako G, Gourgiotis L, Lori CG, Pucino F, Sarlis NJ. Effects of thyroid hormone suppression therapy on adverse clinical outcomes in thyroid cancer. Ann Med. 2002;34:554–64.

80. Biondi B, Filetti S, Schlumberger M. Thyroid-hormone therapy and thyroid cancer: a reassessment. Nat Clin Pract Endocrinol Metab. 2005;1:32–40.

81. Cooper DS, Specker B, Ho M, et al. Thyrotropin suppression and disease progression in patients with differentiated thyroid cancer: results from the National Thyroid Cancer Treatment Cooperative Registry. Thyroid. 1998;8:737–44.

82. Jonklaas J, Sarlis NJ, Litofsky D, et al. Outcomes of patients with differentiated thyroid carcinoma following initial therapy. Thyroid. 2006;16:1229–42.

83. Pujol P, Daures JP, Nsakala N, Baldet L, Bringer J, Jaffiol C. Degree of thyrotropin suppression as a prognostic determinant in differentiated thyroid cancer. J Clin Endocrinol Metab. 1996;81:4318–23.

84. Biondi B, Cooper DS. Benefits of thyrotropin suppression versus the risks of adverse effects in differentiated thyroid cancer. Thyroid. 2010;20:135–46.

85. Kowalczyk P, Roskosz J, Jurecka-Tuleja B, Gubala E, Czernik E, Jarzab B. L-thyroxine therapy in differentiated thyroid carcinoma: criteria for evaluation of TSH suppression. Wiad Lek. 2001;54:268–76.

86. Giovanella L. Highly sensitive thyroglobulin measurements in differentiated thyroid carcinoma management. Clin Chem Lab Med. 2008;46:1067–73.
87. Schlumberger M, Challeton C, De Vathaire F, et al. Radioactive iodine treatment and external radiotherapy for lung and bone metastases from thyroid carcinoma. J Nucl Med. 1996;37:598–605.
88. Zhu RS, Yu YL, Lu HK, Luo QY, Chen LB. Clinical study of 312 cases with metastatic differentiated thyroid cancer treated with large doses of 131I. Chin Med J (Engl). 2005;118:425–8.
89. Rodrigues G, Ghosh A. Synchronous bony and soft tissue metastases from follicular carcinoma of the thyroid. J Korean Med Sci. 2003;18:914–6.
90. Girelli ME, Casara D, Rubello D, et al. Metastatic thyroid carcinoma of the adrenal gland. J Endocrinol Invest. 1993;16:139–41.
91. Shaha AR, Shah JP, Loree TR. Differentiated thyroid cancer presenting initially with distant metastasis. Am J Surg. 1997;174:474–6.
92. Sampson E, Brierley JD, Le LW, Rotstein L, Tsang RW. Clinical management and outcome of papillary and follicular (differentiated) thyroid cancer presenting with distant metastasis at diagnosis. Cancer. 2007;110:1451–6.
93. Kitamura Y, Shimizu K, Nagahama M, et al. Immediate causes of death in thyroid carcinoma: clinicopathological analysis of 161 fatal cases. J Clin Endocrinol Metab. 1999;84:4043–9.
94. Hoftijzer H, Heemstra KA, Morreau H, et al. Beneficial effects of sorafenib on tumor progression, but not on radioiodine uptake, in patients with differentiated thyroid carcinoma. Eur J Endocrinol. 2009;161:923–31.
95. Tulloch-Reid M, Skarulis MC, Sherman SI, Sarlis NJ, Santarpia L. Long-term eradication of locally recurrent invasive follicular thyroid carcinoma after taxane-based concomitant chemoradiotherapy. Anticancer Res. 2009;29:4665–71.
96. Casara D, Rubello D, Saladini G, et al. Different features of pulmonary metastases in differentiated thyroid cancer: natural history and multivariate statistical analysis of prognostic variables. J Nucl Med. 1993;34:1626–31.
97. Ronga G, Filesi M, Montesano T, et al. Lung metastases from differentiated thyroid carcinoma. A 40 years' experience. Q J Nucl Med Mol Imaging. 2004;48:12–9.
98. Lin JD, Chao TC, Hsueh C. Follicular thyroid carcinomas with lung metastases: a 23-year retrospective study. Endocr J. 2004;51:219–25.
99. Porterfield JR, Cassivi SD, Wigle DA, et al. Thoracic metastasectomy for thyroid malignancies. Eur J Cardiothorac Surg. 2009;36:155–8.
100. Muresan MM, Olivier P, Leclere J, et al. Bone metastases from differentiated thyroid carcinoma. Endocr Relat Cancer. 2008;15:37–49.
101. Lopez-Penabad L, Chiu AC, Hoff AO, et al. Prognostic factors in patients with Hurthle cell neoplasms of the thyroid. Cancer. 2003;97:1186–94.
102. Zettinig G, Fueger BJ, Passler C, et al. Long-term follow-up of patients with bone metastases from differentiated thyroid carcinoma – surgery or conventional therapy? Clin Endocrinol (Oxf). 2002;56:377–82.

Medullary Thyroid Carcinoma

Nicole M. Tyer and Run Yu

Introduction

Medullary thyroid cancer (MTC) is a malignancy that arises from the calcitonin-producing parafollicular cells of the thyroid gland. MTC is a rare type of thyroid cancer, constituting only 5–10% of cases. Of nearly 54,000 cases of thyroid cancer reported to The US National Cancer Base from 1985 to 1995, 2,000 are MTC [1].

Seventy-five percent of MTC cases are sporadic, while the remaining are associated with inherited germ-line mutations in the RET protooncogene [2, 3]. MTC can also coexist with other neoplasia, constituting the MEN-2A and MEN-2B syndromes; these interesting familial syndromes will be discussed in further detail in other sections of this chapter.

Following anaplastic thyroid cancer, MTC has the second worst prognosis of all thyroid cancers; average 10-year survival is 50–80%, but this rate varies greatly based on age and TNM stage at the time of diagnosis [4–7]. Unfortunately, half of all MTC patients present with metastases;

10-year survival in these patients is only 20%. Like other thyroid cancers, MTC occurs more frequently in women, with a female to male ratio of two to one [8].

History of Medullary Thyroid Carcinoma

In 1951, Horn described seven cases of an unusual thyroid carcinoma that was unlike the well-known papillary and follicular carcinomas previously understood [9]. In 1959, Hazard further described the carcinoma as a proliferation of parafollicular cells against an amyloid stroma, and named it "medullary thyroid carcinoma" [10]. During the 1960s, Sipple noted an association between MTC, pheochromocytoma, and mucosal neuromas [11]. In the meantime, Copp discovered calcitonin and described its production by parafollicular cells [12], and Williams described the oncologic progression of normal C-cells into frank carcinoma via C-cell hyperpla-

N.M. Tyer
Department of Medicine, Cedars-Sinai
Medical Center, Los Angeles, CA, USA

R. Yu (✉)
Divisions of Endocrinology, Diabetes, and Metabolism,
Carcinoid and Neuroendocrine Tumor Center,
Department of Medicine, Cedars-Sinai Medical Center,
8700 Beverly Blvd, Los Angeles, CA 90048, USA
e-mail: run.yu@cshs.org

G.D. Braunstein (ed.), *Thyroid Cancer*, Endocrine Updates 30,
DOI 10.1007/978-1-4614-0875-8_9, © Springer Science+Business Media, LLC 2012

sia (CCH) [13]. In the 1980s, the calcitonin gene was mapped to chromosome eleven. When gene analysis flourished in the mid-1990s, *RET* was discovered on chromosome ten [14], and is now known to be associated with several types of cancers including MTC [15, 16].

Histology and Function of the Thyroid Gland

Microscopically, the thyroxine-producing follicular cells comprise 99.9% of thyroid cells and align circumferentially around the thyroglobulin colloid. Parafollicular cells comprise only 0.1% of thyroid cells; they are scattered throughout the thyroid gland, but are most numerous at the junction of the upper third and lower two-thirds. Because they are responsible for synthesizing, storing, and secreting calcitonin, parafollicular cells possess extensive endoplasmic reticulum; this endoplasmic reticulum stains clear and therefore parafollicular cells are also referred to as "clear cells" or "C-cells" [10].

Follicular cells develop as early as the 3rd week of gestation, and are derived from a diverticulum of the foregut, whereas parafollicular cells develop around the 12th week of gestation, and are derived from neural crest tissue. This embryologic dichotomy has implications for the development of MTC and its unique treatment as a neuroendocrine tumor [17].

Pathology of Medullary Thyroid Cancer

C-Cell Hyperplasia

In normal thyroid tissue, C-cells are only seen sporadically around the thyroid follicle. When C-cells proliferate at an accelerated rate, CCH results. Histologically, CCH is defined by the presence of more than six C-cells per thyroid follicle, or more than 50 C-cells visualized in one low power field (100×) [18, 19].

Frank medullary thyroid carcinoma is always preceded by CCH; the presence of CCH usually, but not always, implies progression to MTC [20, 21]. In fact, 20–30% of healthy individuals may have CCH evident on thyroid biopsy, and CCH is also commonly seen in autoimmune thyroiditis and follicular thyroid cancers. When C-cells become prolific, they are more likely to disrupt and invade the follicular basement membrane. Disruption of the basement membrane is what defines medullary thyroid carcinoma from CCH [18, 19]. The extent of CCH and rate of progression to MTC are associated with the type of *RET* mutation, which will be discussed more thoroughly in the upcoming pages.

Pathology

Grossly, MTC is firm in consistency and gray-white to tan-pink in color; it is well circumscribed but not encapsulated. Microscopically, MTC consists of many cells separated by fibrous stroma [20, 21]. Unlike normal parafollicular cells which are usually round, MTC cells can be polygonal, round, or most often, spindle shaped. Because of their extensive endoplasmic reticulum for calcitonin production, the cytoplasm stains eosinophilic with conventional H&E staining; likewise, the cells also stain positive for calcitonin and carcinoembryonic antigen (CEA) on immunohistochemical staining. Extensive calcification and amyloid deposition also help distinguish the tumor. Mitotic figures are rarely seen.

Secretory Products

Parafollicular cells primarily secrete calcitonin. Other secretory products include CEA, somatostatin, proopiomelanocortin (POMC), ACTH, vasoactive intestinal peptide (VIP), gastrin-releasing peptide, neurotensin, prostaglandins, kinins, serotonin, histaminase, chromogranin A (CgA) [especially in patients with concomitant pheochromocytoma], and neuron-specific enolase [22–24]. Patients with elevated calcitonin and/or VIP levels may present with diarrhea and flushing, and patients with elevated ACTH levels may present with typical Cushingoid signs and symptoms.

Because it is nonspecific, CEA is generally not used for initial diagnosis of MTC, but serial CEA levels can be followed after treatment. Serum CEA concentration and CEA doubling times (DT) directly correlate with MTC disease severity: higher concentration of CEA or shorter DT implicates a poorer overall prognosis [25].

Calcitonin

Biochemistry of Calcitonin

Calcitonin is a small peptide produced by the parafollicular cells of the thyroid gland in mammals, birds, and fish. *CALC – 1*, the gene that encodes calcitonin, is located on the tip of the short arm of chromosome eleven (11p15.3–15.5). *CALC – 1* encodes a primary transcript (pre-mRNA) that undergoes tissue-specific slicing into one of two end products: CGRP-1 (calcitonin gene-related peptide-1) or CT (calcitonin) [26]. In neuronal cells, exons 1–3 are joined with exons 5–6 for translation into CGRP-1, a neurotransmitter that acts both centrally and peripherally. In thyroid cells, exons 1–4 form the calcitonin precursor mRNA (pre-pro-calcitonin), which undergoes translation and post-translational processing to yield calcitonin.

Function of Calcitonin

The exact physiologic role of calcitonin is not fully understood. Elevated serum calcium levels stimulate release of calcitonin which directly and indirectly lowers serum calcium [27]. Calcitonin directly lowers serum calcium by blocking calcium absorption in the intestine and by inhibiting osteoclast activity in the bones. Calcitonin indirectly lowers serum calcium by inhibiting phosphate reabsorption in the kidney tubule. Calcitonin is also released in response to gastrin and pentagastrin suggesting its role as a satiety hormone; this concept has been studied in rats and monkeys, but has not yet been fully elucidated in human models.

Measuring CT Levels

Radioimmunoassay (RIA) can be used for measuring CT, but is not entirely specific because it measures both calcitonin and calcitonin precursors [28]. The newer immunoradiometric assay (IRMA) is able to specifically measure CT, and is currently available and recommended [29, 30]. Finally, a two-site chemiluminescence immunoassay is able to detect very low levels of calcitonin (0.35 ng/L) via two mouse monoclonal antibodies that sandwich the mature calcitonin [31].

In patients highly suspicious for MTC despite low calcitonin levels, a "pentagastrin stimulation test" is recommended [32]. After an overnight fast, pentagastrin (0.5 μg per kg of body weight diluted in 5 mL of normal saline) is infused over 3 min while the patient lies supine. Serum CT levels are drawn at 0 and 5 min. In 95% of normal patients, basal and stimulated CT levels remain below 10 ng/L and 30 ng/L, respectively. Both basal and stimulated CT levels are elevated in patients with MTC, sometimes as much as 5–10 times normal. Unfortunately, pentagastrin is not currently available in the United States; calcium stimulation test is an acceptable alternative [33].

Administering pentagastrin may induce nausea, dizziness, tachycardia or bradycardia, and substernal tightness; therefore, the test is contraindicated in patients with underlying coronary disease, uncontrolled hypertension, or asthma [34]. Pentagastrin should also not be used in pregnant women or in patients with duodenal ulcer. In attempts to avoid the extensive side effects of pentagastrin, other calcitonin-stimulating tests have been tried using omeprazole or TRH; so far, these tests show poor sensitivity and are not currently recommended [35].

Elevated Calcitonin Levels

Calcitonin levels are high in neonates, but slowly decline during the 1st year of life; this is an important consideration in appropriately developing and interpreting MTC screening techniques for infants. Calcitonin is generally higher in men than in women, and can even fluctuate 20–30% within the same patient [36]. Calcitonin may be elevated during lactation and in disease states associated with hypercalcemia including renal failure, respiratory failure, and some malignancies including pheochromocytoma, carcinoid, melanoma, and solid tumors of the lung, breast, pancreas, and prostate [37, 38]. A blunted rise in calcitonin (peak: basal < two fold difference) to pentagastrin stimulation distinguishes these cancers from MTC [33]. Additionally, calcitonin may also be elevated in patients with thyroiditis or benign CCH, and even in some healthy individuals.

RET Proto-Oncogene

The RET proto-oncogene was first cloned in 1985, and is now known to be responsible for the development of MTC, although the exact causative pathway is currently not clear [39–42]. *RET*, located on chromosome 10 (10q11.2), encodes 21 exons which undergo alternative splicing to form various tyrosine kinase receptor proteins that assist in cell trafficking, differentiation, and signal transduction [43, 44]. RET tyrosine kinase receptors are expressed on thyroid gland C-cells, parathyroid cells, adrenal medulla cells, and neuronal cells. When a ligand binds to the extracellular domain of RET, two RET proteins dimerize, followed by cross-autophosphorylation, and subsequent phosphorylation of intracellular substrates, resulting in signal transduction. Activating mutations in *RET*, such as those seen in MTC, abnormally enhance the RET tyrosine kinase receptor activity and lead to tumorigenesis in specific organs.

Each RET protein consists of an extracellular domain, a transmembrane domain, and an intracellular domain (Fig. 9.1). The extracellular domain, derived from the N-terminus of the RET protein, includes a cadherin-like region and a cysteine-rich region [44]. Mutations in the cysteine-rich region of the extracellular domain

lead to MEN-2A or familial medullary thyroid cancer (FMTC) [34]. The intracellular domain, derived from the carboxy-terminus of the RET protein, consists of two tyrosine kinase subdomains, TK1 and TK2. Mutations in TK1 result in FMTC while mutations in TK2 result in MEN-2B [45].

Genotype–Phenotype Relationship of RET AND Tumor Expression

As alluded to above, strict correlations exist between specific *RET* mutations and phenotype expression of MTC (Table 9.1) [16, 46–48].

Germ-Line Mutations

Patients with FMTC harbor mutations in either the extracellular or intracellular region of the RET tyrosine kinase receptor (Fig. 9.1) [34]. Half of FMTC patients have a mutation in exon 10 (codons 618, 620) of *RET* which encodes the cysteine-rich domain of the extracellular portion of the RET protein [26, 45]. The other half of FMTC patients have various mutations in exon 11 (codons 630, 631, 634), 13 (codons 768, 790, 791), 14 (codons 804, 844), or 15 (codon 891). Interestingly, patients with mutations in exons 13, 14, or 15 usually present at a later age (6–16 years) and are less likely to have lymph node metastases at the time of initial presentation [47, 49].

Patients with MEN-2A usually have mutations in the extracellular cysteine-rich region of the RET tyrosine kinase receptor [34]. More than 80% of patients with MEN-2A have a specific substitution (Arg→Cys) in codon 634 on exon 10 in the cysteine-rich extracellular domain [26, 45]. If present, this codon 634 mutation confers a 50% risk of developing pheochromocytoma and an 8% risk of developing parathyroid neoplasia. All families with MEN-2A and cutaneous lichen amyloidosis harbor the 634 mutation, and all families with MEN-2A and Hirschsprung's disease have a mutation in codon 609, 618, or 620 [34].

Patients with MEN-2B usually have mutations in the tyrosine kinase domain (TK2) of the

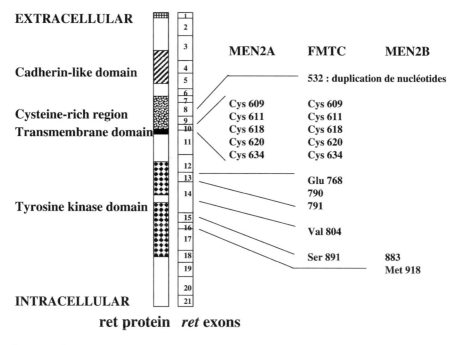

Fig. 9.1 Structure of RET gene and protein. From Leboulleux et al. [34], used with permission

Table 9.1 Genotype–phenotype correlation between RET mutations and MTC syndromes

FMTC	Exon 10	Codon 618, 620
	Exon 11	Codon 630, 631, 634
	Exon 13	Codon 768, 790, 791
	Exon 14	Codon 804, 844
	Exon 15	Codon 891
MEN-2A	Exon 10	Codon 634 (Arg→Cys) MEN-2A with or without cutaneous lichen amyloidosis
	Exon 10	Codon 609, 618, 620 MEN-2A with Hirschsprung's Disease
MEN-2B	Exon 16	Codon 918 (Met→Thr)
	Exon 15	Codon 883

intracellular region of the RET receptor. Ninety-five percent of patients with MEN-2B have a single substitution (Met→Thr) at codon 918 on exon 16, altering the substrate recognition pocket of the catalytic probe [26, 41, 45]. Rarely, a mutation in codon 883 on exon 15 results in MEN-2B [50]. De novo mutations are common in MEN-2B, and usually arise on the paternal allele [45, 51].

Sporadic Mutations

New germ-line mutations in *RET* are found in 6–10% of apparently sporadic MTC [52]. Sporadic MTC occurs most commonly due to deletion of a normal *RET* allele, amplification of a mutant *RET* allele, or a mutation in codons 618, 634, 768, 804, or 883 [53].

Other Mutations

Polymorphisms of *RET* in codons 691 and 836 are poorly understood but are thought to lead to malignant transformation; this is an active area of research [54].

MTC Syndromes

MTC can exist independently or in association with a genetic syndrome. In this section, we will first discuss sporadic MTC, and then delve into a deeper discussion about each of the genetic MTC syndromes including familial MTC, MEN-2A, and MEN-2B. All genetic MTC syndromes are inherited in an autosomal dominant fashion which confers a 50% risk in progeny of affected patients.

Sporadic Medullary Thyroid Carcinoma

Seventy five percent of MTC cases are sporadic; these cases are usually unifocal and present with a solitary thyroid nodule during the fourth decade of life [34]. If the nodule is large enough to press the esophagus, the patient may present with dysphagia; if the nodule invades the laryngeal nerve, the patient may present with hoarseness, cough, or dyspnea. Lymph node metastases are present in 10–20% of cases at the time of presentation. Sporadic MTC confers the best prognosis of all types of MTC.

Six to ten percent of patients with apparently sporadic MTC harbor a de novo germ-line *RET* mutation [52]. Although some clinicians choose only to pursue genetic testing in patients with family history of *RET* mutations, the American Thyroid Association currently provides Grade A recommendation to perform *RET* genetic analysis in all patients diagnosed with MTC, including those with apparently sporadic MTC [55, 56].

Familial Medullary Thyroid Carcinoma

Familial MTC denotes the best prognosis of the inherited MTC syndromes [19, 49]. Like sporadic MTC, familial MTC is isolated and is not associated with other clinical entities such as pheochromocytoma or parathyroid adenomas. Unlike sporadic MTC, though, familial MTC is usually multifocal and bilateral and presents in the second to third decade of life. Like other inherited MTC syndromes, FMTC is inherited in an autosomal dominant fashion. It can be due to a mutation in the extracellular or intracellular region of the RET tyrosine kinase receptor as described in the previous section.

Sometimes it is challenging to differentiate FMTC from MEN-2A, especially if MTC appears isolated; the distinction is important because patients with MEN-2A express associated anomalies which may require screening and treatment [55, 56]. *RET* genetic testing and family history (including more than 10 affected family members, many of whom are over the age of 50) helps distinguish FMTC from MEN-2A.

Multiple Endocrine Neoplasia-2A Syndrome

MEN-2A (Sipple syndrome) encompasses MTC, pheochromocytoma, and parathyroid adenomas. MTC is multifocal, bilateral, and portends a poorer prognosis than sporadic or familial MTC [39]. As discussed earlier, MEN-2A is most often due to a single substitution (Arg→Cys) in the extracellular region of the RET tyrosine kinase receptor; like other familial MTC syndromes, it is inherited in an autosomal dominant fashion.

MTC in MEN-2A develops during early childhood, usually before the age of 6 and often before the age of 2 [57]. For progeny of patients with MEN-2A, genetic testing for a *RET* mutation should be performed shortly after birth; if positive, prophylactic thyroidectomy should be contemplated [55, 56]. Prophylactic thyroidectomy is discussed in the next section.

In MEN-2A, MTC develops with nearly 100% penetrance, pheochromocytomas develop in 50% of patients, and parathyroid adenomas develop in 10–30% of patients [58]. Prior to surgery, pheochromocytoma should be excluded by measuring plasma or urine metanephrines [59]. CgA levels are frequently elevated in patients with pheochromocytoma, but false positive results are seen in patients on antacid treatment (e.g., proton pump inhibitors) or with renal failure. Parathyroid adenomas, if present, can be resected at the time of thyroidectomy.

MEN-2A is also associated with cutaneous lichen amyloidosis (due to a mutation in *RET* codon 634) [60] and Hirschsprung's disease (due to a mutation in *RET* codon 609, 618, or 620) [61]; these clinical entities should be sought, if clinically suspected. Additionally, enlarged corneal nerves [46] and notalgia (a pruritic and pigmented papular rash on the upper portion of the back) are observed in some patients with MEN-2A [62].

Multiple Endocrine Neoplasia-2B

MEN-2B confers the worst prognosis of all types of MTC. Malignancies are multifocal, bilateral, and present extremely early in life, usually during infancy [57, 63]. Ninety-five percent of patients with MEN-2B have a single substitution mutation (Thr→Met) at codon 918 on exon 16 on *RET* [41]. De novo mutations, which usually occur on the paternal allele, are also common in MEN-2B [45, 51]. Progeny of patients with MEN-2B should have RET genetic testing at birth and, if positive, undergo prophylactic thyroidectomy within the 1st month of life. In addition to MTC, which develops with nearly 100% penetrance, patients with MEN-2B also develop pheochromocytomas (50%) and gastrointestinal mucosal ganglioneuromas (Fig. 9.2) [64]. Patients with MEN-2B may have a Marfinoid body habitus. Clinical findings in different forms of MTC are summarized in Table 9.2.

Diagnosis of Medullary Thyroid Carcinoma

More than half the patients eventually diagnosed with MTC present with a solitary thyroid nodule or thyroid mass [2, 4]. More than three-quarters of these patients will have regional lymph node spread or frank metastases at the time of diagnosis. These patients can be otherwise asymptomatic, or have symptoms of local invasion including hoarseness or dysphagia [66]. Systemic symptoms such as diarrhea and flushing may be present, especially if calcitonin and/or VIP levels are elevated, and Cushingoid symptoms may be present if ACTH levels are elevated. Though only 4% of thyroid nodules are cancerous [67], those with high clinical suspicion should undergo fine-needle aspiration. If present, FNA usually reveals malignancy, but can only specifically identify MTC in half the samples.

Because MTC is aggressive, some endocrinologists perform routine calcitonin measurements in all patients who present with a solitary thyroid nodule [68, 69]. On the other hand, because MTC is relatively rare (only one out of every 200 thyroid nodules is MTC), other endocrinologists do not perform routine CT screening. Most European physicians routinely measure CT levels, whereas most American physicians currently do not. Current literature suggests that it is still controversial to routinely measure CT in all patients who present with a solitary thyroid nodule [70]. If FNA results suggest MTC or are inconclusive, CT should be measured for accurate diagnosis and preoperative planning.

Less than half the MTC cases are detected via laboratory screening in asymptomatic kindreds of patients with FMTC or MEN syndrome [2, 4]. Because morbidity and mortality in patients with MEN syndrome are relatively high, family members of these patients should be screened with

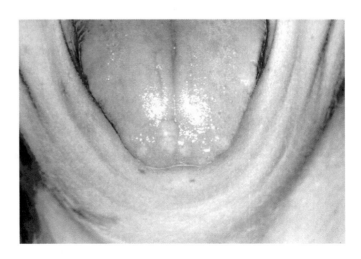

Fig. 9.2 Mucosal ganglioneuromas on the tongue of a patient with MEN-2B Syndrome

Table 9.2 Comparison of clinical findings in different forms of MTC. Adapted from Schlumberger and Pacini [65]

Clinical entity	Sporadic MTC	FMTC	MEN-2A	MEN-2B
Muticentricity/bilaterality	~30%	100%	100%	100%
Age at presentation	< 40 years	< 20 years	< 20 years, usually < 6	< 1 year
Inheritance pattern	None	AD	AD	AD
CCH	Rare	100%	100%	100%
MTC	100%	100%	100%	100%
Pheochromocytoma	0%	0%	10–60%	50%
Hyperparathyroidism	0%	0%	10–30%	0%
Cutaneous lichen amyloidosis	0%	0%	< 5%	0%
Ganglioneuromatosis	0%	0%	0%	100%
Marfinoid body habitus	0%	0%	0%	100%

AD Autosomal dominant

annual CT levels. CT levels greater than 100 pg/mL are interpreted as "suspicious for MTC" and further work-up pursued.

Genetic testing is increasingly feasible and accessible, making early detection of genetic diseases easier. Some studies suggest genetic analysis for *RET* mutations via polymerase chain reaction (PCR) amplification and direct DNA sequencing is 100% sensitive and 100% specific [71, 72]. Identification of a *RET* mutation implicates a more than 90% risk of developing MTC throughout one's lifetime; detection of a *RET* mutation may lead to prophylactic thyroidectomy before an aggressive MTC is able to develop [73].

The American Thyroid Association provides Grade A recommendation that all MTC patients undergo genetic screening for *RET* mutations. Children of patients with MEN-2B should undergo *RET* analysis at birth, and children of patients with MEN-2A or FMTC should undergo *RET* analysis before the age of six [55, 56]. Even 6–10% of apparently sporadic cases of MTC demonstrate de novo germ-line *RET* mutations, thus making genetic testing worthwhile in all patients with MTC [52]. The risk of a familial MTC syndrome in an apparently sporadic MTC patient with a negative *RET* screen and negative CT stimulation test in first-degree relatives is less than 1% and negligible, respectively [55].

There is no "gold standard" imaging modality used to diagnose MTC (Table 9–3). MTC does not concentrate iodine and appears "cold" on thyroid iodine scintigraphy. Ultrasound is performed for all thyroid nodules, and can assist in performing fine-needle aspiration [34]. CT

scan may show calcifications, but is most helpful in looking for extrathyroidal metastases, especially in the lung and mediastinum. MRI is best for suspected metastases in the abdomen, especially the liver, while bone scintigraphy is best for assessing bone metastases. Unlike in other malignancies, the utility of FDG-PET is unreliable as FDG uptake in MTC is generally low. Other novel imaging modalities such as ^{18}F-dihydroxyphenylalanine, immunoscintigraphy with labeled monoclonal antibodies against CEA, and gastrin receptor scintigraphy have all been studied, and appear promising, but are not yet widely available [74].

Prophylactic Thyroidectomy in Asymptomatic MEN Patients

Prophylactic thyroidectomy in asymptomatic MEN-2 patients is debatable. Some studies suggest early prophylactic thyroidectomy in all kindreds of patients with MEN-2A or MEN-2B; after aggressive thyroidectomy, few patients will develop MTC later in life [74, 75]. At the Seventh International Workshop on MEN in 1999, MTC was classified into various risk groups based on the type of *RET* mutation. The American Thyroid Association recommends prophylactic total thyroidectomy in all infants with high-risk MEN-2B (Codon 918 mutation) before the 1st year of life, and in all children with MEN-2A (Codon 634 mutation) before the 6th year of life [55, 56, 76]. Lower-risk patients, including those with family history of FMTC, can defer prophylactic thyroidectomy, but only with aggressive follow-up including annual CT measurements and neck ultrasound [49, 77].

First-Line Treatment

Surgery

Total thyroidectomy with complete cervical lymph node dissection is the treatment of choice for all patients with MTC [78–81]. After excluding pheochromocytoma, which would necessitate a prior adrenalectomy, all patients with MTC should proceed to surgery as soon as possible. Lymph node metastases are present in up to 80% of patients with a palpable neck mass at the time of surgery [82]. Reoperation for residual (or recurrent) disease portends a 5–14% risk of injury to adjacent organs, including recurrent laryngeal nerve injury, hypoparathyroidism, and thoracic duct injury [83–85]. With presence of locoregional lymph node metastases and reoperation injury rate both high, most surgeons prefer an initial early aggressive approach including total thyroidectomy and complete cervical lymph node dissection.

During surgery, the parathyroid glands are identified and preserved if at all possible; if normal in appearance, they are left in place or transplanted into an intact sternocleidomastoid muscle or nondominant forearm muscle [65, 66, 86]. In patients with MEN-2A, three of four parathyroid glands are removed to help mitigate development of future parathyroid adenomas which will develop in 10% of these patients [65].

Treatment for Persistent or Residual Disease

External Beam Radiation Therapy

External beam radiation therapy (EBRT) is generally not recommended for treatment of MTC except in two specific situations: (1) patients with inoperable disease and (2) patients with residual local disease despite surgical resection [87]. In general, overall survival is equal in patients who are treated with surgery alone compared to surgery plus external beam radiation. One report retrospectively compared 80 patients who received surgery alone to 35 patients who received surgery plus EBRT. Relapse rate and total survival were equal in both groups, though the patients who receive surgery plus EBRT had a worse initial prognosis due to tumor burden [88].

Targeted Radiotherapy

C-cells do not take up or store iodine; therefore, radioactive iodine treatment is of no value in MTC and is not discussed further. ^{131}I-MIBG, however, is taken up by a minority of MTC patients and can be considered; one study shows an overall response rate of 40% with ^{131}I-MIBG radiotherapy in patients who take up ^{131}I-MIBG [89].

Patients with widely metastatic disease despite surgery can be evaluated for radioimmunotherapy with radio-labeled anti-CEA or radio-labeled octreotide. In one report, 29 patients with metastatic MTC were treated with anti-CEA monoclonal antibodies (MAb's) [90]. These high-risk patients have short CT doubling times, bone marrow involvement of MTC, and are incurable with surgery alone. The patients were divided into two groups: one group received murine anti-CEA MAb and one group received humanized anti-CEA MAb. There was no difference in survival between the two groups, but both groups demonstrated longer survival duration than a similarly matched high-risk untreated group of patients (110 versus 61 months). Another study also showed promising results. Fifteen patients with advanced disease were given ^{131}I-labeled anti-CEA MoAbs; seven patients had a 55% reduction in tumor burden and eleven patients experienced stabilization of disease lasting 3–26 months [91].

Radioisotope-labeled octreotide has also been studied. In a study published in 2004, 21 patients with metastatic MTC, a positive OctreoScan, and residual or progressive disease after surgery received 2–8 cycles of ^{90}Y-labeled octreotide [92]. Two patients obtained a complete response and

12 patients experienced stabilization of disease; average response duration was 3–40 months. Half the patients received no benefit from [90] Y-labeled octreotide. Currently, radiolabeled anti-CEA MoAb and radiolabeled octreotide radioimmunotherapy are only available through clinical trials.

Chemotherapy

Because MTC is a relatively uncommon disease with variable degrees of expression, chemotherapy trials are small, heterogeneous, and difficult to compare. Most studies use "traditional chemotherapies" including a combination of doxorubicin, 5-fluorouracil (5-FU), cis-platin, and/or dacarbazine (DTIC) [87]. All studies are small (less than ten patients each) with a heterogeneous group of patients, making results difficult to interpret. Conventional chemotherapy regimen used in other cancers – doxorubicin and 5-FU – has not achieved reduction in tumor bulk or cure for patients with MTC. It also has significant adverse side effects and is therefore not currently recommended as first-line therapy for MTC.

Other neuroendocrine tumors such as carcinoid tumor and islet cell carcinomas show response to 5-FU and DTIC; this regimen was tried in a small (seven patients) trial. Four patients achieved a clinically significant response, but the remission was partial and short-lived [93]. Another small (seven patients) trial evaluated DTIC, cyclophosphamide, and vincristine; four patients developed partial response or stabilization of disease while three patients progressed on chemotherapy [94].

Novel chemotherapy agents are also being investigated. Heat shock protein (Hsp) 90 facilitates cellular proliferation as a molecular chaperone; 17-allylaminogeldanamycin, an Hsp 90 inhibitor, is under investigation and appears promising [95]. Given the role of RET tyrosine kinase receptor in the development of MTC, tyrosine kinase inhibitors are a logical agent for treatment of MTC [96, 97]. Preliminary results from phase II clinical trials demonstrate promising but somewhat limited efficacy of monotherapy by those tyrosine kinase inhibitors that harbor specific activity against RET (vandetanib, sorafenib, and sunitinib) [98, 99]. It is still not clear if these novel chemotherapeutic agents will significantly improve MTC treatment.

For now, chemotherapy is not recommended as first-line treatment for MTC but may be considered in patients with short CT doubling time without other viable treatment options [87]. CT levels are often used to evaluate response rates, but this can be misleading as CT levels do not always directly correlate with tumor burden [87]. If one chooses to proceed with conventional chemotherapy, the combination of 5-FU and DTIC is first-line, based on its low adverse effect profile, though results of this chemotherapeutic regimen are partial at best. Patients should be encouraged to enroll in clinical trials evaluating novel targeted therapies.

Biologic Agents

Somatostatin decreases calcitonin secretion in vitro and in vivo, thereby making it an obvious therapeutic agent for calcitonin-secreting MTC [100–102]. Multiple case reports and small trials have shown that octreotide, a somatostatin analog, unreliably decreases CT levels and/or CT-related symptoms such as diarrhea and flushing. If given, octreotide is administered twice to thrice daily, subcutaneously. Despite early promise, somatostatin analogs show little to no benefit of treating MTC but may occasionally improve symptoms of diarrhea and flushing [87].

Other neuroendocrine tumors, such as carcinoid tumor, show response to recombinant interferon alpha (rINF-α (alpha)). In one study, seven MTC patients received rINF-α (alpha) and octreotide; though six patients reported significant symptomatic relief, a reduction in tumor burden was not shown [103].

Immunotherapy

In a preclinical trial, labetuzumab, a humanized anti-CEA monoclonal antibody, inhibited growth of human MTC xenografts alone or in combination with DTIC [104]. Another immunotherapy, autologous dendritic cells pulsed with tumor cell lysate derived from allogeneic MTC, has been tried in patients with MTC with limited efficacy [105].

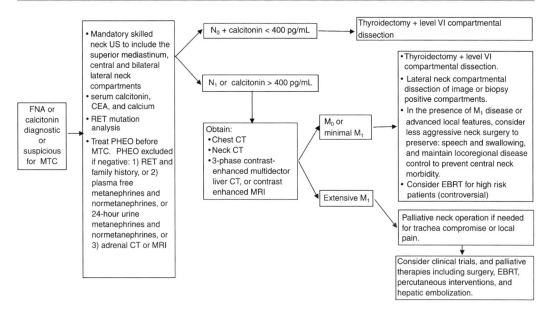

Fig. 9.3 Initial treatment algorithm of MTC as proposed by the American Thyroid Association. From Kloos et al. [56], used with permission

Treatment of Metastatic Lesions

Bone surgery is indicated when bone metastases result in unstable or painful bones and joints. Likewise, surgical resection is considered for brain, lung, and liver metastases; unfortunately though, most metastases in MTC are small and diffuse and therefore not easily amenable to surgical removal. Embolization or chemoembolization can also be considered for liver metastases [106].

The algorithm for initial evaluation and treatment of MTC recently established by the American Thyroid Association is shown in Fig. 9.3 [56].

Follow-Up

Biochemical Follow-Up

Normalization of CT and CEA levels after surgery usually indicates cure; therefore, serial CT and CEA measurements are an effective way to follow patients. After complete surgical resection, CT levels normalize within 72 h [107] while CEA levels normalize in 2–3 months [108]. The optimal time frame is not defined, but most physicians measure CT and CEA levels every 6 months for 2 years, and then annually thereafter.

There is debate between whether basal or stimulated CT levels should be measured. Some physicians argue that obtaining a stimulated CT level is cumbersome and has little clinical consequence. Most physicians, however, prefer to measure stimulated CT levels as it is much more sensitive than measuring basal CT levels. A preoperative CT level less than 50 pg/mL portends a postoperative normalization of CT [109]. Half the patients who present with palpable disease have persistently elevated CT even after total thyroidectomy and complete cervical lymph node dissection [110]. Fortunately, most of these patients have a relatively indolent course without clinically significant recurrence; follow-up, however, becomes challenging. If CT levels rise dramatically from the already elevated baseline, or palpable disease develops, prompt investigation including ultrasound-guided FNA and imaging should commence [56].

CEA is elevated in several malignancies and is not recommended for initial diagnosis of MTC. However, postoperative CEA levels are measured serially in follow-up; a rapid rise in CEA should prompt re-evaluation for disease recurrence or progression [25].

Radiographic Follow-Up

To investigate an elevated CT level (CT > 150 pg/mL), imaging should be obtained [56], but the optimal radiographic choice is not well defined (Table 9.3) [111–113]. If there is a palpable neck mass, ultrasound is performed, preferably with FNA [56]. To investigate suspected metastases in the lung or abdomen, CT or MRI are preferred. Even with high-resolution CT scan or MRI, liver metastases may be too small to identify radiographically so some physicians recommend diagnostic laparoscopy with direct visualization of the liver [83, 114]. Bone scintigraphy and skeletal MRI are both successfully used to evaluate bone metastases. Both PET and technetium-M ^{99}-DMSA scans are fairly sensitive at detecting sizable tumors, but have poor sensitivity for occult tumors, and are generally not recommended for MTC [113, 115].

Postoperative Recurrence

Total thyroidectomy with complete cervical lymph node dissection portends biochemical cure (normocalcitonemia) in most children with MEN-2A or FMTC who are diagnosed via genetic testing [74, 75]. In MTC patients who present with a solitary thyroid nodule, however, recurrence

rates reach 50% [110]. In a study of 56 patients thought to be "cured" after surgery, 44% developed elevated CT level, 10% developed elevated CEA level, and 29% developed imaging-defined relapse [113]. Important prognostic factors include age, postoperative CT levels, and TNM stage of disease [4, 5, 7, 113, 116].

Each component of the TNM stage helps determine prognosis [113]. Large tumor size portends a poorer prognosis. Patients with large tumor size (T4) have a 70% risk of relapse despite the presence or absence of nodal involvement or metastases. Nodal involvement is also an important prognostic indicator. T1 disease patients are divided into two groups: those with positive lymph nodes (N1) or those without (N0). In patients with T1N0 stage (small tumor without lymph nodes), relapse rate is very low. In patients with T1N1 (small tumor with even just one positive lymph node), relapse rate is 37% [113]. The presence or absence of metastases also plays a major prognostic role in patients with MTC; distant metastases are the main cause of death in patients with MTC. Half the patients have distant metastases on presentation; organs most often involved are lung, bone, and liver. Ten-year survival after the detection of a distant metastasis is only 20%.

Postoperative CT levels are also prognostically significant. Nearly half the patients with initially palpable disease will have an elevated CT level postoperatively [110]. If CT normalizes after surgery, there is only a 9% relapse rate. If CT does not normalize after surgery, relapse rate is more than 50% [113].

Table 9.3 Sensitivities of imaging modalities for detecting local or recurrent gross MTC in patients with elevated postoperative calcitonin levels. Adapted from Giraudet et al. [111]. Used with permission

	PET(%)	US(%)	CT(%)	MRI(%)	Bone scan(%)
Neck	32	98	61		
Mediastinal LN	70		100		
Lung	34		100		
Liver	25	81	82	100	
Bone	30			51	65

PET Positron emission tomography
US Ultrasound
CT Computed tomography
MRI Magnetic resonance imaging

Re-operation

Re-operation poses significant risk and is currently only recommended for patients with inadequate initial surgery or for patients who develop palpable disease after initial surgery. In one study, 32 patients with elevated CT levels after total thyroidectomy and complete cervical lymph node dissection underwent re-operation; 28% of patients achieved biochemical cure while 40% demonstrated a reduction in CT [117]. Additional studies in a more carefully selected patient population demonstrated CT reduction in up to 90% of patients [83]. Unfortunately, re-operation of the neck is technically challenging, with complication rates reaching 14%; however, this number greatly varies on the time frame in which repeat surgery is performed. Patients are at risk for thoracic duct injury, permanent hypoparathyroidism, and recurrent laryngeal nerve injury; all of these injuries carry their own long-term sequelae. Complication rates are lower in patients who undergo repeat surgery within 1 week of initial neck surgery.

Ultimately, the risk of surgical complication must be compared with the benefit of achieving biochemical cure before recommending re-operation in patients with an elevated postoperative CT level. If there is a palpable lesion or radiographic evidence of neck recurrence, repeat surgery should be considered; in others, the decision is not clear [56]. It is not uncommon to see patients in clinical practice who had an inadequate initial surgery; these patients who initially received partial thyroidectomy or total thyroidectomy without complete cervical lymph node dissection should undergo repeat surgery.

Conclusion

MTC is a calcitonin-secreting carcinoma of the thyroid gland, found in association with interesting genetic patterns. Our understanding of the disease has greatly increased with the discovery of the *RET* and the genotype–phenotype relationship of its various mutations, but MTC remains a challenging disease. Surgical resection is the best treatment for MTC, and prophylactic thyroidectomy is recommended for children with MEN-2A and MEN-2B very early in life, sometimes even during infancy. Novel treatments, including tyrosine kinase receptor inhibitors, biologic agents, and monoclonal antibodies, are still under study and may prove to be efficacious in the future.

References

1. Horner M, Ries L, Krapcho M, et al. SEER cancer statistics review, 1975 – 2006. National Cancer Institute. http://seer.cancer.gov/csr/1975_2006/. Accessed 156 Jan 2010.
2. Saad M, Ordonez N, Rashid R, et al. Medullary carcinoma of the thyroid. A study of the clinical features and prognostic factors in 161 patients. Medicine. 1984;63:319–42.
3. Olson JE, Hughes J, Alpern HD. Family members of patients with sporadic medullary thyroid carcinoma must be screened for hereditary disease. Surgery. 1992;112:1074–8.
4. Dottorini M, Assi A, Sironi M, et al. Multivariate analysis of patients with medullary thyroid carcinoma. Prognostic significance and impact on treatment of clinical and pathologic variables. Cancer. 1996;77:1556–65.
5. Modigliani E, Cohen R, Campos J. Prognostic factors for survival and for biochemical cure in medullary thyroid carcinoma; results in 899 patients. Clin Endocrinol. 1998;48:265–73.
6. Kebebew E, Ituarte P, Siperstein A, et al. Medullary thyroid carcinoma. Clinical characteristics, treatment, prognostic factors, and comparison of staging systems. Cancer. 2000;88:1139–48.
7. Clark J, Fridman T, Odell J, et al. Prognostic variables and calcitonin in medullary thyroid cancer. Laryngoscope. 2005;115:1445–50.
8. Guyetant S, Josselin N, Savagner F. C-cell hyperplasia and medullary thyroid carcinoma: clinicopathological and genetic correlations in 66 consecutive patients. Mod Pathol. 2003;16:756–63.
9. Horn R. Carcinoma of the thyroid: description of a distinctive morphological variant and report of seven cases. Cancer. 1951;4:697–707.
10. Hazard J, Hawk W, Crile G. Medullary (solid carcinoma of the thyroid – a clinicopathological entity. J Clin Endocrinol Metab. 1959;19:152–61.
11. Sipple J. The association of pheochromocytoma with carcinoma of the thyroid gland. Am J Med. 1961; 31:163–6.
12. Copp D, Cameron E. Demonstration of a hypocalcemic factor (calcitonin) in commercial parathyroid extract. Science. 1961;134:2038.
13. Williams E. A review of 17 cases of carcinomas of the thyroid and pheochromocytomas. J Clin Pathol. 1965; 18:288–92.

14. Mathew C, Chin K, Easton D, et al. A linked genetic marker for multiple endocrine neoplasia syndrome type 2A on chromosome 10. Nature. 1987;328: 527–8.
15. Eng C. The RET proto-oncogene in multiple endocrine neoplasia type 2 and Hirschsprung's disease. N Engl J Med. 1996;335:943–51.
16. Eng C, Clayton D, Schuffenecker I, et al. The relationship between specific RET proto-oncogene mutation and disease phenotype in multiple endocrine neoplasia type 2: international RET Mutation Consortium Analysis. JAMA. 1996;276:1575–9.
17. Varga I, Pospisilova V, Gmitterova K, et al. The phylogenesis and ontogenesis of the human pharyngeal region focused on the thymus, parathyroid, and thyroid glands. Neuro Endocrinol Lett. 2008;29:837–45.
18. Wolfe H, Delellis R. Familial medullary thyroid carcinoma and C-cell hyperplasia. Clin Endocrinol Metab. 1981;10:351–65.
19. Wolfe H, Melvin K, Cervi-Skinner S, et al. C-cell hyperplasia preceding medullary thyroid carcinoma. N Engl J Med. 1973;289:437–41.
20. Hedinger C, Williams E, Sobin L. Histological typing of thyroid tumours. In: WHO, editor. International classification of tumours. 2nd ed. Berlin: Springer; 1988.
21. Rosai J, Carcangiu M, DeLellis R. Tumors of the thyroid gland. In: Rosai J, Carcangiu M, DeLellis R, editors. Atlas of tumor pathology. 3rd ed. Armed Forces Institute of Pathology: Washington, DC; 1992.
22. More A, Gicquel C, Abdelmoumene N, et al. Cushing's syndrome in medullary thyroid carcinoma. J Endocrinol Invest. 1995;18:180–5.
23. Sawicki B. Evaluation of the role of mammalian thyroid parafollicular cells. Acta Histochem. 1995;97: 389–99.
24. Guignat L, Bidart J, Nocera M, et al. Chromogranin A and the alpha-subunit of glycoprotein hormones in medullary thyroid carcinoma and phaeochromocytoma. Br J Cancer. 2001;84:808–12.
25. Mendelsohn G, Wells S, Baylin S. Relationship of carcinoembryonic antigen and calcitonin to tumor virulence in medullary thyroid carcinoma. Cancer. 1984;54:657–62.
26. Lips C, Hoppener J, Thijssen J. Medullary thyroid carcinoma: role of genetic testing and calcitonin measurement. Ann Clin Biochem. 2001;38:168–79.
27. Pondel M. Calcitonin and calcitonin receptors: bone and beyond. Int J Exp Pathol. 2000;81:405–22.
28. Tobler P, Tschopp F, Dambacher M, et al. Identification and characterization of calcitonin forms in plasma and urine of normal subjects and medullary thyroid carcinoma patients. J Clin Endocrinol Metab. 1983;57: 749–54.
29. Body J, Heath H. Estimates of circulating monomeric calcitonin: physiological studies in normal and thyroidectomized man. J Clin Endocrinol Metab. 1983;57: 897–903.
30. Motte P, Vauzelle P, Gardet P, et al. Construction and clinical validation of a sensitive and specific assay for serum mature calcitonin using monoclonal anti-peptide antibodies. Clin Chim Acta. 1988;174:35–54.
31. Grauer A, Raue F, Ziegler R. Clinical usefulness of a new chemiluminescent two-site immunoassay for human calcitonin. Exp Clin Endocrinol Diabetes. 1998;106:289–91.
32. Demers L, Spencer C. Laboratory medicine practice guidelines. Laboratory support for the diagnosis and monitoring of thyroid disease. Thyroid. 2003;13: 4–126.
33. Baloch Z, Carayon P, Conte-Devolx B. Laboratory medicine practice guidelines: laboratory support for the diagnosis and monitoring of thyroid disease. Thyroid. 2003;13:3–126.
34. Leboulleux S, Baudin E, Travagli J, et al. Medullary thyroid carcinoma. Clin Endocrinol. 2004;61: 299 310.
35. Vitale G, Ciccarelli A, Caraglia M, et al. Comparison of two provocative tests for calcitonin in medullary thyroid carcinoma:omeprazole vs. calcitonin. Clin Chem. 2002;48:1505–10.
36. Deftos L, Weisman M, Williams G, et al. Influence of age and sex on plasma calcitonin in human beings. N Engl J Med. 1980;302:1351–3.
37. Hillaryd C, Coombes R, Greenberg P, et al. Calcitonin in breast and lung cancer. Clin Endocrinol. 1976;5:1–8.
38. Whang K, Steinwald P, White J. Related serum calcitonin precursors in sepsis and systemic inflammation. J Clin Endocrinol Metab. 1998;83:3296–301.
39. Mulligan L, Kwok J, Healy C, et al. Germline mutation of the RET proto-oncogene in multiple endocrine neoplasia syndrome type 2A. Nature. 1993;363:458–60.
40. Donis-Keller H, Dou S, Chi D, et al. Mutations in the RET proto-oncogene are associated with MEN2A and FMTC. Hum Mol Genet. 1993;2:851–6.
41. Hofstra R, Landsvater R, Ceccherini I, et al. A mutation in the RET proto-oncogene associated with multiple-endocrine neoplasia syndrome type 2B and sporadic medullary thyroid carcinoma. Nature. 1994;367:375–6.
42. Eng C, Mulligan L. Mutations of the RET proto-oncogene in the multiple endocrine neoplasia type 2 syndromes, related sporadic tumours, and Hirschsprung disease. Hum Mutat. 1997;9:97–109.
43. Manie S, Santor M, Fusco A, et al. The RET receptor: function in development and dysfunction in congenital malformation. Trends Genet. 2001;17:580–9.
44. Hansford J, Mulligan L. Multiple endocrine neoplasia type 2 and RET: from neoplasia to neurogenesis. J Med Genet. 2000;37:817–27.
45. Carlson K, Bracamontes J, Jackson C, et al. Parent-of-origin effects in multiple endocrine neoplasia type 2B. Am J Hum Genet. 1994;55:1076–82.
46. Yip L, Cote G, Shapiro S, et al. Multiple endocrine neoplasia type 2. Evaluation of the genotype-phenotype relationship. Arch Surg. 2003;138:409–16.
47. Machens A, Niccoli-Sire P, Hoegel J, et al. Early malignant progression of hereditary medullary thyroid cancer. N Engl J Med. 2003;349:1517–25.

48. Kouvaraki M, Shapiro S, Perrier N, et al. RET proto-oncogene: a review and update of genotype-phenotype correlations in hereditary medullary thyroid cancer and associated endocrine tumors. Thyroid. 2005;15: 531–44.
49. Lombardo F, Baudin E, Chiefari E, et al. Familial medullary thyroid carcinoma: clinical variability and low aggressiveness associated with RET mutation at codon 804. J Clin Endocrinol Meta. 2002;87:1674–80.
50. Menko F, van der Luijt R, de Valk I. Atypical MEN type 2B associated with two germline RET mutations on the same allele not involving codon 918. J Clin Endocrinol Metab. 2002;87:393–7.
51. Schuffenecker I, Ginet N, Goldgar D, et al. Prevalence and parental origin of de novo RET mutations in MEN 2A and FMTC. Am J Hum Genet. 1997;60:233–7.
52. Hubner R, Houlston R. Molecular advances in medullary thyroid cancer diagnostics. J Clin Pathol Mol Pathol. 2006;54:206–14.
53. Huang S, Koch C, Vortmeyer A, et al. Duplication of the mutant RET allele in trisomy 10 or loss of the wild-type allele in multiple endocrine neoplasia type 2-associated pheochromocytoma. Cancer Res. 2000;60:6223–6.
54. Robledo M, Gil L, Pllan M. Polymorphisms G691S/S904S of RET as genetic modifiers of MEN2A. Cancer Res. 2003;63:1814–7.
55. Brandi M, Gagel R, Angeli A, et al. Guidelines for diagnosis and therapy of MEN type 1 and type 2. J Clin Endocrinol Metab. 2001;86:5658–71.
56. Kloos R, Eng C, Evans D, et al. Medullary thyroid cancer: management guidelines of the American Thyroid Association. Thyroid. 2009;19:565–93.
57. Skinner M, DeBenedetti M, Moley J, et al. Medullary thyroid carcinoma in children with multiple endocrine neoplasia types 2A and 2B. J Pediatr Surg. 1996; 31:177–81.
58. Shimotake T, Iwai N, Yanagihara J, et al. The natural history of multiple endocrine neoplasia type 2A – A clinical analysis. Jpn J Surg. 1990;20:290–3.
59. Lenders J, Pacak K, Walther M, et al. Biochemical diagnosis of pheochromocytoma. Which test is best? JAMA. 2002;287:1427–34.
60. Pacini F, Fugazzola L, Bevilacqua G, et al. Multiple endocrine neoplasia type 2A and cutaneous lichen amyloidosis: description of a new family. J Endocrinol Invest. 1993;16:295–6.
61. Decker R, Peacock L, Watson P, et al. Hirschsprung disease in MEN 2A: increased spectrum of RET exon 10 genotypes and strong genotype-phenotype correlation. Hum Mol Genet. 1998;7:129–34.
62. Gagel R, Levy M, Donovan D, et al. Multiple endocrine neoplasia type 2a associated with Cutaneous lichen Amyloidosis. Ann Intern Med. 1989;111:802–6.
63. Gill J, Reyes-Mugica M, Iyengar S, et al. Early presentation of metastatic medullary carcinoma in multiple endocrine neoplasia, type IIA: Implications for therapy. J Pediatr. 1996;129:459–64.
64. Lebouleux S, Travagli J, Caillou B. Medullary thyroid carcinoma as part of multiple endocrine neoplasia type 2B syndrome. Influence of the stage on the clinical course. Cancer. 2002;94:44–50.
65. Schlumberger M, Pacini F. Thyroid tumors. Paris: Nucleon; 1999.
66. Quayle F, Moley J. Medullary thyroid carcinoma: including MEN 2A and MEN 2B syndromes. J Surg Oncol. 2005;89:122–9.
67. Pacini F, Burroni L, Ciuoli C, et al. Thyroid nodules: pathogenesis, diagnosis and treatment. Baillieres Best Pract Res Clin Endocrinol Metab. 1994;14:559–75.
68. Vierhapper H, Raber W, Bieglmayer C, et al. Routine measurement of plasma CA in nodular thyroid diseases. J Clin Endocrinol Metab. 1997;82:1589–993.
69. Mayr B, Brabant G, von zur Muhlen A. Incidental detection of familial medullary thyroid carcinoma by calcitonin screening for nodular thyroid disease. Eur J Endocrinol. 1999;141:286–9.
70. Elisei R, Bottici V, Luchetti F, et al. Impact of routine measurement of serum calcitonin on the diagnosis and outcome of medullary thyroid cancer: experience in 10,864 patients with nodular thyroid disorders. J Clin Endocrinol Metab. 2004;89:163–8.
71. Lips C, Landsvater R, Hoppener J, et al. Clinical screening as compared with DNA analysis in families with multiple endocrine neoplasia syndrome type 2A. N Engl J Med. 1994;331:870–1.
72. Utiger R. Medullary thyroid carcinoma, genes, and the prevention of cancer. N Engl J Med. 1994; 331:870–1.
73. Freyer G, LIgneau B, Schlumberger M, et al. Quality of life in patients at risk of medullary thyroid carcinoma and followed by a comprehensive medical network; trends for future evaluations. Ann Oncol. 2001;12:1461–5.
74. Gagel R, Tashjian A, Cummings T, et al. The clinical outcome of prospective screening for multiple endocrine neoplasia type 2A. An 18-year experience. N Engl J Med. 1988;318:478–84.
75. Wells S, Skinner M. Prophylactic thyroidectomy, based on direct genetic testing, in patients at risk for the multiple endocrine neoplasia type 2 syndromes. Exp Clin Endocrinol Diabetes. 1998;106:29–34.
76. Cote G, Gagel R. Lessons learned from the management of a rare genetic cancer. N Engl J Med. 2003;349:1566–8.
77. Frohnauer M, Decker R. Update on the MEN 2A c804 RET mutation: is prophylactic thyroidectomy indicated? Surgery. 2000;128:1052–8.
78. Russell C, Heerden J, Sizemore G, et al. The surgical management of medullary thyroid carcinoma. Ann Surg. 1983;197:42–8.
79. Duh Q, Sancho J, Greenspan F, et al. Medullary thyroid carcinoma. The need for early diagnosis and total thyroidectomy. Arch Surg. 1989;124:1206–10.
80. Kallinowski F, Buhr H, Meybier H, et al. Medullary carcinoma of the thyroid. Therapeutic strategy derived from fifteen years of experience. Surgery. 1993; 114:491–6.
81. Cohen M, Moley J. Surgical treatment of medullary thyroid carcinoma. J Intern Med. 2003;253:616–26.

82. Moley J, DeBenedetti M. Patterns of nodal metastases in palpable medullary thyroid carcinoma. Ann Surg. 1999;229:880–8.

83. Moley J, Dilley W, DeBenedetti M. Improved results of cervical reoperation for medullary thyroid carcinoma. Ann Surg. 1997;225:734–43.

84. Hundahl S, Cady B, Cunningham M, et al. Initial results from a prospective cohort study of 5583 cases of thyroid carcinoma treated in the United States during 1996. U.S. and German Thyroid Cancer Study Group. Cancer. 2000;89:202–17.

85. Rosato L, Avenia N, Bernante P, et al. Complications of thyroid surgery: Analysis of a multicentric study on 14,934 patients operated on in Italy over 5 years. World J Surg. 2004;28:271–6.

86. Herfarth K, Bartsch D, Doherty G, et al. Surgical management of hyperparathyroidism in patients with multiple endocrine neoplasia type 2A. Surgery. 1996;120:966–73.

87. Orlandi F, Caraci P, Mussa A, et al. Treatment of medullary thyroid carcinoma: an update. Endocr Relat Cancer. 2001;8:135–47.

88. Tubiana M, Haddad E, Schlumberger M, et al. External radiotherapy in thyroid cancer. Cancer. 1985;55:2062–71.

89. Clarke S, Lazarus C, Edwards S, et al. Scintigraphy and treatment of medullary carcinoma of the thyroid with iodine-131-metaiodobenzylguanidine. J Nucl Med. 1987;28:1820–5.

90. Chatal J, Campion L, Kraeber-Bodere F, et al. Survival improvement in patients with medullary thyroid carcinoma who undergo pretargeted anti-carcinoembryonic-antigen radioimmunotherapy: a collaborative study with the French Endocrine Tumor Group. J Clin Oncol. 2007;166:1705–11.

91. Juweid M, Hajjar G, Swayne L, et al. Phase I/II trial of ^{131}I-MN-14 F(ab)2 anti-carcinoembryonic antigen monoclonal antibody in the treatment of patients with metastatic medullary carcinoma. Cancer. 1999;85:1828–42.

92. Bodei L, Handkiewicz-Junak D, Grana C, et al. Receptor radionuclide therapy with 90-Y-DOTATOC in patients with medullary thyroid carcinomas. Cancer Biother Radiopharm. 2004;19:65–71.

93. Orlandi F, Caraci P, Berruti A, et al. Chemotherapy with dacarbazine and 5-fluorouracil in advanced medullary thyroid cancer. Ann Oncol. 1994;5:763–5.

94. Wu L, Averbuch S, Ball D, et al. Treatment of advanced medullary thyroid carcinoma with a combination of cyclophosphamide, vincristine, and dacarbazine. Cancer. 1994;73:432–6.

95. Geogakis G, Younes A. Heat-shock protein 90 inhibitors in cancer therapy: 17AAG and beyond. Future Oncol. 2005;1:273–81.

96. Cohen M, Hussain H, Moley J. Inhibition of medullary thyroid carcinoma cell proliferation and RET phosphorylation by tyrosine kinase inhibitors. Surgery. 2002;132:960–6.

97. Ezzat S, Huang P, Dackiw A, et al. Dual inhibition of RET and FGFR4 restrains medullary thyroid cancer cell growth. Clin Cancer Res. 2005;11:1336–41.

98. Cakir M, Gross A. Medullary thyroid cancer: molecular biology and novel molecular therapies. Neuroendocrinology. 2009;90:323–48.

99. Sugawara M, Geffner D, Martinez D, et al. Novel treatment of medullary thyroid cancer. Curr Opin Endocrinol Diabetes Obes. 2009;16:367–72.

100. Gordin A, Lamberg A, Prelkonen R, et al. Somatostatin inhibits the pentagastrin induced release of serum calcitonin in medullary carcinoma of the thyroid. Clin Endocrinol. 1978;8:289–95.

101. Pacini F, Elisei R, Anelli S, et al. Somatostatin in medullary thyroid cancer. In vitro and in vivo studies. Cancer. 1989;63:1189–95.

102. Diez J, Iglesias P. Somatostatin analogs in the treatment of medullary thyroid carcinoma. J Endocrinol Invest. 2002;25:773–8.

103. Vitale G, Tagliaferri P, Caraglia M, et al. Slow release lanreotide in combination with interferon alpha-2b in the treatment of symptomatic advanced medullary thyroid carcinoma. J Clin Endocrinol Metab. 2000; 85:983–8.

104. Stein R, Goldenberg D. A humanized monoclonal antibody to carcinoembryonic antigen, labetuzumab, inhibits tumour growth and sensitizes human medullary thyroid cancer xenografts to dacarbazine chemotherapy. Mol Cancer Ther. 2004;3: 155901564.

105. Bachleitner-Hofmann T, Friedl J, Hassler M, Hayden H, Dubsky P, Sachet M, et al. Pilot trial of autologous dendritic cells loaded with tumor lysate(s) from allogeneic tumor cell lines in patients with metastatic medullary thyroid carcinoma. Oncol Rep. 2009; 21(6):1585–92.

106. Roche A, Girish B, de Baere T, et al. Trans-catheter arterial chemoembolization as first-line treatment for hepatic metastases from endocrine tumors. Eur Radiol. 2003;13:136–40.

107. Fugazzola L, Pinchera A, Luchetti F. Disappearance rate of serum calcitonin after total thyroidectomy for medullary thyroid carcinoma. Int J Biol Markers. 1994;9:21–4.

108. MacDonald J. Carcinoembryonic antigen screening: pros and cons. Semin Oncol. 1999;26:556–60.

109. Cohen R, Campos J, Salaun C, et al. Preoperative calcitonin levels are predictive of tumor size and postoperative calcitonin normalization in medullary thyroid carcinoma. J Clin Endocrinol Metab. 2000;85:919–22.

110. Stepanas A, Samaan N, Hill C, et al. Medullary thyroid carcinoma: Importance of serial calcitonin measurement. Cancer. 1979;43:825.

111. Giraudet A, Vanel D, Leboulleux S, et al. Imaging medullary thyroid carcinoma with persistent elevated calcitonin levels. J Clin Endocrinol Metab. 2007;11: 4185–90.

112. Frank-Raue K, Raue F, Buhr H, et al. Localization of occult persisting medullary thyroid carcinoma before microsurgical reoperation: high sensitivity of selective venous catheterization. Thyroid. 1992;2:113–7.

113. Pellegriti G, Leboulleux S, Baudin E, et al. Long-term outcome of medullary thyroid carcinoma in patients with normal postoperative medical imaging. Br J Cancer. 2003;88:1537–42.

114. Tung W, Vesely T, Moley J. Laparoscopic detection of hepatic metastases in patients with residual or recurrent medullary thyroid cancer. Surgery. 1995;118:1024–9.

115. de Groot J, Links T, Jager P, et al. Impact of 18 F-fluoro-2-deoxy-D-glucose positron emission tomography (FDG-PET) in patients with biochemical evidence of recurrent or residual medullary thyroid cancer. Ann Surg Oncol. 2004;11:786–94.

116. Kebebew E, Kikuchi S, Duh Q, et al. Long-term results of reoperation and localizing studies in patients with persistent or recurrent medullary thyroid cancer. Arch Surg. 2000;135:895–901.

117. Moley J, Wells S, Dilley W. Reoperation for recurrent or persistent medullary thyroid cancer. Surgery. 1993;114:1090–5.

Anaplastic Thyroid Carcinoma

10

Marina Vaysburd

Introduction

Anaplastic thyroid carcinoma (ATC) is a rare aggressive malignancy characterized by a rapidly progressive clinical course nearly always culminating in a fatal outcome. Rare reports of successful treatment and anecdotal accounts of long-term survivors of ATC contribute to the therapeutic nihilism related to ATC, although promising new treatment approaches are emerging.

Epidemiology

ATC is a rare malignancy, accounting for only 1–2% of thyroid carcinomas. In the United States, the incidence of ATC is approximately 300 cases per year, and is similar to other developed countries [1, 2]. Almost all of ATC occurs in individuals above 50 years of age, and most patients present in the seventh decade of life. Slight female to male predominance has been noted, in the 1.5–2 range [1, 2]. The incidence of ATC has been declining in the last 20 years, perhaps reflecting more accurate classification of thyroid neoplasms, higher detection rates, and more

aggressive treatment of DTC, which is considered to be a precursor to ATC [2, 3].

Etiology and Molecular Features

ATC may occur as de novo cancer, or arise from a pre-existing differentiated thyroid carcinoma (DTC), most commonly follicular type. However, only a minority of ATC (~10%) is found in the absence of co-existing differentiated carcinoma, and most ATC occurs in the background of DTC, suggesting that DTC is a precursor lesion. This clinical observation is further supported by genetic findings, suggesting a sequence of gene alterations that accompanies transformation from normal thyroid cells to DTC and on to ATC; similar to well-described transition of colonic mucosa to adenoma and on to colon carcinoma (Figs. 10.1 and 10.2). This accumulation of chromosomal abnormalities and ensuing gene dysregulation lead to loss of cell cycle control, signal transduction activation, and is likely the underlying reason for aggressive clinical behavior. It is likely that multiple pathways of genetic alterations could lead to development of ATC, as not all ATC have identical genetic profiles. Most common genetic abnormalities in ATC involve *RET, p53, RAS, BRAF,* and *β-catenin* genes. As molecular rearrangements in thyroid carcinoma are becoming better described, findings from the DTC specimens, transgenic animal models, and cell cultures demonstrate several early translocations that lead to transformation from normal thyroid epithelium

M. Vaysburd (✉)
Division of Hematology/Oncology, Department of
Medicine, Cedars-Sinai Medical Center, 200 N. Robertson
Blvd #300, Beverly Hills, CA 90211, USA
e-mail: Marina.vaysburd@cshs.org

G.D. Braunstein (ed.), *Thyroid Cancer*, Endocrine Updates 30,
DOI 10.1007/978-1-4614-0875-8_10, © Springer Science+Business Media, LLC 2012

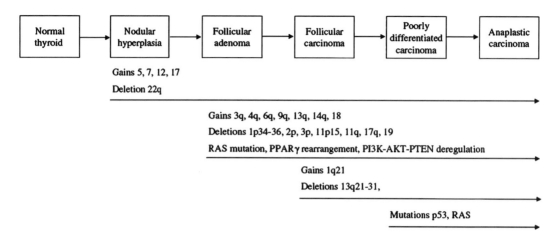

Fig. 10.1 Tumor progression model for follicular thyroid carcinoma. From Wreesman et al. with permission

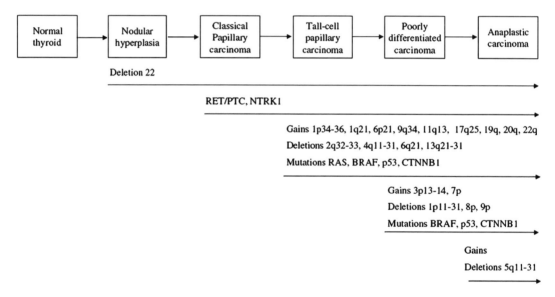

Fig. 10.2 Tumor progression model for papillary thyroid carcinoma. From Wreesman et al. with permission

to either thyroid adenomas or hyperplasia and on to DTC, most prominently affecting *RET* and *RAS* oncogenes and *p53* tumor-suppressor gene (Fig. 10.3) [4, 5]. These "early" genetic abnormalities are nearly always present in ATC, in the background of additional and more complex chromosomal aberrations. Accumulation of increasing number of genetic alterations leads the way to chromosomal instability and is likely responsible for loss of differentiation and clinical transition to ATC.

Pathology

Accurate pathologic identification for ATC is critical as treatment and prognosis can be significantly different from other tumors arising in the thyroid region. Fine-needle aspiration (FNA) is reported to be ~90% accurate [6]. Cytologic features of ATC are usually easily recognizable, provided adequate sample has been obtained. Main reasons for nondiagnostic FNA are: tumor regressive changes (necrosis, hemorrhage, and leukocytic

	Papillary carcinoma				Follicular tumors				Anaplastic carcinoma
	CPTC	FVPTC	TCV	PDPTC	FTA	MIFTC	WIFTC	PDFTC	UTC
Empty nuclei[a]	+	+	+	+	–	–	–	–	–
Papillary growth	+	–	+	+	–	–	–	–	–
Follicular growth	±	+	±	±	+	+	+	±	–
Mitotic activity	–	–	–	++	–	–	–	++	+++++
Necrosis	–	–	–	++	–	–	–	++	+++++
Nuclear polymorphism	–	–	–	++	–	–	–	++	+++++
Encapsulation	–	+	–	–	+	+	+	–	–
Capsular invasion	–	±	–	–	–	+	+++	–	–
Vascular invasion	±	±	–	+	–	+	+++	+	+
Multicentricity	+	–	+	–	–	–	–	–	–
Lymphatic metastasis	++	–	++	++	–	–	–	+	+++
Hematogenous metastasis	–	–	++	++	–	±	++	+++	+++++
Recurrence	10%	10%	40%	50%	0%	10%	40%	60%	100%
Death of disease	5%	5%	25%	40%	0%	10%	40%	60%	100%
RET/PTC	30%	<5%	30%	10%	0%	0%	0%	0%	0%
BRAF	40%	<5%	60%	70%	0%	0%	0%	0%	60%
RAS	<5%	40%	UNK	50%	30%	40%	50%	60%	70%
P53	<5%	<5%	30%	40%	0%	<5%	<5%	40%	80%
CTNNB1	<5%	<5%	UNK	25%	0%	0%	0%	25%	65%
PI3K-AKT–PTEN	24%	24%	24%	UNK	31%	55%	55%	UNK	58%
PPARγ	0%	30%	UNK	UNK	30%	40%	40%	UNK	0%

Fig. 10.3 Clinicopathologic and genetic features of most common thyroid cancer subtypes. a – including optically clear nuclei, nuclear overlap, nuclear enlargement, irregularly shaped nuclei, nuclear grooves, and nuclear pseudoinclusions. Abbreviations: *PTC* papillary thyroid carcinoma, *FTC* follicular thyroid carcinoma, *FTA* follicular thyroid adenoma, *CPTC* classical PTC, *FVPTC*, follicular-variant PTC, *MIFTC*, minimally invasive FTC, *TCV*, tall cell variant, *PDFTC*, poorly differentiated FTC, *PDPTC* poorly differentiated PTC; *UTC* undifferentiated thyroid carcinoma, *WIFTC*, widely invasive FTC, UNK unknown, + present, – not present, ± sometimes present. From Wreesman et al. [4] with permission

infiltration), extensive tumor fibrosis, and distinct differentiated and anaplastic patterns in the same tumor [6]. When ATC is suspected based on clinical grounds, such as a rapidly enlarging fixed neck mass, and FNA is inconclusive, further diagnostic maneuvers, such as core biopsy, should be pursued promptly, because the window of curability for ATC is narrow, and cure, if it can be accomplished at all, can only occur in the setting of complete surgical removal, which is rarely possible except for the earliest and smallest presentations of ATC.

Cytologic features associated with ATC include giant or spindled cells often described as bizarre in appearance with variable size and shapes, and malignant nuclear features (Fig. 10.4). Numerous mitotic figures, irregular nuclear

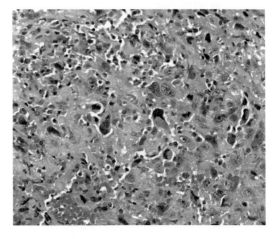

Fig. 10.4 Typical H&E appearance of ATC. Undifferentiated tumor with bizarre cells showing enlarged, pleomorphic hyperchromatic nuclei. (Photo courtesy of Dr. David Frishberg)

membranes with coarse dark chromatin are present. Necrosis and neutrophil infiltration are common, while cartilaginous or osseous metaplasia can also be encountered [7]. Differential diagnosis consideration include primary thyroid lymphoma, DTC, squamous cell carcinoma, and metastases from another primary site. Thyroid transcription factor (TTF-1) expression is absent in ATC cells, but may be present on the admixed DTC cells. In the analysis of 35 ATC cases, TTF1 expression was only found in two cases, and thyroglobulin in one case, thus distinguishing ATC from DTC. At the same time, several epithelial markers are usually expressed, including cytokeratin [7, 8]. Similarly, distinction from lymphoma and medullary thyroid cancer can be accomplished by lack of staining for lymphoid antigens and calcitonin respectively.

Clinical Presentation and Work-Up

Most patients with ATC typically present in the sixth or seventh decade of life. The hallmark of clinical presentation is a history of rapidly enlarging low anterior neck mass, which is hard on palpation and fixed to underlying structures. ATC is known for rapid local, regional, and metastatic spread. In the Surveillance Epidemiology End Results database (SEER) from 1973 to 2000, only 39 (7.5%) of 516 patients presented with localized disease, while 222 (43%) patients presented with distant metastases [1]. Enlarging neck mass, dysphagia, and dysphonia are the most common presenting symptoms [9]. The majority of patients present with masses >5 cm, some up to 20 cm [9]. Local extension is into the surrounding structures of the upper aerodigestive system (trachea, larynx, and esophagus), as well as muscle and fat in approximately 70% of the patients [10]. Spread to the regional lymph nodes occurs early and frequently (~80%) [9]. Distant metastases, most frequently to lungs, are present in up to 50–80% of the patients [9, 10].

The goal of diagnostic tests should be to determine the extent of the disease and the necessity for immediate clinical intervention. Because of the aggressive infiltrative behavior of ATC, patients are at risk for airway compromise, and the need for tracheostomy has to be addressed promptly. Laryngoscopy and esophagoscopy may be necessary to establish the invasion of the airway and esophagus, respectively.

Imaging studies are also very helpful in evaluation of the disease spread (Fig. 10.5). Computed tomography (CT) scan of the neck, chest, abdomen,

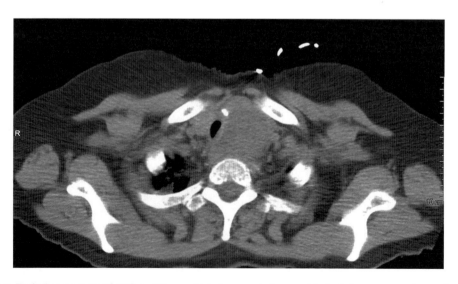

Fig. 10.5 Typical appearance of ATC on CT scan. Note large central mass with deviation, compression, and probable invasion of trachea

and pelvis should be performed for staging and surgical planning. Positron emission tomography (PET) scanning with 18FDG is extremely helpful in finding metastatic disease, not disclosed by other imaging studies. PET scanning requires high FDG metabolism in tumor cells, and experience in using PET in ATC confirms high degree of FDG uptake in ATC primary, nodal, and metastatic lesions [11]. Compared to normal tissue, ATC lesions appear to have up to ten times increase in expression of glucose transporter GLUT1 correlating with increase in FDG uptake [12, 13]. In paraffin-embedded tissue specimens for DTC and ATC, levels of GLUT1 predicted for tumor aggressiveness, suggesting that FDG–PET may emerge not only as diagnostic, but also as a prognostic tool. In addition, as new treatment approaches for ATC evolve, FDG–PET may be used to monitor disease response to treatment and to differentiate between active disease and post-treatment effect. In a study of 16 patients, FDG–PET scanning appeared to change clinical management in eight patients (50%) [11]. However, as PET has a resolution of ~0.5 cm, small metastases can be missed on PET imaging and, therefore, it should be combined with CT. In contrast to DTC, which typically demonstrate I-131 uptake, because of the loss of differentiation, ATC does not uptake I-131, and consequently I-131 scanning does not have a role in ATC.

Staging and Prognosis

American Joint Committee on Cancer (AJCC) staging version 6th edition classifies all ATC as stage IV. This is further subdivided into stage IVA-intrathyroid anaplastic carcinoma – surgically resectable, IVB-extrathyroid anaplastic carcinoma – surgically unresectable, and IVC-distant metastases.

Alternatively, Sugitani et al. [14] have devised a prognostic system based on their review of 47 ATC patients. Using multivariate analysis, they found that four prognostic factors were the most important and independent for predicting death from ATC: (1) presence of acute symptoms, (2) tumor size >5 cm, (3) distant metastasis at

Table 10.1 Prognostic score for ATC

Prognostic score	Survival (days)
0	310
1	280
2	143
3	62
4	42

Sugitani et al. [14]

presentation, and (4) WBC >10,000/mm^3. Based on this information, they proposed a prognostic system in which absence or presence of each of these factors is assigned the value of 0 or 1, respectively. Depending on the score 0–4, five distinct prognostic groups could be identified and the score correlated with survival (Table 10.1). No patients whose PI was three survived more than 6 months, and all patients whose PI was four died within 3 months. Patients whose PI was ≤1 had a 62% survival rate at 6 months. It is also likely, that many anecdotal reports of long-term survivors of ATC include patients whose small ATC was incidentally discovered at the time of thyroidectomy for another diagnosis, and consequently were serendipitously completely excised before local invasion or metastases could develop, or patients whose more favorable tumors were misclassified as ATC. However, the author is aware of one long-term survivor who presented at the age of 62 with a 6 week history of a small neck lump. FNA revealed ATC, and within 5 days of presentation she underwent total thyroidectomy which confirmed 1.5 × 1.3 cm ATC without evidence of extrathyroid extension and 0.1 cm surgical margin. She then underwent a course of postoperative radiation therapy, and is currently without evidence of disease 13 years later. Retrospective review of pathology material confirmed histopathologic features of ATC.

Treatment

Comprehensive review of the ATC treatment reports published during 1975–2002 dramatically demonstrates disappointing outcomes with less than 10% long-term survivors (>2 years) and many reports with 100% fatal outcomes [15].

Similarly, in the SEER database including patients treated during 1971–2000, ATC-specific 1-year mortality was 80.3%, with favorable factors predictive of 1-year survival being age <60 years, disease limited to thyroid, and use of surgery and radiation therapy [1]. At the same time, even though cure of ATC is rare, preserving quality of life by controlling local disease should also be considered an important goal of therapy. Due to the aggressive natural course of ATC, most patients die of uncontrolled local symptoms, which means that attempt at local control should be made even in the presence of distant metastases. While there is no established standard and mortality is nearly 100%, the treatment of localized ATC with curative or long-term disease control intent requires a multimodality approach combining surgery, radiation therapy, chemotherapy, and most recently biologic therapy.

Surgery

For rare patients whose disease has not spread beyond the thyroid, complete surgical resection offers hope for cure. Even with complete surgical resection, recurrence and metastatic spread are common. In the review of 21 cases of ATC managed at Roswell Park Cancer Institute between 1968 and 1992 by Tan, complete surgical resection was accomplished in five patients, and two of these patients survived >10 years, while the third patient is alive 2 years after treatment. In contrast, only one of the remaining patients who did not have complete resection survived beyond 1 year after postoperative radiation therapy [9]. In the 50-year ATC experience from Mayo Clinic, 96 out of 134 patients (72%) underwent primary surgical treatment with complete resection achieved in 29 cases (30% of the surgical patients); with "minimal residual disease" seen in 25 [16]. No statistically significant correlation between extent of operation or completeness of resection and survival was found. There were 13 long-term survivors (>1 year), all treated surgically with complete tumor resection achieved in eight, and only minimal residual disease in three. The main argument against aggressive surgical treatment is potential excessive morbidity related to the extent of surgery required to achieve disease clearance. Invasion of the trachea, esophagus, and larynx is thought to preclude complete surgical resection mostly due to morbidity associated with procedures required. Published consensus on the treatment of ATC recommends complete surgical resection in selected patients if it can be accomplished without resection of vital structures (larynx, pharynx, and esophagus) and should be attempted only if all gross cervical and mediastinal disease can be resected without excessive morbidity [15, 17]. A neck dissection should be performed only in the setting of complete macroscopic resection [15]. However, recent advances in surgical technique may allow for reduction in surgical morbidity, and more aggressive resections with attempt of total disease clearance may be considered by expert surgeons in very select patients with limited extrathyroid disease. The role of surgical debulking (incomplete resection) is not well established. One study has noted survival benefit to debulking and radiation therapy versus biopsy and radiation, while other studies show no survival benefit of debulking surgery [18–20].

Despite uncertain survival benefit, debulking may play an important role in surgical palliation of local symptoms in patients with unresectable and/or metastatic disease. Prevention of asphyxiation can be accomplished by debulking and tracheostomy. The airway compromise is usually caused by the presence of the tumor bulk in the central neck compartment, either due to compression of the trachea, direct invasion, vocal cord paralysis, laryngeal edema, or a combination of these factors. Patients with acute airway compromise require either tracheostomy or crycothyrotomy. These procedures are best performed with fiberoptic intubation in the operating room because of the technical difficulty and challenge of identifying the trachea related to presence of the hard and fixed central mass and the severely deviated or compressed trachea [21]. These surgical procedures can be associated with significant complications, and the pursuit of surgical intervention has to be carefully considered in the context of clinical situation, further treatment options available, and patient and family wishes.

Radiation Therapy

Radiation therapy has emerged as an alternative or adjunct (to surgery) modality to achieve local control in ATC. Early reports using radiation therapy during the 1970s and 1980s demonstrate improvement in local control and short-term survival but no effect on the cure rate [22, 23]. Some authors have called ATC a radioresistant tumor, but such description is probably inaccurate [2]. Several studies demonstrate response of ATC to radiation, with one series of 91 patients showing 80% total response rate and 39% complete clinical response to radiation [23]. In many cases, lack of response to radiation is related to insufficiently high radiation dose administered, frequently caused by technical difficulty of delivering doses >45–50 Gy to central neck limited by spinal cord tolerance (45–50 Gy), particularly using conventional 2D radiation therapy.

With the emergence of 3D conformal radiation therapy in the 1990s and intensity-modulated radiation therapy (IMRT) early in this decade, it is now possible to administer doses >60 Gy to central neck without exceeding spinal cord tolerance (Fig. 10.6). Even in the early radiation studies it was noted that patients who received higher radiation doses had better survival. In a series of 37 patients with ATC treated with radiation, mean survival of 6 months was associated with doses >30 Gy, as compared to mean survival of 2 months in patients treated with lower doses [24]. Another study demonstrated a similar relationship between the dose and survival with median survival of 0.6 months in patients treated with <30 Gy in contrast to median survival of 3.3 months in patients treated with higher dose, with 50% of the patients having metastatic disease at presentation [22]. Furthermore, achieving local control even in the presence of metastatic disease was associated with median survival of 7.5 months

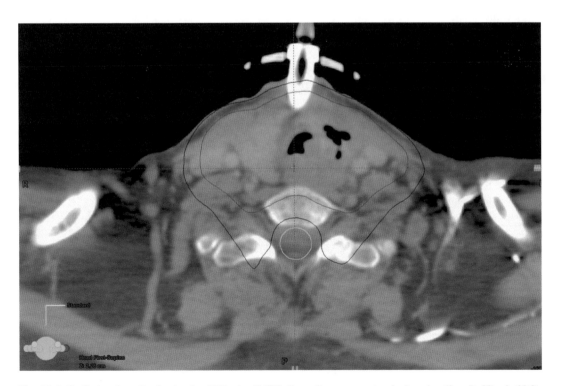

Fig. 10.6 Radiation dose distribution for ATC using IMRT. *Green line* represents spinal cord outline. *Red line* is 66 Gy dose, *blue line* is 45 Gy dose. Note sparing of the spinal cord

compared to 1.6 months in patients who did not achieve local control. Efficacy of radiation therapy can be further enhanced by the use of altered fractionation schedules, namely accelerated fractionation and hyperfractionation. Accelerated fractionation implies delivery of the same total radiation dose in shorter total treatment time by administering multiple doses per day with the goal of reducing repopulation in rapidly proliferating tumors, which is particularly relevant to ATC. Hyperfractionation delivers the same total dose of radiation but divided over a larger number of treatment fractions while keeping the same treatment time, aiming to increase local control without increase in toxicity. Kim et al. reported administered total 57.6 Gy given as 1.6 Gy BID with low dose doxorubicin resulting in median survival of 12 months, but with all patients eventually dying from disease [25]. The approach of hyperfractionated, progressively accelerated treatment in combination with doxorubicin chemotherapy in a prospective study involving 55 patients was undertaken by a group in Sweden [26]. Total dose of 46 Gy was given as 1 Gy BID, followed by 1.3 Gy BID, with 30 Gy given preoperatively and 16 Gy postoperatively, followed by 1.6 Gy BID with the total 46 Gy given preoperatively. There were five (9%) long-term survivors, and perhaps more importantly 33 (60%) who achieved local control, resulting in relatively low (24%) rate of death from local failure. These studies demonstrate that radiation therapy can clearly impact local control in ATC, and lead to improvement in quality of life. At the same time, radiation toxicity, including mucositis, skin reactions, fatigue, and nausea can be significant, and may prevent some patients from completing the treatment, thus incurring toxicity without clinical benefit. Given that radiation therapy appears to have more impact on local control and quality of life than survival, decision to proceed with radiation treatment has to be made while also considering potential side effects in the background of overall dismal prognosis of ATC. Nevertheless, radiation therapy should be strongly considered in fit patients, even in the presence of metastatic disease as local control can be a meaningful goal of treatment.

Chemotherapy and Chemoradiotherapy

High propensity of ATC for metastatic dissemination suggests an important role for systemic therapy. Unfortunately, results of chemotherapy in ATC have been disappointing. Doxorubicin is considered to be one of the first agents investigated in this disease. A review of single-agent doxorubicin experience in ATC disclosed a 22% response rate [27]. In an attempt to improve these results several multiagent combinations have been evaluated, including various combinations of bleomycin, etoposide, cisplatin, paclitaxel, and gemcitabine but none demonstrating clear evidence of efficacy in ATC [28, 29]. Addition of chemotherapy to radiation therapy, either in definitive or postoperative therapy, appears to allow modest improvement in local control, most likely because of radiosensitizing properties of the agents used [26]. Multimodality experience at Erasmus Medical Center for 55 patients treated since 1988 with surgery (whenever possible), radiation therapy, and systemic therapy consisting of doxorubicin at 50 mg/m [2] every 3 weeks to a maximum of 550 mg/m [2] demonstrated 1-year survival of 9% with median survival of only 3 months [30]. Best results were seen in patients who were able to achieve R0 (microscopically negative margin) or R1 (complete removal of gross tumor with microscopic margin involvement) resection and completed chemoradiation, including three patients who survived for longer than 5 years. Grade 3 pharyngeal/esophageal toxicity was noted in 46% patients receiving chemoradiation. Most patients received "modern" radiation therapy and, as in previous studies, dose correlated with survival as patients receiving >40 Gy had median survival of 5.4 months versus 1.7 months in those with <40 Gy. Another contemporary experience from the Institut Gustave-Roussy included 30 selected patients with favorable prognostic factors (80% M0, 50% R0 resections, median age 59) treated with surgery and sequential combination chemotherapy and radiation [31]. Patients received two cycles of doxorubicin (60 mg/m [2]) and cisplatin

(120 mg/m [2]) before and four cycles after radiation. RT consisted of two daily fractions of 1.25 Gy, 5 days/week to a total dose of 40 Gy to the cervical lymph node areas and the superior mediastinum, with boost to 50–55 Gy in select patients. This study in favorably selected patients demonstrated 1-year survival of 46% and 3-year survival of 27% with associated acute grade 3/4 mucositis in 33% patients and grade 4 neutropenia in 70%. Overall, it does not appear that chemotherapy yields meaningful therapeutic benefits in the absence of local treatment, radiation, surgery, or both, but marginally improves outcome in the multimodality setting.

Novel Therapies

Biologic therapy holds perhaps the greatest promise for cure in anaplastic thyroid carcinoma. High prevalence of genetic abnormalities and our increasing understanding of molecular underpinnings of ATC suggest that molecular targets can be exploited to overcome this aggressive malignancy. Gene alterations frequently encountered in ATC, including *p53, RAS, β-catenin*, epidermal growth factor receptor (EGFR), and many others are becoming targets of novel therapies that began to emerge in the twenty-first century [32]. For example, in one case report, a patient who progressed after combined modality treatment was given a course of erlotinib (oral EGFR inhibitor) and demonstrated dramatic clinical and radiographic disease shrinkage [33]. Fosbretabulin (also known as combretastatin A4) is a vascular disrupting agent originally isolated from the bark of the African bush willow tree, *Combretum caffrum*. Although the exact mechanism of fosbretabulin action has not been completely elucidated, its antitumor effects are thought to be related to its effects on the tumor vasculature [34]. Activity of fosbretabulin in combination with chemotherapy in ATC has been shown in nude mouse xenograft model experiments [35]. A phase II trial of single-agent fosbretabulin in 26 patients with ATC progressive after initial combined modality therapy yielded no complete or partial responses, with 27% of patients achieving stable disease, thus suggesting that fosbretabulin may best work in combination with other agents [36]. Because forsbretabulin is not myelosuppressive and its main toxicity is cardiovascular (hypertension, ischemia, and QT prolongation) and it does not overlap with many other cytotoxic agents, it can be combined with traditional chemotherapy. This has led to development of ongoing trial with fosbretabulin in combination with carboplatin and paclitaxel.

Another promising biologic agent in ATC is sorafenib, a multikinase inhibitor of the BRAF, which is frequently mutated in ATC. Sorafenib exerts significant antitumor activity in an orthotopic xenograft model of ATC [37]. A phase II trial of sorafenib in ATC patients is ongoing, but an early report in the first 15 patients who progressed after conventional therapy disclosed two patients with partial response and four with stable disease [38].

Conclusion

Several studies incorporating traditional cytotoxic drugs and novel agents including fosbretabulin, sorafenib, imatinib, gefitinib, pazopanib, and several others have been completed or are ongoing. Given the rarity of ATC enrollment of patients in clinical trials of ATC is crucial to future development of successful therapy for this currently near universally fatal disease. Therefore, patients and clinicians should be strongly encouraged to seek participation in a clinical trial. A current list of clinical trials can be found at http://www.clinicaltrials.gov.

References

1. Kebebew E, Greenspan FS, Clark OH, Woeber KA, McMillan A. Anaplastic thyroid carcinoma. Treatment outcome and prognostic factors. Cancer. 2005;103(7): 1330–5.
2. Ain KB. Anaplastic thyroid carcinoma: behavior, biology, and therapeutic approaches. Thyroid. 1998; 8(8):715–26.
3. Chiacchio S, Lorenzoni A, Boni G, Rubello D, Elisei R, Mariani G. Anaplastic thyroid cancer: prevalence, diagnosis and treatment. Minerva Endocrinol. 2008; 33(4):341–57.

4. Wreesmann VB, Singh B. Clinical impact of molecular analysis on thyroid cancer management. Surg Oncol Clin N Am. 2008;17(1):1–35.

5. Zitzelsberger H, Bauer V, Thomas G, Unger K. Molecular rearrangements in papillary thyroid carcinomas. Clin Chim Acta. 2009;411(5–6):301–8.

6. Us-Krasovec M, Golouh R, Auersperg M, Besic N, Ruparcic-Oblak L. Anaplastic thyroid carcinoma in fine needle aspirates. Acta Cytol. 1996;40(5): 953–8.

7. Guarda LA, Peterson CE, Hall W, Baskin HJ. Anaplastic thyroid carcinoma: cytomorphology and clinical implications of fine-needle aspiration. Diagn Cytopathol. 1991;7(1):63–7.

8. Miettinen M, Franssila KO. Variable expression of keratins and nearly uniform lack of thyroid transcription factor 1 in thyroid anaplastic carcinoma. Hum Pathol. 2000;31(9):1139–45.

9. Tan RK, Finley 3 RK, Driscoll D, Bakamjian V, Hicks Jr WL, Shedd DP. Anaplastic carcinoma of the thyroid: a 24-year experience. Head Neck. 1995;17(1):41–7. discussion 47–8.

10. Giuffrida D, Gharib H. Anaplastic thyroid carcinoma: current diagnosis and treatment. Ann Oncol. 2000; 11(9):1083–9.

11. Bogsrud TV, Karantanis D, Nathan MA, et al. 18 F-FDG PET in the management of patients with anaplastic thyroid carcinoma. Thyroid. 2008;18(7):713–9.

12. Lazar V, Bidart J-M, Caillou B, et al. Expression of the Na/I symporter gene in human thyroid tumors: a comparison study with other thyroid-specific genes. J Clin Endocrinol Metab. 1999;84:3228–34.

13. Ciampi R, Vivaldi A, Romei C, et al. Expression analysis of facilitative glucose transporters (GLUTs) in human thyroid carcinoma cell lines and primary tumors. Mol Cell Endocrinol. 2008;291:57–62. Epub 2008 May 14.

14. Sugitani I, Kasai N, Fujimoto Y, Yanagisawa A. Prognostic factors and therapeutic strategy for anaplastic carcinoma of the thyroid. World J Surg. 2001;25(5):617–22.

15. Are C, Shaha AR. Anaplastic thyroid carcinoma: biology, pathogenesis, prognostic factors, and treatment approaches. Ann Surg Oncol. 2006;13(4):453–64. Epub 2006 Feb 15.

16. McIver B, Hay ID, Giuffrida DF, Dvorak CE, Grant CS, Thompson GB, et al. Anaplastic thyroid carcinoma: a 50-year experience at a single institution. Surgery. 2001;130(6):1028–34.

17. Cobin RH, Gharib H, Bergman DAL. AACE/AAES medical/surgical guidelines for clinical practice: management of thyroid cancer. Endocr Pract. 2001;7: 203–20.

18. Sugino K, Ito K, Mimura T, et al. The important role of operations in the management of anaplastic thyroid carcinoma. Surgery. 2002;131:2458.

19. Venkatesh YSS, Ordonez NG, Schultz PN, et al. Anaplastic carcinoma of the thyroid. A clinicopathological study of 121 cases. Cancer. 1990;66:321–30.

20. Demeter JG, De Jong SA, Lawrence AM, Paloyan E. Anaplastic thyroid carcinoma: risk factors and outcome. Surgery. 1991;110:956–63.

21. Shaha AR. Airway management in anaplastic thyroid carcinoma. Laryngoscope. 2008;118(7):1195–8.

22. Levendag PC, De Porre PM, van Putten WL. Anaplastic carcinoma of the thyroid gland treated by radiation therapy. Int J Radiat Oncol Biol Phys. 1993; 26:125–8.

23. Junor EJ, Paul J, Reed NS. Anaplastic thyroid carcinoma: 91 patients treated by surgery and radiotherapy. Eur J Surg Oncol. 1992;18:83–8.

24. Kobayashi T, Asakawa H, Umeshita K, et al. Treatment of 37 patients with anaplastic carcinoma of the thyroid. Head Neck. 1996;18(1):36–41. Jan–Feb.

25. Kim JH, Leeper RD. Treatment of locally advanced thyroid carcinoma with combination doxorubicin and radiation therapy. Cancer. 1987;60:2372–5.

26. Tenvall J, Lundell G, Wahlberg P, et al. Anaplastic thyroid carcinoma: three protocols combining doxorubicin, hyperfractionated radiotherapy and surgery. Br J Cancer. 2002;86:1848–53.

27. Ahuja S, Ernst H. Chemotherapy of thyroid carcinoma. J Endocrinol Invest. 1987;10:303–10.

28. De Besi P, Busnardo B, Toso S, et al. Combined chemotherapy with bleomycin, adriamycin and platinum in advanced thyroid carcinoma. J Endocrinol Invest. 1991;14:475–80.

29. Ain KB, Egorin MJ, DeSimone PA. Treatment of anaplastic thyroid carcinoma with paclitaxel: phase 2 trial using ninety-six-hour infusion. Collaborative Anaplastic Thyroid Cancer Health Intervention Trials (CATCHIT) Group. Thyroid. 2000;10(7):587–94.

30. Swaak-Kragten AT, de Wilt JH, Schmitz PI, Bontenbal M, Levendag PC. Multimodality treatment for anaplastic thyroid carcinoma–treatment outcome in 75 patients. Radiother Oncol. 2009;92(1):100–4. Epub 2009 Mar 26.

31. De Crevoisier R, Baudin E, Bachelot A, et al. Combined treatment of anaplastic thyroid carcinoma with surgery, chemotherapy, and hyperfractionated accelerated external radiotherapy. Int J Radiat Oncol Biol Phys. 2004;60(4):1137–43.

32. Wiseman SM, Masoudi H, Niblock P, et al. Anaplastic thyroid carcinoma: expression profile of targets for therapy offers new insights for disease treatment. Ann Surg Oncol. 2007;14(2):719–29. Epub 2006 Nov 10.

33. Hogan T, Jing Jie Yu, Williams HJ, Altaha R, Liang Xiaobing, Qi HE. Oncocytic, focally anaplastic, thyroid cancer responding to erlotinib. J Oncol Pharm Pract. 2009;15(2):111–7. Epub 2009 Mar 10.

34. Siemann DW, Chaplin DJ, Walicke PA. A review and update of the current status of the vasculature-disabling agent combretastatin-A4 phosphate (CA4P). Expert Opin Investig Drugs. 2009;18(2): 189–97.

35. Yeung SC, She M, Yang H, Pan J, Sun L, Chaplin D. Combination chemotherapy including combretastatin A4 phosphate and paclitaxel is effective against

anaplastic thyroid cancer in a nude mouse xenograft model. J Clin Endocrinol Metab. 2007;92(8):2902–9. Aug. Epub 2007.

36. Mooney CJ, Nagaiah G, Fu P, et al. A phase II trial of fosbretabulin in advanced anaplastic thyroid carcinoma and correlation of baseline serum-soluble intracellular adhesion molecule-1 with outcome. Thyroid. 2009;19(3):233–40.

37. Kim S, Yazici YD, G, et al. Sorafenib inhibits the angiogenesis and growth of orthotopic anaplastic thyroid carcinoma xenografts in nude mice. Mol Cancer Ther. 2007;6(6):1785–92.

38. Nagaiah G, Fu P, Wasman K, et al. Phase II trial of sorafenib (bay 43–9006) in patients with advanced anaplastic carcinoma of the thyroid (ATC). J Clin Oncol. 2009;27:15s. suppl; abstr 6058.

Thyroid Lymphoma

Basil Rapoport and Sandra M. McLachlan

Introduction

Although the incidence (or at least the clinical presentation) of thyroid malignancies has been increasing in recent years, clinically significant thyroid cancers remain far less common than autoimmune thyroid diseases, Graves' disease, and Hashimoto's thyroiditis. Further, of the different pathological types of thyroid cancer, thyroid lymphomas are rare, representing less than 5% of thyroid neoplasms. Therefore, thyroid lymphomas are only encountered infrequently in clinical practice, for example, approximately two patients per year in a major referral center [1]. Nevertheless, awareness and recognition of this condition is important because it is typically symptomatic and it may be amenable to therapy. Lymphomatous involvement of the thyroid gland can be localized to the gland ("primary") or may be one component of more widespread lymphoma. This distinction may sometimes be blurred when the disease is primarily located in the thyroid but is also present to a limited extent in other regions, such as in lymph nodes adjacent to the thyroid. Viewed from another perspective, less than 1% of non-Hodgkin lymphomas present with primary thyroid involvement [2].

Clinical Presentation

Most patients with thyroid lymphoma are elderly, in their 60s or 70s, and present with a mass in the thyroid or diffuse thyroid enlargement. Women are affected more commonly than men, as with Hashimoto's thyroiditis. An important clinical feature of the disease is that there is typically relatively rapid enlargement of the lesion, a finding that should increase awareness of the risk of thyroid lymphoma. Presentation of thyroid lymphoma may be associated with hypothyroidism and an elevated serum TSH level [1]. Local pressure symptoms in the neck are common, particularly with diffuse rather than focal lymphomatous enlargement. Tracheal compression that can be associated with stridor or dyspnea is particularly serious and requires urgent therapy [3]. Other symptoms may include hoarseness, pain, and dysphagia. Anaplastic thyroid neoplasia may present with similar symptoms and signs and should, therefore, be included in the differential diagnosis. In some patients with aggressive diffuse large B-cell lymphomas (see below), systemic symptoms characteristic of disseminated lymphoma, such as fever, night sweats, and weight loss, may be present [1].

Pathology

The pathological classification of lymphomas, such as the R.E.A.L. and WHO classifications [4], is constantly evolving and is beyond the

B. Rapoport (✉) • S.M. McLachlan
Division of Endocrinology, Diabetes, and Metabolism, Department of Medicine, Cedars-Sinai Medical Center, B-131, 8700 Beverly Blvd, Los Angeles, CA 90048, USA
e-mail: rapoportb@cshs.org; Mclachlan@cshs.org

scope of the present chapter. Almost all thyroid lymphomas are of the B-cell variety. In a large review of 108 cases (79 women and 29 men) [5], all were B-cell lymphomas. Of these, the most common subtype was diffuse large B-cell lymphoma (71%), approximately half of which also had mixed features with marginal zone B-cell lymphoma. With one exception (follicle center lymphoma), the remaining patients had marginal zone B-cell lymphoma of mucosa-associated lymphoid tissue (MALT). In other series, rare forms of lymphoma presenting with primary involvement of the thyroid are described, including Hodgkin's disease and Burkitt's lymphoma [1, 6]. Histological evidence of Hashimoto's thyroiditis is reported in many cases, but with a wide variation in different series (for example 32–94%) [5, 6]. Primary T-cell lymphomas are extremely rare, with fewer than 20 cases reported in the English literature [7–9]. The phenotype of two of these cases has been determined to be CD3+, CD4+, CD8–, with other features suggesting a Th1 T-cell origin [7]. In T-cell, unlike in primary B-cell thyroid lymphomas, there is no female preponderance. Nevertheless, both B-cell and T-cell thyroid lymphomas are associated with Hashimoto's thyroiditis [8].

Pathogenesis

The association between primary thyroid lymphoma and Hashimoto's thyroiditis, as mentioned above, has long been recognized. Long-term follow-up studies (17–22 years) of large numbers of Hashimoto patients revealed an incidence of thyroid lymphoma of 0.48% in Japan [10] and 0.14% in Sweden [11]. The relative risk of a Hashimoto's thyroiditis patient developing thyroid lymphoma was 67-fold greater than in the normal population [11]. Graves' disease is not associated with a similar risk [10]. The precise process by which Hashimoto's thyroiditis can evolve into a B-cell lymphoma is unknown but it seems reasonable to speculate that it is the end result of chronic antigenic stimulation of intrathyroidal B-cells. Autoimmune involvement of the thyroid is associated with B- and T-cell infiltration, quantitatively to a much greater extent in Hashimoto's

thyroiditis than in Graves' disease. In many respects, the thyroid acquires features similar to a lymph node, with well-formed lymphoid follicles with germinal centers. Indeed, B-cells from the Hashimoto gland have been demonstrated to secrete autoantibodies to thyroglobulin and thyroid peroxidase (at the time, the microsomal antigen) [12]. Analysis of the heavy (H) and light (L) chain genes of thyroid peroxidase autoantibodies isolated from thyroid-infiltrating B-cells reveals their antigen-binding regions to be heavily mutated relative to their germline precursors, consistent with their high affinity for antigen [13]. These observations indicate that there is antigen-driven affinity maturation of intrathyroidal B-cells, a process involving stimulation of B-cell division. Thyroid peroxidase autoantibodies are encoded by germline genes from different families, indicating intrathyroidal B-cell polyclonality, as reflected in the polyclonality of autoantibodies in patients' sera. Intense antigen-driven stimulation of B-cell proliferation can be envisioned to predispose to a genetic alteration in a single B-cell, leading to the origin of an unrestrained, clonal B-cell lymphoma. Molecular evidence supporting the evolution of Hashimoto's thyroiditis into thyroid lymphoma, particularly of the MALT variety, has been obtained by analysis of immunoglobulin H chain genes [14]. Indeed, there may be near nucleotide sequence identity between immunoglobulin H chain genes in thyroid lymphomas and Hashimoto's thyroiditis regions in the same patient [15]. Environmental factors such as viruses, including Epstein–Barr virus (EBV) [16] may contribute to malignant transformation of Hashimoto B-cells.

Diagnosis

Clinical suspicion of thyroid lymphoma requires confirmation by subsequent diagnostic tests. Blood tests are rarely helpful. Patients may be euthyroid, hypothyroid, and, very rarely, hyperthyroid [1]. The presence of thyroid peroxidase or thyroglobulin autoantibodies does not distinguish between thyroid lymphoma and Hashimoto's thyroiditis. In aggressive diffuse large-cell B-cell thyroid lymphomas, particularly with extranodal involvement, serum LDH and beta-microglobulin levels may be elevated. Radionucleide scans and ultrasonography do not provide specific evidence for thyroid lymphoma.

Tissue samples are required for diagnosis, commonly obtained by fine-needle aspiration (FNA) biopsy, but sometimes requiring open surgical biopsy [17]. Standard microscopic cytopathological examination may reveal marked loss of epithelial cells as well as lymphoepithelial lesions and is frequently inconclusive. Therefore, examination of additional cytologic aspirates may be required to distinguish lymphoma from Hashimoto's thyroiditis. Lymphocytes can be characterized by flow cytometry for their surface markers using monoclonal antibodies, but these, too, do not provide high diagnostic specificity. In equivocal cases, the greater clonality of lymphoma cells versus tissue-infiltrating B-cells in Hashimoto's thyroiditis can be used as a diagnostic tool. One method to apply this principle is to determine the ratio of B-cells expressing kappa versus lambda light chains [18]. However, the limitation of this approach is evident from a study utilizing polymerase chain reaction (PCR) in which Hashimoto thyroiditis germinal center B-cells had a kappa/lambda ratio extending beyond the 0.8–2.2 range regarded as normal and none of the patients followed up for 3 years developed lymphoma [19]. Another molecular approach that can be applied is to determine the clonality of immunoglobulin H chain genes using Southern blotting [20] or, more recently and more effectively, PCR [21–24]. Nevertheless, diagnostic caution is warranted because some Hashimoto thyroids have clonal immunoglobulin H chain gene bands on PCR analysis and such clonality in these glands does not predict evolution into lymphoma, at least during a follow-up period of 10–13 years [25].

Therapy and Prognosis

The purpose of this review is not to discuss therapy of lymphomas in general, but to focus on lymphoma restricted to the thyroid. According to the Ann Arbor classification of non-Hodgkin's lymphoma, this category is described as stage IE ("I" referring to involvement in one location and "E" indicating extranodal involvement). Optimal treatment requires a team including an endocrinologist, radiation and medical oncologists, and, in some instances an endocrine or oncology surgeon. It is generally agreed that modern therapy does not require surgical debulking or total thyroidectomy [6, 17]. Thyroid lymphomas are sensitive to radiation and chemotherapy. Surgery is only indicated when open biopsy is necessary. When noninvasive treatment is not sufficiently rapid to alleviate compressive symptoms in the neck a palliative tracheal stent may be preferable to surgery for airway obstruction [17].

Because of the rarity of thyroid lymphoma, there are no prospective, randomized clinical trials comparing monotherapy (radiation or chemotherapy) or combined chemoradiation. However, data on such trials have been reported for extranodal lymphomas involving regions other than the thyroid. An excellent evidence-based evaluation of therapy is provided in reference [17]. The most commonly used chemotherapy protocol involves cycles of CHOP, namely the combination of cyclophosphamide (Cytoxan), doxorubicin (Adriamycin), vincristine (Oncovin), and prednisolone. Other chemotherapeutic reagents that have been used include vindesine and bleomycin. Because of the relatively indolent course of the MALT subtype of thyroid lymphoma, radiation therapy alone is associated with a relatively low relapse rate and a 10-year survival rate of 90% [26]. In a more recent study of IE and IIE non-Hodgkin's lymphoma involving a number of sites including the thyroid, localized moderate-dose radiation therapy resulted in a 5-year survival rate of 98% and a disease-free survival rate of 77% [27]. Thyroid MALT lymphomas had better outcomes than most other sites. Surgical resection alone for stage IE MALT thyroid lymphomas may be effective but its efficacy relative to radiation therapy is controversial in the absence of adequate data. Diffuse, large B-cell lymphomas of the thyroid and mixed histological varieties have a more aggressive course and combined chemoradiation therapy is typically the preferred form of therapy [27].

In terms of future developments in the treatment of lymphoma localized to the thyroid, there are no data on the use of rituximab, a monoclonal antibody against CD20 expressed on the surface of B-cells. This reagent is certainly effective in disseminated non-Hodgkin's lymphoma, but its potential serious side effects make it unlikely to substitute for radiation or chemotherapy in thyroid lymphoma, especially of the MALT variety. In terms of evaluation following therapy, FDG–PET has recently been reported to be a useful and sensitive modality for assessing disease activity in thyroid lymphoma. Its ability to detect disease recurrence was found to be superior compared to CT in a limited number of patients [28].

Summary

Thyroid lymphoma is a rare thyroid neoplasm that, when isolated to the thyroid (stage IE), is pathogenetically associated with Hashimoto's thyroiditis. Clinical suspicion is typically aroused by relatively rapid enlargement of a Hashimoto gland that may be associated with local compression symptoms in the neck. Diagnosis requires tissue analysis, initially by FNA biopsy and in some instances by open surgical biopsy. When the diagnosis remains uncertain, clonality of the B-cells in the biopsy tissue may be determined by molecular analysis of immunoglobulin genes. The pathology of thyroid lymphoma varies. The great majority are non-Hodgkin's B-cell lymphomas, represented primarily by (1) diffuse large B-cell, (2) MALT, and (3) mixed varieties. MALT lymphomas are relatively indolent, typically respond to local radiation therapy, and have an excellent prognosis. The more aggressive diffuse large B-cell lymphomas can be treated with either local radiation, chemotherapy, or a combination of both modalities.

References

1. Thieblemont C, Mayer A, Dumontet C, Barbier Y, Callet-Bauchu E, Felman P, et al. Primary thyroid lymphoma is a heterogeneous disease. J Clin Endocrinol Metab. 2002;87:105–11.
2. Ansell SM, Grant CS, Habermann TM. Primary thyroid lymphoma. Semin Oncol. 1999;26:316–23.
3. Miller BS, Gauger PG. Thyroid lymphoma arising from Hashimoto's thyroiditis. J Clin Endocrinol Metab. 2006;91:3711–12.
4. Harris NL, Jaffe ES, Diebold J, Flandrin G, Muller-Hermelink HK, Vardiman J. Lymphoma classification: from controversy to consensus - the R.E.A.L. and WHO Classification of lymphoid neoplasms. Ann Oncol. 2000;11(1):3–10.
5. Derringer GA, Thompson LD, Frommelt RA, Bijwaard KE, Heffess CS, Abbondanzo SL. Malignant lymphoma of the thyroid gland: a clinicopathologic study of 108 cases. Am J Surg Pathol. 2000;24:623–39.
6. Ruggiero FP, Frauenhoffer E, Stack Jr BC. Thyroid lymphoma: a single institution's experience. Otolaryngol Head Neck Surg. 2005;133:888–96.
7. Koida S, Tsukasaki K, Tsuchiya T, Harasawa H, Fukushima T, Yamada Y, et al. Primary T-cell lymphoma of the thyroid gland with chemokine receptors of Th1 phenotype complicating autoimmune thyroiditis. Haematologica. 2007;92:e37–40.
8. Yang H, Li J, Shen T. Primary T-cell lymphoma of the thyroid: case report and review of the literature. Med Oncol. 2008;25:462–6.
9. Motoi N, Ozawa Y. Malignant T-cell lymphoma of the thyroid gland associated with Hashimoto's thyroiditis. Pathol Int. 2005;55:425–30.
10. Kato I, Tajima K, Suchi T, Aozasa K, Matsuzuka F, Kuma K, et al. Chronic thyroiditis as a risk factor of B-cell lymphoma in the thyroid gland. Jpn J Cancer Res. 1985;76:1085–90.
11. Holm LE, Blomgren H, Lowhagen T. Cancer risks in patients with chronic lymphocytic thyroiditis. N Engl J Med. 1985;312:601–4.
12. McLachlan SM, McGregor A, Rees Smith B, Hall R. Thyroid-autoantibody synthesis by Hashimoto thyroid lymphocytes. Lancet. 1979;1(8108):162–3.
13. McLachlan SM, Rapoport B. The molecular biology of thyroid peroxidase: cloning, expression and role as autoantigen in autoimmune thyroid disease. Endocr Rev. 1992;13:192–206.
14. Yamauchi A, Tomita Y, Takakuwa T, Hoshida Y, Nakatsuka S, Sakamoto H, et al. Polymerase chain reaction-based clonality analysis in thyroid lymphoma. Int J Mol Med. 2002;10:113–7.
15. Moshynska OV, Saxena A. Clonal relationship between Hashimoto thyroiditis and thyroid lymphoma. J Clin Pathol. 2008;61:438–44.
16. Lam KY, Lo CY, Kwong DL, Lee J, Srivastava G. Malignant lymphoma of the thyroid. A 30-year clinicopathologic experience and an evaluation of the presence of Epstein-Barr virus. Am J Clin Pathol. 1999;112:263–70.
17. Mack LA, Pasieka JL. An evidence-based approach to the treatment of thyroid lymphoma. World J Surg. 2007;31:978–86.
18. Hyjek E, Isaacson PG. Primary B cell lymphoma of the thyroid and its relationship to Hashimoto's thyroiditis. Hum Pathol. 1988;19:1315–26.
19. Chen HI, Akpolat I, Mody DR, Lopez-Terrada D, De Leon AP, Luo Y, et al. Restricted kappa/lambda light

chain ratio by flow cytometry in germinal center B cells in Hashimoto thyroiditis. Am J Clin Pathol. 2006;125:42–8.

20. Wozniak R, Beckwith L, Ratech H, Surks MI. Maltoma of the thyroid in a man with Hashimoto's thyroiditis. J Clin Endocrinol Metab. 1999;84:1206–9.

21. Lovchik J, Lane MA, Clark DP. Polymerase chain reaction-based detection of B-cell clonality in the fine needle aspiration biopsy of a thyroid mucosa-associated lymphoid tissue (MALT) lymphoma. Hum Pathol. 1997;28:989–92.

22. Hsi ED, Singleton TP, Svoboda SM, Schnitzer B, Ross CW. Characterization of the lymphoid infiltrate in Hashimoto thyroiditis by immunohistochemistry and polymerase chain reaction for immunoglobulin heavy chain gene rearrangement. Am J Clin Pathol. 1998;110:327–33.

23. Kato K, Ohshima K, Shiokawa S, Shibata T, Suzumiya J, Kikuchi M. Rearrangement of immunoglobulin heavy and light chains and VH family in thyroid and salivary gland lymphomas. Pathol Int. 2002;52:747–54.

24. Hummel M, Oeschger S, Barth TF, Loddenkemper C, Cogliatti SB, Marx A, et al. Wotherspoon criteria combined with B cell clonality analysis by advanced polymerase chain reaction technology discriminates covert gastric marginal zone lymphoma from chronic gastritis. Gut. 2006;55:782–7.

25. Saxena A, Alport EC, Moshynska O, Kanthan R, Boctor MA. Clonal B cell populations in a minority of patients with Hashimoto's thyroiditis. J Clin Pathol. 2004;57:1258–63.

26. Laing RW, Hoskin P, Hudson BV, Hudson GV, Harmer C, Bennett MH, et al. The significance of MALT histology in thyroid lymphoma: a review of patients from the BNLI and Royal Marsden Hospital. Clin Oncol (R Coll Radiol). 1994;6:300–4.

27. Tsang RW, Gospodarowicz MK, Pintilie M, Wells W, Hodgson DC, Sun A, et al. Localized mucosa-associated lymphoid tissue lymphoma treated with radiation therapy has excellent clinical outcome. J Clin Oncol. 2003;21:4157–64.

28. Basu S, Li G, Bural G, Alavi A. Fluorodeoxyglucose positron emission tomography (FDG-PET) and PET/computed tomography imaging characteristics of thyroid lymphoma and their potential clinical utility. Acta Radiol. 2009;50:201–4.

Surgical Management of Thyroid Cancer

12

C. Suzanne Cutter, Kenneth W. Adashek,
Michel Babajanian, and Babak Larian

History of Thyroid Surgery

Surgery on the thyroid gland was first performed around 500 a.d. Later, Abū al-Qāsim, a surgeon innovator also known as Albucasis, wrote a 30-volume treatise on numerous instruments he developed as well as procedures he performed. Prior to his death in 1013 a.d., he performed the first thyroid surgery that was successful. It was not until 1511 that, through the drawings of Leonardo Da Vinci, the thyroid was regarded as a gland and not just tissue overlying the trachea [1].

Prior to 1850, thyroid surgery was plagued with morbidity and mortality related to hemorrhage, lack of anesthesia, and infection. Later, the safety of thyroid surgery changed dramatically with the introduction of techniques for:

1. Hemostasis originally described by Abu al-Qasim but brought to modern surgery by Harvey in 1929
2. Anesthesia in 1842 by Crawford Long
3. Antisepsis with carbolic acid by Joseph Lister in 1867

These developments drove Billroth's mortality rate down from 36.1% in 1860 to 8.3% by 1881. During his career, Theodor Kocher reported a 0.5% mortality rate and wrote extensively about his experiences. He was the first to describe clinical abnormalities following total versus partial thyroidectomies, and he conducted extensive investigations in thyroid pathophysiology. Fortunately, in 1891, George Murphy demonstrated that injection of thyroid extract effectively treated the symptoms Kocher described [1]. In 1909, Kocher was awarded the Nobel Prize in medicine for his significant contributions to the understanding of thyroid gland physiology, pathology, and surgery [2]. Through Theodor Billroth's experiences in the 1870s, tetany was recognized as an additional complication of total thyroidectomy. Two key discoveries brought surgical technique closer to avoiding this complication. Sandstrom first described the human parathyroid glands in 1880 [3]. His discovery led to the anatomical understanding of parathyroid gland blood supply in 1907 by Halstead and Evans [1]. With the further understanding of the parathyroids' role in calcium physiology, these discoveries led to the development of surgical techniques that spared the glands in order to maintain calcium homeostasis. Two of Billroth's assistants, Mikulicz and Wolfler, initiated surgical focus on preservation of the recurrent laryngeal nerves (RLNs) by preserving the posterior thyroid attachments to the trachea [1]. In contrast, Kegel and Dunleavy brought attention to the importance of the superior laryngeal nerve (SLN) to vocal range after they performed a thyroidectomy on an operatic soprano that ended her promising career.

C.S. Cutter • K.W. Adashek • M. Babajanian •
B. Larian (✉)
Department of Surgery, Cedars-Sinai Medical Center,
Los Angeles, CA, USA
e-mail: Larianb@yahoo.com

G.D. Braunstein (ed.), *Thyroid Cancer*, Endocrine Updates 30,
DOI 10.1007/978-1-4614-0875-8_12, © Springer Science+Business Media, LLC 2012

Contemporary advancements continue to build on these discoveries. The advent of electrocautery followed by the ultrasonic shears encourages hemostasis and decreases operating time. Minimally invasive techniques have decreased the trauma and improved the cosmesis of the procedure. Finally, intraoperative nerve monitoring provides an additional defense against dreaded RLN injury which impact airway integrity as well as phonation. Postoperative parathyroid hormone levels help predict likelihood of postoperative hypocalcemia.

Locoregional Thyroid Anatomy

Overview of Anatomy

Anatomically, the neck has a significant number of critical structures compressed into an abbreviated space. The thyroid lies in the space between the cervical strap muscles and the trachea just inferior to the thyroid cartilage (Fig. 12.1). Layers of pretracheal fascia surround the thyroid and form the posterior suspensory ligament of Berry posteriorly which attaches the thyroid to the cricoid cartilage and first two tracheal rings (Fig. 12.2). The thyroid capsule is closely adherent to the gland and forms the septum that connects its left and right lobes. On the posterior surface of each lobe lies an inferior and superior parathyroid gland (Fig. 12.1). Compared to the 15–25 g thyroid, the parathyroid glands are miniscule portions of caramel-colored tissue, weigh only 30–70 mg, and are difficult to distinguish from surrounding adipose tissue. The thyroid and parathyroid share a set of inferior thyroid arteries (Fig. 12.2). There are also pairs of superior thyroid arteries and three pairs – superior, middle, and inferior – of thyroid veins. Two pairs of nerves are in close relationship with the thyroid: bilateral RLNs and bilateral SLNs. The RLNs branch from the vagus nerves to innervate the intrinsic muscles of the larynx except the cricothyroid muscle. After the vagus nerves descend to the thoracic inlet, each RLN branches off loops around vascular structures – aorta on the left and

subclavian on the right – before they return superiorly to the neck, pass adjacent to the inferior thyroid artery, travel within the tracheoesophageal groove, and enter into the larynx posterolaterally. The ultimobranchial body develops bilaterally from the fourth brachial pouch and carry neural crest cells into the developing thyroid gland to form the parafollicular cells (C-cells) that secrete calcitonin. The point at which the ultimobranchial body joins the thyroid in a large percentage of cases leaves a remnant of tissue known as the tubercle of Zuckerkandl. This tissue is often intimately associated and, at times wraps around, the RLN. Thus, dissection in this area can be challenging and with increased risk. Injury to either of two key structures – RLN or parathyroid glands – may result in the most challenging postoperative complications: paralysis of the vocal cords and hypocalcemia.

Recurrent Laryngeal Nerve Anatomy

Injury to one RLN compromises apposition of the vocal cords which may lead to hoarseness and, if bilateral injury, airway compromise. Bilateral injury usually requires tracheostomy. Unfortunately, the RLN pathway (Fig.12.2) and relationship to surrounding structures is subject to significant variation:

- Inferior thyroid artery [4] course:
  - Left: anterior in 50%, posterior in 10%, and splits anterior and posterior in 30%
  - Right: anterior in 20%, posterior in 50%, and splits anterior and posterior in 30%
- Rarely (<1%), there is nonrecurrence of the nerve which is most commonly associated with a subclavian artery anomaly (e.g., retropharyngeal right subclavian artery) when the right nerve is affected and situs inversus when the left nerve is affected

This variability in combination with the tissue of the tubercle of Zuckerkandl makes detachment of the thyroid parenchyma adjacent to the trachea particularly precarious. During this portion of the surgery, the pace slows significantly and thermal dissection instruments are avoided. In some cases, thyroid tissue surrounds the nerve and

Fig. 12.1 Central neck anatomy. The thyroid gland is shown with overlying strap muscles and underlying parathyroid glands. In the plane beneath all these structures lies the lymph nodes that comprise level VI. The close relationship of the thyroid with the innominate artery and thymus gland are also shown. From Carty, Sally, Cooper, David S et al. Thyroid Volume 19, Number 11, 2009. Used with permission

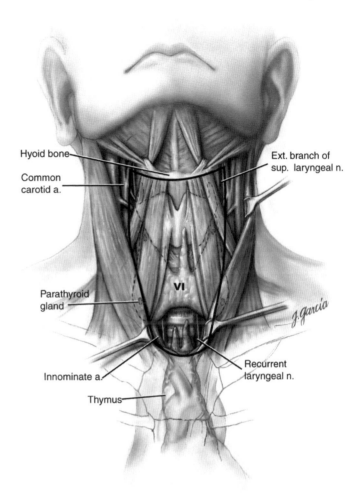

must be carefully dissected. The SLN is in close proximity to the superior thyroid artery and uncommonly may be found in association with the thyroid parenchyma at the superior pole.

Parathyroid Gland Anatomy

The inferior thyroid artery is the principal blood supply to both superior and inferior parathyroid glands. Most patients (80%) have four parathyroid glands, but some have either three (13%) or five (6%) glands. Superior parathyroid glands develop from the fourth pharyngeal pouch in close association with the lateral lobes of the thyroid and as such have a less variable location.

They are most reliably located at the level of the cricoid cartilage, usually dorsolateral to the intersection of the RLN and the inferior thyroid artery. In contrast, the inferior parathyroid glands develop from the third pharyngeal pouch in close association with the thymus. They descend together during development which results in significant variation (Fig. 12.3) in the final location of the inferior parathyroid glands once the associated thymic tail involutes. Usually found at the inferior poles of the thyroid (whether posterior, anterior, or lateral aspects) in 61%, the inferior parathyroid glands are also found in the thyrothymic ligament of the thymic tail in 26%, in the region of the superior parathyroid glands in 7%, within the carotid sheath in 1–2%, as well as

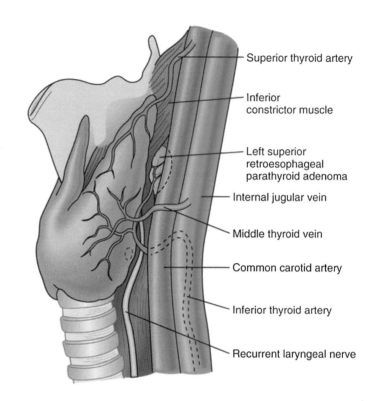

Fig. 12.2 Left thyroid vasculature and the recurrent laryngeal nerve anatomy. Anatomic relationship of the left thyroid, thyroid vasculature, recurrent laryngeal nerve, superior parathyroid, common carotid artery, and internal jugular vein are shown. Aberrantly located parathyroid glands can be found behind the esophagus, as well as within the carotid sheath, the thymus, and the mediastinum. From Townsend: Sabiston Textbook of Surgery, 18th ed. Copyright© 2007 Saunders, An Imprint of Elsevier Used with permission

- Superior thyroid artery
- Inferior constrictor muscle
- Left superior retroesophageal parathyroid adenoma
- Internal jugular vein
- Middle thyroid vein
- Common carotid artery
- Inferior thyroid artery
- Recurrent laryngeal nerve

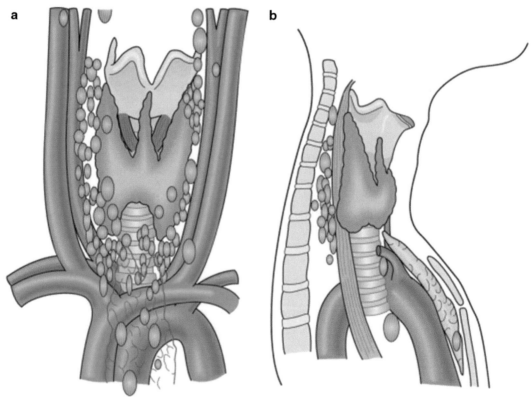

a

b

Fig. 12.3 Possible locations of enlarged parathyroid glands in the neck and superior mediastinum with the use of an anteroposterior projection (**a**) and a lateral projection (**b**). From Udelsman R, Donovan PI: Remedial parathyroid surgery: Changing trends in 130 consecutive cases. Ann Surg 244:471–479, 2006. http://www.lww.com. Used with permission

within the tracheoesophageal groove [4]. As much as 8% of parathyroid glands have been found within the thyroid parenchyma. Further, the four glands are closely adherent to the posterior thyroid capsule. Thus, the parathyroid glands are in jeopardy during thyroid surgery either through devascularization with ligation of the inferior thyroid artery, resection with the thyroid specimen, or during central lymph node dissection (CLND). To avoid postoperative disturbances in calcium physiology, in situ visualization of the parathyroid glands associated with the resected portions of the thyroid as well as reimplantation of any inadvertently resected glands is protective.

Lymph Node Anatomy

Metastatic disease to the lymph nodes travels along lymphatics of the thyroid gland and into the deep cervical lymph nodes usually found at level VI (Fig. 12.4). Lymphatic drainage from each thyroid lobe is involved in a ramified network of interconnections with some connections to the retropharyngeal and superior mediastinal lymph nodes found in level VII (Fig. 12.5) [5]. There are four principal lymphatic trunks for the thyroid which drain into several levels of cervical lymph nodes (Fig. 12.4) (1) inferomedial lymphatics drain into the pre- and paratracheal lymph nodes in level VI which is the most

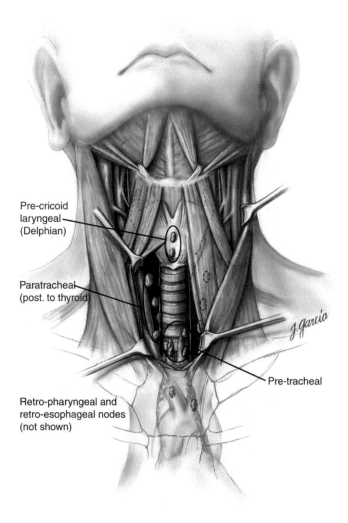

Fig. 12.4 Cervical Lymph Node Levels. Thyroid lymph node drainage occurs most commonly to the central cervical lymph nodes known as level VI. Lymphatic metastasis may also occur in other lymph node levels, including II–IV and VI. Sally E. Carty, David S. Cooper, et al. Consensus Statement on the Terminology and Classification of Central Neck Dissection for Thyroid Cancer. Thyroid Volume 19, Number 11, 2009. Used with permission

Pre-cricoid laryngeal (Delphian)

Paratracheal (post. to thyroid)

Pre-tracheal

Retro-pharyngeal and retro-esophageal nodes (not shown)

Fig. 12.5 American Thyroid Association terminology for central neck lymph nodes. Precricoid, known Delphian, paratracheal, pretracheal, retrotracheal, and retroesophageal lymph nodes are shown. From Sally E. Carty, David S. Cooper, et al. Consensus Statement on the Terminology and Classification of Central Neck Dissection for Thyroid Cancer. Thyroid Volume 19, Number 11, 2009. Used with permission

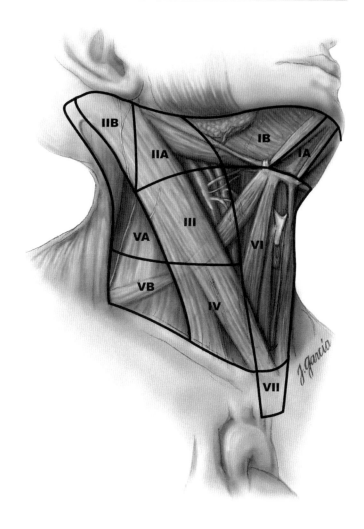

common route of metastasis; (2) superomedial lymphatics drain into the prelaryngeal node, known as the "Delphian node" (Fig. 12.4); (3) superolateral lymphatics drain into the nodes of the upper internal jugular vein in level II; and (4) inferolateral lymphatics drain into the supraclavicular nodes mainly in level V as well as the jugulosubclavian nodes [6]. There are other occasions where the drainage will not occur as predicted and malignant lymph nodes lie outside the central compartment. Once optimized, techniques such as sentinel node biopsy (SNB), radio-guided surgery (RGS), and lymphosonography may add to the specificity of lymph node dissection.

Role of Preoperative Studies to Guide Surgical Therapy

Of the imaging modalities available, neck sonography is one of the most beneficial for surgeon and patient. Not only does it provide anatomical detail about the lesion, adjacent critical structures, and other regional pathology, but it also allows diagnostic biopsy. Image-guided fine needle aspiration (FNA) may obviate surgery for benign lesions and hasten surgery for malignant lesions, recurrent cysts, and indeterminate FNA pathology results. CT and MRI are useful adjuncts to evaluate bulky, locally advanced lesions as

Table 12.1 Indications for diagnostic studies and impact on surgical planning

Diagnostic study	Indications	Surgical planning advantages	Surgical planning disadvantages
Ultrasonography	Solid, cystic, or complex lesions Thyroid enlargement	Delineates anatomical features Allows diagnostic biopsy and aspiration Helps in assessment of lateral nodal compartment	May be inadequate to assess central compartment Operator dependent
CT or MRI	Bulky lesions Extension beyond neck	Thorough evaluation of: • Central compartment • Upper thoracic cavity • Retrotracheal area	May delay surgery. Iodine uptake from contrast may impact RAI
Nuclear Medicine	Suppressed thyrotropin Follicular histology on FNA	Functional lesions usually obviate invasive procedures	Inadequate anatomic information
PET/CT	Suspected metastatic disease High risk patients 1. High-risk disease 2. Adverse histology (e.g., columnar cell, tall cell, and insular variants) 3. Rising Tg levels with no known anatomic source 4. Hurthle cell carcinoma	Identifies clinically occult non-iodine avid tumor metastasis	May not identify slow-growing lesions
Laryngoscopy	Assess vocal cord function, especially if voice change	Reliable vocal cord assessment, even if asymptomatic	None
Thyroglobulin Level	Baseline	Combined pre- and postoperative assessment reflects completeness of resection	

CT computed tomography, *MRI* magnetic resonance imaging, *RAI* radioactive iodine, *PET/CT* positron emission tomography/computed tomography, *Tg* thyroglobulin

well as central lymphadenopathy. Use of iodine-based contrast for imaging studies leads to iodine uptake by thyroid tissue. This additional uptake may impact postoperative radioactive iodine (RAI) therapeutic dosing, and, therefore, such contrast should be avoided. Radionuclide studies have a limited role in preoperative surgical planning since the study establishes functional versus anatomical delineation, except in recurrent cancers, where they may play a role in identifying approximate locations. FDG-PET may be used to evaluate suspected disease when indicated radionuclide studies are normal. It has been advocated for monitoring high-risk disease or for following up elevated thyroglobulin [7] in non-iodine-avid tumors. Although laboratory evaluation is an essential part of the diagnostic process, there is little direct benefit to planning the surgical approach. In additional, nearly all patients with

thyroid cancer are euthyroid. However, baseline preoperative laboratory studies as part of a comprehensive history and physical examination are essential elements in the assessment of surgical candidacy (Table 12.1).

Thyroid Surgery and Controversies

Primary Surgery for Well-Differentiated Thyroid Cancers

The spectrum of thyroid cancers histologies is classified based on degree of differentiation. Papillary (PTC) and follicular (FTC) thyroid cancers are well-differentiated thyroid carcinoma (WDTC) histologies that arise from follicular epithelial cells and behave in a benign fashion when compared to undifferentiated histologies. Most of the thyroid cancer literature is written from the perspective of the most common histology, PTC. Occult and otherwise silent papillary lesions are found in cadaver studies with a surprising frequency as high as 34%. Prognosis worsens for tall cell, columnar cell, and diffuse sclerosing PTC histologic variants. The presence of follicular cells on biopsy of a thyroid lesion requires surgical excision to confirm the architectural features. At a minimum, follicular malignancy is characterized by microscopic breach of the tumor capsule. Features of more aggressive FTC subtypes include tumors with extensive necrosis or mitoses as well as invasion of vascular structures or surrounding tissues.

Options for surgical management of thyroid cancer as defined by the American Thyroid Association (ATA) Guidelines include total thyroidectomy, subtotal thyroidectomy, hemithyroidectomy, and completion thyroidectomy. Total thyroidectomy entails complete removal of all thyroid tissue from the bilateral thyroid beds including tracheal attachments. Subtotal thyroidectomy allows for a remnant of the thyroid at the tracheal attachments to remain while removing the majority of the gland. This allowance provides an opportunity to avoid RLN dissection and thereby preserve RLN integrity. Hemithyroidectomy, also known as thyroid lobectomy, preserves the unaffected lobe of the thyroid through removal of only the affected lobe including its tracheal attachments as well as the pyramidal lobe. Patients who have previously undergone thyroid surgery that is less than a total thyroidectomy may undergo completion thyroidectomy to fully evacuate any remaining thyroid tissue that remains. If, in the original surgery, no exploration of the contralateral side has been performed, completion thyroidectomy can be straightforward. If, however, dense scarring has formed in the contralateral side, then the surgery becomes more precarious for the surgeon and puts the patient at increased risk of RLN and parathyroid injury. Surgeons experienced in reoperative surgery are best prepared both for this surgical challenge as well as to minimize risk to the patient. Completion thyroidectomy is optimally performed

within 2 weeks of the initial surgery to avoid formation of dense scarring.

Hemithyroidectomy Versus Total Thyroidectomy

The decision to pursue total over hemithyroidectomy for WDTC has been the subject of repetitive study. Early experience at Memorial Sloan Kettering Cancer Center (MSKCC) identified that in patients with WDTC, age >45 years, metastatic disease, lesions >4 cm, and histology were factors associated with a decreased 20-year overall survival of 43% [8]. Lymph node status was not significant. Yet, a more recent outcome analysis of the Surveillance, Epidemiology, and End-Results (SEER) database demonstrated that lymph node status did significantly affect outcome [9]. Nevertheless, when type of surgical intervention was compared over the same 20-year period, MSKCC found similar survival for patients with low risk lesions – defined as age younger than 45 years, tumors <4 cm in size, low-grade histology, absence of distant metastasis, and absence of extrathyroidal extension – treated with total (99%) versus hemi- (100%) thyroidectomy [10]. Thus, the MSKCC approach is to stratify patients into risk groups to determine surgical approach: hemithyroidectomy for low risk, total thyroidectomy for intermediate risk, and total thyroidectomy with adjuvant therapy for high-risk patients. The overall disadvantage of hemithyroidectomy is that postoperatively, patients are poorly suited for RAI if indicated. Hay et al. from the Mayo Clinic compared low- and high-risk patients based on both recurrence and survival rates over a 20–25-year period [11]. They found that although low-risk patients had similar survival rates independent of surgical approach, recurrence rates increased significantly in patients undergoing hemithyroidectomy (Fig. 12.6). In high-risk patients, both a recurrence and survival advantage were detected with total thyroidectomy. Thus, based on recurrence risk, all patients with PTC would benefit from total thyroidectomy. This finding was confirmed in a retrospective study of

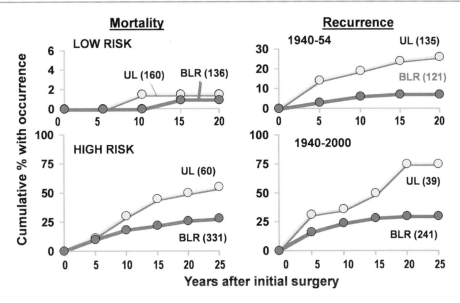

Fig. 12.6 Impact of BLR (Bilateral Lobar Resection or Total Thyroidectomy) versus UL (Hemithyroidectomy) on mortality and recurrence in low and high-risk papillary thyroid cancer treated at Mayo Clinic (1940–2000). Hay ID, McConahey WM, Goellner JR 2002 Managing patients with papillary thyroid carcinoma: insights gained from the Mayo Clinic's experience of treating 2,512 consecutive patients during 1940 through 2000. Trans Am Clin Climatol Assoc. 113:241–260. Used with permission

50,000 patients with PTC >1 cm where both recurrence and survival advantages were realized after total thyroidectomy [12]. Several PTC features have been identified as independent risk factors associated with a worse outcome, suggesting that hemithyroidectomy is inadequate therapy. Although some patients with a history of ionizing radiation exposure may present with only a small, single nodule, total thyroidectomy is the appropriate therapy. These patients are 30–40% more likely to harbor malignancy and as many as half have multifocal disease [13]. Patients with nodules 4 cm or greater seem to harbor malignancy more frequently than FNA confirms. In these patients, the false negative rate is 34%, and 40% of indeterminate lesions later prove to be malignant [13]. Also, the worsened prognosis observed in patients with locally advanced lesions, positive margins, and high-risk histologic WDTC variants – tall cell, columnar cell, and diffuse sclerosing – are indications for aggressive therapy that includes total thyroidectomy. Patients >45 years are known to have a higher recurrence rates, suggesting that near-total or total thyroidectomy is the treatment of choice [14].

Management of Papillary Thyroid Microcarcinoma

Lesions <1 cm, known as microcarcinomas, are treated with hemithyroidectomy if they are unifocal, intrathyroidal, node-negative, and low-risk histology according to the ATA Taskforce [14]. However, due to the frequency of PTMC multifocality, some surgeons choose to treat these lesions with total thyroidectomy. PTMC is less likely to be associated with metastatic disease, whether lymphatic or distant. Although surgery alone is viewed as adequate therapy for PTMC, a retrospective study demonstrated that young age and referral to an endocrinologist are associated with a more aggressive course of therapy beyond total thyroidectomy, including RAI and suppressive levothyroxine (LT4) [15]. There are inadequate data to support this practice. Yet, there are conflicting data that suggest that not all PTMCs require surgery. More recently, Sugitani et al. concluded a prospective trial demonstrating that almost 95% of PTMCs may be safely observed if they remain unchanged in size and asymptomatic [16]. Even when the remaining 5% increased in size or led to symptoms, most lesions only required hemithyroidectomy.

Medullary Thyroid Carcinoma

Medullary thyroid cancer (MTC) has a histologically distinct cell of origin when compared to PTC and FTC. Calcitonin-secreting C cells derived from the neural crest surround thyroid follicles and give rise to MTC which is characterized histologically by amyloid deposition. Further, when compared to PTC and FTC, the trajectory of disease progression in MTC is far more aggressive. Although MTC represents only a 4% segment of all thyroid cancers, it is the subject of intense study related to its association with familial syndromes. Inherited MTC syndromes account for 20–25% of all MTC cases. They include multiple endocrine neoplasia (MEN) 2A (Sipple's syndrome), MEN 2B, and familial MTC (FMTC). MEN 2A is the most common MEN 2 subtype and is characterized by MTC, pheochromocytoma, and primary hyperparathyroidism in association with a RET mutation. The more aggressive MEN 2B is characterized by MTC, pheochromocytoma, and developmental anomalies (musculoskeletal defects, facial neuromas, urinary ganglioneuromas, and gastrointestinal ganglioneuromas). To distinguish it from MEN-related syndromes, FMTC is MTC occurring in individuals with several family members affected by MTC but neither the individual nor family members are affected by MEN. In the 2009 ATA MTC guidelines, FMTC is defined as "a clinical variant of MEN in which MTC is the only manifestation" [17]. In patients affected by MEN syndromes, MTC will develop in 90% of MEN 2A. Association of MTC with mutations in the RET protooncogene has increased the understanding of disease progression and provided pathways of cancer prevention in affected patients. In fact, the ATA has developed a risk stratification system that is based on the types of RET mutations a child sustains and determines at what age the child undergoes prophylactic thyroidectomy. In contrast, adults found to have sporadic MTC without local invasion or clinically apparent lymphadenopathy should undergo total thyroidectomy with prophylactic CLND. This surgical approach is also recommended for MTC patients with limited metastasis, whether cervical lymph nodes or a distant site (Table 12.2).

Minimally Invasive Thyroid Surgery

Many thyroidectomy techniques have been described as being minimally invasive. The three main approaches are: minimally invasive thyroidectomy (MIT), minimally invasive video-assisted thyroidectomy, and robotic trans-axillary thyroidectomy. Each may be used to perform any type of thyroid resection including hemi-, subtotal, total, and even completion thyroidectomy.

It is clear that minimally invasive procedures are technology driven, and the advent of endoscopic technology is the precursor of these types of procedures. One other important factor was development of newer vessel sealing technologies. The Harmonic Scalpel is one such tool that has been subject of hot debate and investigation. This instrument uses high-frequency mechanical energy to cut and coagulate blood vessels less than 3 mm in diameter. It does not transmit electricity in the tissue, as seen in traditional cautery systems, and thus has been reported to have less lateral heat dispersement, limiting heat injury to the surrounding tissue or nerves [18]. The safety and reliability of this technique is well reported for thyroid vessels, and is equivalent to conventional tying of vessels or using metal hemoclips. The other advantage that has been reported is decreasing the length of operative time [19]. In particular, the trans-axillary thyroidectomy, discussed below, is completely technology dependent and driven.

MIT is essentially a thyroidectomy done through a smaller incision, measuring 3–4 cm. This technique only differs from the standard technique in that the incision is smaller, the degree of dissection is less, and there is more retraction to visualize and access the entire thyroid bed. The instrumentation and completeness of the surgery are the same as traditional thyroidectomy.

Table 12.2 Determinants of surgery extent by thyroid cancer differentiation

2009 ATA Guidelines: surgical goals
- Remove all thyroidal and extra-thyroidal disease, including affected lymph nodes
- Minimize surgery and disease-related morbidity
- Permit accurate staging
- Facilitate postoperative RAI treatment when indicated
- Permit accurate long-term surveillance for recurrence
- Minimize the risk of disease recurrence and metastatic spread

Cancer differentiation	Thyroid lobectomy	Near-total thyroidectomy	Total thyroidectomy	Completion thyroidectomy
Well-differentiated thyroid carcinoma (WDTC) (Papillary, Follicular)[a]	Lesions <1 cm if: • Absence of prior neck irradiation • Unifocal • Intrathyroidal • Absence of cervical nodal metastasis	T1 lesions >1 cm or T2 lesions. Lobectomy criteria are met.	Lesions >4 cm. Presence of high risk features with: • Clinical LAD • Family history • Hard, fixed, or enlarging mass • Vocal cord paralysis Aggressive histology	If postoperative diagnosis known preoperatively would have indicated near-total or total thyroidectomy. Lobectomy criteria no longer met postoperatively. Prior to RAI. Note: RAI is not a recommended alternative to completion thyroidectomy
Medullary[b]			All lesions. If advanced, cytoreduction surgery for local control plus: • Preserve critical organs and structures to maintain speech, swallowing, and parathyroid function • Consider tracheostomy	An alternative to surveillance if MTC final pathology following lobectomy or near-total thyroidectomy and at least one of the following: • Multicentricity • CCH • Extrathyroidal extension • Positive margins • RET positive • MEN 2 family history
Anaplastic			Cytoreduction surgery for local control plus: • Preserve critical organs and structures to maintain speech, swallowing, and parathyroid function • Consider tracheostomy	Cytoreduction surgery for local control plus: • Preserve critical organs and structures to maintain speech, swallowing, and parathyroid function. Consider tracheostomy
Indeterminate	Usually	Additional margin w/small lesion	>4 cm	If suspicion high; otherwise, ongoing surveillance

WDTC well-differentiated thyroid carcinoma, *LAD* lymphadenopathy, *MTC* medullary thyroid carcinoma, *RLN* recurrent laryngeal nerve, *CCH* C cell hyperplasia
[a]Based on Revised American Thyroid Association Management Guidelines for Patients with Thyroid Nodules and Differentiated Thyroid Cancer (Cooper, et al, Thyroid, 2009)
[b]Based on Medullary Thyroid Cancer: Guidelines of the American Thyroid Association (Kloos, et al, Thyroid, 2009)

Minimally invasive video-assisted thyroidectomy (MIVAT) is also called endoscopically assisted thyroidectomy. The incision measures less than 2 cm, and as such, access to all areas of the thyroid gland is very limited. Thus, the success of this technique depends on an appreciation of anatomic characteristics and their variability within the neck as well as endoscopic visualization. Identification of the RLN, SLN, and parathyroid glands are essentially the initial steps of MIVAT after accessing the thyroid bed via the small incision. Since endoscopes are used, the degree of dissection required to access the limits of the thyroid gland is reduced. Once these structures are identified, dissected, and separated from the thyroid gland, the gland is removed. Once the thyroid is removed, a central compartment neck dissection can also be performed via the same incision if indicated.

Shimizu and Miccoli first described this type of thyroidectomy in 1999 [20, 21]. Initially, the only advantage appeared to be the size of the incision and cosmesis. However, the clear advantages and disadvantages have become apparent over time. The disadvantages of MIVAT include the need for additional assistants in surgery and specialized equipment. There is a learning curve for this technique that impacts the duration of surgery and complication rates initially [22] (Table 12.3).

However, the incidence of side effects in experienced hands is the same as conventional thyroidectomy: hypocalcemia 0.67%, RLN paralysis 1.2%, and hematoma 0.1% [23].

The most important advantage of minimally invasive surgery is the significant reduction in the patient's pain and resulting analgesic usage [24]. From the patient's perspective, the benefit of the small incision is improved cosmesis. A small incision, however, is important in that it minimizes trauma to surrounding tissues, thus decreasing pain and shortening recovery time. Furthermore, use of the endoscope also minimizes dissection and tissue trauma. Since blood loss during MIVAT is equivalent to conventional thyroidectomy, drains are not generally used.

Tabaqchali et al. noted no difference in the incidence of postoperative bleeding or airway obstruction between patients who had drains and those who did not and further reported that patients with postthyroidectomy drains were more likely to develop wound infections [25]. Avoidance of surgical drains and less pain reduces the need for hospitalization and makes outpatient thyroidectomy feasible [26].

One important consideration is the efficacy of MIVAT. One may ask if this minimal access approach allows for a comparable surgical resection. Studies indicate that one month postoperative thyroglobulin level and ^{131}I uptake are the same for both traditional thyroidectomy and MIVAT [27]. The incidence of conversion to open procedure is 5% [28]. In the initial reports, MIVAT was only indicated for small benign nodules. A broadened set of indications as well as contraindications are defined (Table 12.4) but are constantly evolving.

Robotic trans-axillary thyroidectomy (RTAT) or axillo-breast thyroidectomy was popularized in the Far East. The technique involved approaching the thyroid bed through incisions in bilateral axilla and breast areas to avoid cervical scars. The operative time for this procedure was longer, but the complication rates, although initially appeared higher, are now reported to be the same (Fig. 12.7) [29].

The addition of the robotic technology to TAT surgery has allowed a reduction of limita-

Table 12.4 Surgical decision-making includes the understanding of indications and contraindications for MIVAT [23]

Surgical decision-making	
Indications	Nodule <3 cm
	Thyroid volume <25 cc
	Low grade follicular carcinoma
	Papillary carcinoma
Contraindications	
• Absolute	Previous neck surgery
	Large goiter
	Local metastases
• Relative	Previous radiation therapy
	Hyperthyroidism
	Thyroiditis
	Short neck in obese patient

Table 12.3 Incidence of MIVAT complications and operative time decline with increased operative experience [22]

No. of cases	A (1–25)	B (25–50)	C (50–100)
Duration (min)	102	85	63
Hypocalcemia	4		2
Nerve Palsy	2		0

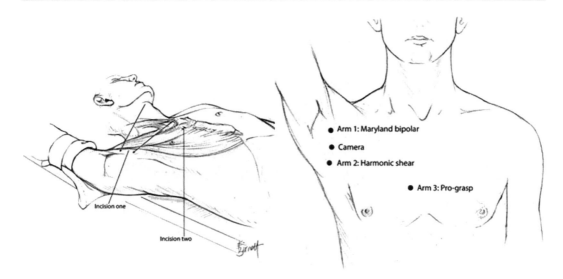

Fig. 12.7 Transaxillary robotic thyroidectomy. Patient positioning and operating port sites are shown. Head and Neck Volume 32 Issue 1, Pages 121–126 Published Online: 8 Dec 2009. Copyright© 2010 Wiley Periodicals, Inc., A Wiley Company. Used with permission

tions of conventional endoscopy by (1) improving freedom of motion through the use of multiarticulated instruments; (2) providing the surgeon with an ergonomically favorable position at a site remote from the patient; (3) providing a three-dimensional, stable, magnified image; and (4) downscaling (translating motion into a smaller motion in the operative field), which enables the surgeon to perform precise movements and allows the dampening of physiologic tremors [30]. Most of the data come from our colleagues in Hong Kong and Korea, where they report faster operating times and low complication rates. Just like any other technique, the success, efficacy, and risks of the procedure are experience dependent [29]. The pain associated with RTAT appears to be similar in scale to traditional thyroidectomy with the added advantage of concealed incisions. Kang et al. report that they have not had to convert to an open procedure in the 338 robotic cases, and were able to perform central compartment neck dissections when necessary. They also explain the potential for additional complications due to location of access ports, although present, to be very low and include Horner's syndrome and temporary arm paralysis. Robotic thyroidectomy received FDA approval in 2009, and the indications for it are sure to evolve.

EMG Monitoring of the RLN

The path of the RLN from the thoracic cavity and behind the thyroid gland to enter the larynx exposes it to risk of injury during any thyroid surgery. The consequences of injury to the nerve can be transient or permanent while the patient's experience ranges from imperceptible to severely debilitating. Bilateral vocal cord paralysis is a devastating complication, potentially requiring tracheostomy placement. Identification of RLN during surgery is well documented to decrease the incidence of postoperative nerve dysfunction [31, 32]. The use of RLN monitoring (RLNM) is an adjunct to visual identification of the nerve to avoid permanent injury. The EMG signal is detected via a special endotracheal tube equipped with vocal cord EMG sensor electrodes. When placed between the true vocal cords during intubation and attached to an EMG monitor, the system provides visual and auditory alerts to the surgeon with each stimulation of the RLNs, whether kinetic, thermal, or electrical. As an adjunct, it can provide a measure of safety in challenging cases in which visual identification of the nerve is limited due to anatomic variation, scarring, or encasement by tumor.

The reported incidence of RLN paralysis is somewhat variable but fairly low, ranging 0.5–2.4% for permanent paralysis ranges and 2.6–5.9% for temporary paresis [33]. In view of such rates, specifically of permanent paralysis, a study enrolling a large number of patients would be required to assess the impact of RLNM. The most comprehensive assessment of RLNM was undertaken in a multi-institutional German study in which 29,998 RLNs at 63 medical centers were assessed. The study demonstrated a statistically significant reduction in nerve injury when RLNM was used by medium-volume surgeons and in patients with Graves' disease [34]. Dralle et al. indicate that fewer than 45 RLNs (or roughly 23 total thyroidectomies or 45 hemithyroidectomies) as the threshold for a low-volume surgeon for whom RLNM helps reduce the incidence of nerve injury. Nevertheless, there is merit to using RLNM by even expert or high-volume surgeons. RLNM provides important feedback regarding nerve traction, particularly when the gland is exteriorized during endoscopic thyroidectomy [26]. Early detection of unanticipated anatomical nerve variants (e.g., non-RLNs or early branching RLNs) may allow surgery to be safer. Also, identification of the nerves can be much easier in patients who are heavily scarred, have undergone previous surgery, or have inflammatory conditions (i.e., thyroiditis) that can obscure the surgical field. In reoperative cases, it is imperative to use RLNM. Finally, nerve function can be assessed intraoperatively by using the nerve stimulator at a lower setting of <0.5 mA which correlates with normal vocal cord movement [35]. The use of RLNM has been the subject of great debate. The monitors are not always reliable, experience a fair amount of signal artifact, and often lack a response even when the nerve is stimulated. Thus, although it is a helpful tool, it is in no way a substitute for anatomic expertise in identification and dissection of the RLN.

Parathyroid Preservation and Autotransplantation

As discussed earlier, superior and inferior thyroid gland anatomy differs as a result of the difference in their embryologic source and resulting pathway to their final positioning. Thorough knowledge of the anatomic relationship of the parathyroid glands to the thyroid capsule, their expected locations, and their variable blood supply from inferior or superior thyroid arteries is essential in preserving the integrity of the parathyroid glands during thyroid surgery. Parathyroid glands that are located more anteriorly (ventrally) on the capsule of thyroid gland are more likely to be injured and devitalized during thyroid surgical manipulations and dissection off the capsule of thyroid [36]. The blood supply to all four glands is derived from the inferior thyroid artery in majority of cases, but can be variable (Table 12.5) [4, 37].

Thus, careful visual identification of the glands, atraumatic dissection, preservation of glandular blood supply with gentle microsurgical techniques, and ligature of the terminal branches of the inferior and superior thyroid arteries as close as possible to the thyroid capsule will optimize the postoperative viability of the parathyroid glands.

Despite meticulous technique, the parathyroid glands can be devascularized or inadvertently resected. The parathyroid vasculature can be minute and easily disrupted. The glands themselves are often very small, closely resemble adjacent adipose tissue, and, as a result, can be easily overlooked. Location within the thyroid capsule or central neck compartment heightens the risk. Studies show that removal of one gland

Table 12.5 Knowledge of parathyroid glands blood supply helps avoid devascularization

Blood supply to parathyroid glands	
Superior parathyroids	Branch of inferior thyroid artery
	Superior thyroid artery
	Branches from anastamotic loop between superior and inferior thyroid arteries
	Direct branches from thyroid gland
Inferior parathyroids	Inferior thyroid artery
	Direct branches from thyroid gland

is not associated with postoperative hypocalce-mia, but resection of at least two or identification of less than three parathyroid glands increases the risk [38, 39]. Large-scale studies have shown that extent of surgery and surgeon expertise are fac-tors contributing to hypocalcemia [40]. As such the increased prevalence of CLND by surgeons with minimal experience in performing this pro-cedure has increased the risk of permanent hypoparathyroidism.

Permanent hypoparathyroidism can be greatly minimized by observing two basic principles of thyroid surgery (1) meticulous technique in identi-fication of the glands and preservation of the blood supply and (2) identification of poorly perfused glands after thyroid removal, or excised glands in the thyroid or CLND specimen. Devascularized glands are then morcelized and reimplanted within the sternocleidomastoid muscle. An autotrans-planted parathyroid gland will take approximately 4 weeks to become functional [41]. Although many studies report a high degree of success with routine autotransplantation, it is not absolute pro-tection against permanent hypoparathyroidism [42–45]. Measurement of postoperative PTH between 6 and 12 h after surgery as either a single measurement or in a series to asses a decline in parathyroid function is an accurate predictor of postoperative hypocalcemia.

Management of Lymph Node Compartments

In WDTC, nodal metastasis is present in as many as 60–80% [46]. The incidence is highest in patients with multifocal primary tumors, larger tumors, extrathyroidal spread, and chil-dren [47–49]. Metastases have been reported in as many as 40–60% of patients with papillary thyroid microcarcinoma (PTMC) – defined as lesions <1 cm [50, 51]. Follicular variant of pap-illary carcinoma usually has lower rates of nodal metastasis than pure papillary. Follicular carci-nomas have a 10–30% risk. The higher rates are usually associated with Hurtle cell carcinoma. Metastastatic lymphadenopathy is the initial presentation of approximately 40% of thyroid malignancies [5].

Despite lymphatic drainage that correlates with the three venous drainage systems of the thyroid – superior, middle, and inferior – there is no correla-tion between the site of the tumor within the thyroid and the sites of its nodal metastasis. Regardless of the site of the tumor within the thyroid, the most common site of metastasis is in the central com-partment (Figs. 12.4 and 12.5). Nevertheless, 18–20% of patients with nodal metastasis have lat-eral but not central neck lymph node involvement. When the lateral neck is involved, jugular nodal metastases are most common in level IV, followed by levels III, V, and II (Fig. 12.5) in order of fre-quency [48, 52]. Contralateral nodal involvement is approximately half the ipsilateral incidence, level for level.

Central Lymph Node Dissection

Recent ATA guidelines describe the boundaries for the CLN compartment: hyoid bone to the axial plane of the innominate artery, the carotid arteries laterally, as well as the expanse of both the superficial and deep layers of the deep cervi-cal fascia. Dissection of this area requires removing the prelaryngeal, pretracheal, as well as the paratracheal nodes [53]. CLND is desig-nated as extended when it includes retropharyn-geal, retroesophageal, paralaryngopharyngeal (superior vascular pedicle), and/or superior mediastinal (inferior to innominate artery) basins. Location of Involved nodes may differ depending on neck laterality. Lymph nodes may surround the RLN on the right side because of its oblique course and likewise lie posterior to the right common carotid artery because of the artery's more ventral and medial location com-pared with the left. Complete dissection allows sparing of the RLNs, external branch of SLNs, as well as the parathyroid glands.

Lateral Lymph Node Dissection

Access to lateral neck lymph nodes is dependent on the incision. A standard thyroidectomy inci-sion may be used with one of the following modifications:

1. Extend the thyroidectomy incision laterally to the anterior border of the trapezius. If necessary, add a small parallel incision 2–3 cm below the angle of the mandible.

2. Extend the thyroidectomy incision upward along the posterior border of the sternocleidomastoid muscle (SCM) toward the mastoid area in a hockey stick fashion.

The lymph node bearing compartment is cleared of tissue, extending from the inferior border of the mandible to the clavicles longitudinally with a transverse expanse from the carotid sheath to the posterior border of the Sternod endomastoid muscle SCM. A complete dissection allows for sparing of the internal jugular, SCM, and cranial nerve XI. In less aggressive cases, level II dissection may not be necessary.

Paratracheal nodal metastasis can go on to invade the trachea, RLN, and esophagus. Even without much invasion, failure to remove macroscopically involved central nodes results in substantial rates of local recurrence (10–30%) [54]. Lateral nodal disease can become quite bulky without invading adjacent structures but ultimately can invade nerves, vessels, and muscle. Radioactive iodine is not very effective for palpable disease, and results in recurrences at least 50% of the time. For these reasons, there is general agreement that therapeutic dissection is indicated for clinically or radiographically positive nodal disease.

With regard to clinically and radiographically negative nodes, the indications for dissection are less clear. Certainly, there is *prognostic* information that can be obtained. Nodal involvement in patients older than 45 worsens the prognosis (increasing both the risk of local recurrence and disease-specific mortality), and this is reflected in the staging system for thyroid cancer, which upgrades stage I or II patients to stage III if nodes are involved. However, is there any *therapeutic* benefit to *prophylactic* dissection of central or lateral nodal compartments?

Prophylactic Lymphadenectomy – Central Compartment (PCLND)

For central nodes, the ATA guidelines for management of differentiated thyroid cancer,

published in 2006, stated that, "routine central neck dissection should be considered for patients with papillary thyroid cancer." [14]. Also, the recently published ATA consensus statement on the terminology and classification of central neck dissection for thyroid cancer suggests that omitting central neck dissection in clinically node-negative patients might be acceptable only in cases of small primary tumors – T1 and T2 [53]. However, the ATA working group also states that the level of evidence supporting their recommendation for routine PCLND is primarily expert opinion. A systematic review of the literature, using evidence-based criteria, found no prospective randomized data to explain the impact of CLND on recurrence or disease-specific mortality in WDTC [55]. Nevertheless, there are some significant reasons to consider routinely doing at least a unilateral PCLND, even in clinically and radiographically negative patients.

As indicated previously, the incidence of central node involvement is as high as 60% in these patients. Very low recurrence rates have been reported in occult cases even without prophylactic dissection [50], as long as all macroscopically involved nodes are removed. One problem is that it may be difficult to reliably determine at operation that central nodes are not macroscopically involved. The size of central nodes and the number of nodes grossly apparent can depend on concomitant problems such as Hashimoto's thyroiditis, and the very fact of metastatic behavior can increase the total number of central compartment nodes [51]. Thus, the distinction between macroscopic and microscopic involvement may not always be precise. Other features favoring PCLND because of higher risk for local recurrence are extrathyroidal extension, older age, and aggressive subtypes, such as multifocal or diffuse sclerosing variants. Another benefit of removing central nodes routinely is that this lowers the postoperative thyroglobulin levels significantly and increases the number of patients with undetectable TG, which can facilitate postoperative therapeutic follow-up.

Thus, there are some potential benefits to routine CLND, but they must be balanced against the risks. Total thyroidectomy without PCLND performed by surgeons experienced in the procedure results in permanent hypoparathyroidism in 1–2% of patients and in permanent nerve injury (RLN and/or external branch of SLN) in 1–2% of patients. A recent review of complications of CLND suggests that the risk of permanent RLN injury remained fairly low (1–3%), whereas the risk of permanent hypoparathyroidism is significantly higher, ranging from 0% to 16%, with an average of approximately 5% even in seasoned hands, when a bilateral CLND is performed [56]. More recently, Shen et al. reported RLN injury rates <1% for total thyroidectomy alone, and a rate of 2.6% for total thyroidectomy plus CLND at initial operation [57].

Although it has generally been accepted that reoperations in the central neck are associated with even *greater* risks of hypoparathyroidism and permanent RLN injury, there are conflicting reports. Pederson found a 1.7% risk for permanent hypoparathyroidism when CLND was done at the time of thyroidectomy and a 6.8% incidence when CLND was done as a reoperation [58]. White reported a range of permanent nerve injury of 2.6–6.8% and permanent hypoparathyroidism of 1.7–8.3% in 290 patients from five series of reoperative CLND. On the other hand, Alvarado and Sywak reported no additional morbidity when unilateral CLND was performed as a secondary procedure [59], and Shen et al. actually found a lower rate of temporary hypocalcemia, the same rate of complications, and the same rate of recurrence in reoperative CLND when compared to initial CLND [57]. It would seem that if PCLND is to be done in the *absence* of macroscopically abnormal central nodes, it would make most sense to routinely dissect only the ipsilateral paratracheal and pretracheal nodes in order to minimize the risks.

Prophylactic Lymphadenectomy – Lateral Compartment (PLLND)

For lateral nodes, recurrence rates as low as 1.5–7.6% have been reported for WDTC patients whose clinically and radiographically negative nodes were not initially dissected, despite the known high incidence of microscopic metastatic disease [60]. The reasons probably include the indolent nature of many of the tumors, the benefit of TSH suppression, and the fact that RAI has some effect on subclinical metastases. There are no clear data to prove that prophylactic lateral node dissection improves survival and, as mentioned earlier, the dissection required to remove these nodes is substantial. Most patients will have disease limited to levels III and IV, but metastasis at two levels bridged by an uninvolved level may occur in 30% of cases [61]. The complication risk includes injury to the spinal accessory, phrenic, vagal, and hypoglossal nerves, as well as to the brachial plexus, cervical sympathetic chain, and thoracic duct. Since a subsequent lateral node dissection would still be in a previously unoperated area, and since an interval lateral node dissection does not worsen prognosis, most authors do not recommend routine prophylactic dissection of the lateral neck in the clinically and radiographically node negative patient.

For either therapeutic or prophylactic node dissection of central or lateral compartments, "berry-picking" of nodal tissues is not advised since this practice is associated with higher recurrence rates and subsequent morbidity from revision surgery [53]. When either a CLND or lateral lymph node dissection (LLND) is done, it should be a compartment-oriented dissection.

Controversy: Sentinel Node Biopsy (SNB)

Studies of SNB followed by compartment dissection, demonstrated that SNB was feasible, repeatable, and detected the sentinel lymph node in 86.5–96.7% depending on technique used – blue dye versus radio-guided [62, 63]. Initial high false negative rates associated with a learning curve are to be expected. Previous SNB studies had false negative rates of 0–33% with gamma probe [64–66] and 0–16.6% with blue dye [67–73]. The combination of blue dye and radio-guided techniques decreased the false negative by 21% to 9% [74]. Complications included laryngoscopy-proven temporary dysphonia in 10.9% of patients.

At this point in time, the benefit of SNB for thyroid cancer is the subject of controversy in the literature. Nevertheless, with continued progress toward accuracy and the clear benefit of minimizing dissection of central compartment's critical structures, SNB would be an ideal modality for thyroid cancer therapy. Until accuracy-related outcome measures improve, we cannot advocate this technique for widespread use.

Aggressive Surgery for Advanced Disease

Upper Aero-Digestive Tract Invasion

Aerodigestive tract invasion (ATI) by well-differentiated papillary and follicular thyroid carcinoma has been reported in approximately 7–16% of all cases of thyroid carcinoma [75]. MTC, although more aggressive, rarely presents with ATI. In contrast, ATI is a frequent clinical presentation in anaplastic carcinoma. Sites of invasion include larynx, trachea, esophagus, strap muscles,

and RLN. This type of tumor invasion is associated with significant morbidity, and a large number of thyroid cancer-related deaths (36%) are due to uncontrolled locoregional disease. Similarly, 39% of patients with AT succumb to distant metastases which attests to the aggressive nature of this type of clinical presentation [76]. A staging system based on the degree of invasion has been devised to assist in surgical planning (Fig. 12.8).

ATI occurs by direct extension or by extracapsular extension of metastatic paratracheal lymph nodes located in the tracheoesophageal groove or paratracheal area. Direct extension not only occurs mostly through points of weakness into structures such as the cricothyroid membrane, and intercartilaginous tracheal spaces, but also occurs through direct destruction of cartilage or muscle. The airway mucosa is a poor barrier for spread of tumor. Esophageal mucosa, on the other hand, is surprisingly resilient and despite circumferential involvement, mucosal invasion is rare.

There are varying opinions in the literature as to the appropriate treatment of aerodigestive tract invasion by WDTC, ranging from radical com-

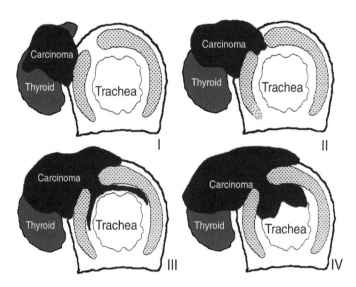

Fig. 12.8 Staging system for upper aerodigestive tract (AT). Stage I – Tumor invades the AT perichondrium or abuts muscle but does not invade into cartilage or deeply into muscle. Stage II – Tumor invades through airway perichondrium and into cartilage or deeply into muscle but not into the submucosa. Stage III – Tumor invades through the airway perichondrium and cartilage or

through the muscle, deforms the submucosa, but does not penetrate the mucosa. Stage IV – Gross transmucosal airway involvement by carcinoma. McCaffrey JC, Aerodigestive Tract Invasion by Well-Differentiated Thyroid Carcinoma: Diagnosis, Management, Prognosis, and Biology. Laryngoscope 2006,116:1–11. Used with permission

plete excision to near complete excision (shave technique). McCaffery, in an extensive study of ATI and surgical treatment, reports equal survival statistics for patients who had radical excision (frozen section negative margin) and those who had shave excision without residual macroscopic disease [77]. However, incomplete resection with residual macroscopic disease led to an extremely reduced survival outcome. Reliance on ^{131}I to manage the remaining measurable disease in these cases, which it clearly cannot, leads to progression of disease. In the absence of gross luminal involvement, a conservative surgical resection that preserves function of the upper AT is the most appropriate choice. An algorithm directing surgical management of lesions involving the AT has been developed (Fig. 12.9). It is imperative that the operating surgeon is not only familiar with the algorithm but also well versed in techniques of

both complex surgical resection and reconstruction of the upper AT. Useful techniques in order of degree of invasiveness are listed below:

- Partial thickness tracheal wall excision (originally described as shave technique)
- Tracheal window
- Tracheal resection and reanastamosis
- Crico-tracheal resection
- Partial laryngectomy
- Partial esophagectomy
- Laryngopharyngoesophagectomy

Surgical Management of Metastatic Thyroid Cancer

While lymph node metastasis occurs commonly, distant metastasis occurs in only 9–10% of patients [78]. A recent literature review of

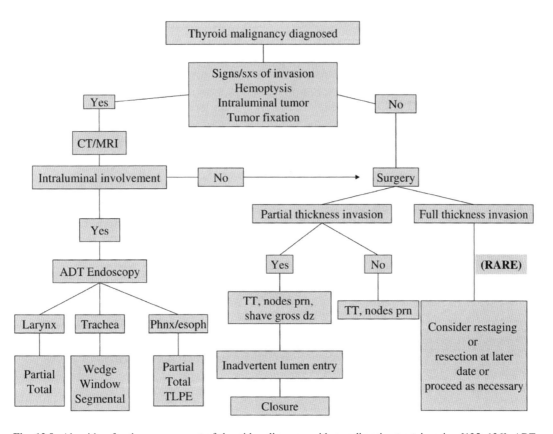

Fig. 12.9 Algorithm for the management of thyroid malignancy with aerodigestive tract invasion [135, 136]. ADT aerodigestive tract, TLPE Laryngopharyngoesophagectomy

PTC with distant metastasis identified the most common sites (in order): lungs, bone, as well as skin, liver, and brain [79]. In their review, the authors also identified individual case reports of distant metastasis to the breast, parotid, adrenal, pituitary, kidney, porta hepatis, orbit, sphenoid sinus, pancreas, and skeletal muscle. Source control and metastectomy are associated with improved survival [80]. Optimal source control includes a total thyroidectomy with CLND.

Incidence of distant thyroid metastasis varies with histology ranging from 10% for PTC to 33% for Hurthle cell carcinoma. Initial presentation with distant metastasis occurs in approximately 4% and is associated with overall long-term survival of approximately 50% [81]. The prognosis is better with WDTC and worse with MTC and anaplastic thyroid carcinoma. Management of thyroid cancer metastasis depends on the extent and pathology. Isolated thyroid cancer metastasis should be excised if resectable including lesions in lung, liver, head and neck, skin, and brain. External beam radiation may be used to treat a localized metastasis that is neither iodine-avid nor resectable. Metastasis to the axial skeleton is less often resected, but it may be feasible to treat these lesions with ablation techniques such as ethanol injection or cryoablation. Reports on ablation approaches to treat thyroid cancer metastatic to the axial skeleton are lacking. Widely distributed metastasis is better treated with RAI and disease-specific survival (DSS) is 66.54% at 5 years [82]. DSS for lesions that are not iodine-avid is 18.33% and chemotherapy is an alternative treatment. Doxorubicin or hormone suppression has been used to treat these lesions resulting in successful palliation but usually not resulting in cure. More recently, targeted therapy has led to disease stabilization. After 20 or more years of follow-up, metastasis are found in the cervical lymph nodes in 35–80% of patients, and only 10–40% of patients have distant metastases [83]. Risk of distant metastasis is long term and has been reported as long as 47 years following hemithyroidectomy [84].

Controversy: Cytoreduction of Anaplastic Carcinoma

Anaplastic thyroid cancer is viewed as uniformly fatal as this very aggressive disease is often discovered at an advanced stage, does not demonstrate a durable response to therapy, and has a median survival of 3–10 months. The AJCC classifies all anaplastic tumors as stage IV, independent of extent. Nevertheless, NCCN guidelines and a recent retrospective review support surgical intervention in a subset of cases. Locally resectable anaplastic cancer should undergo total or near total thyroidectomy with selective resection of involved structures followed by chemoradiation or clinical trial (NCCN. V.1.2009.). For advanced lesions, a retrospective review of 30 patients over 5 years found that maximal debulking surgery followed by adjuvant chemoradiotherapy provided a survival advantage [85]. This advantage was independent of negative prognostic factors (e.g., metastases, type of surgery, and tracheal infiltration) and was not seen in patients treated with neoadjuvant chemoradiation or chemotherapy alone. Maximal debulking included resection of disease adherent to vital structures (e.g., pharynx, esophagus, larynx, or trachea), preservation of vital structures, as well as en bloc resection of adjacent muscles, internal jugular vein, and no more than one RLN if involved by tumor. A recent SEER (surveillance, epidemiology, and end results) study of 261 patients [86] as well as a retrospective study of 50 patients [87] demonstrated a clear survival advantage following surgical resection combined with adjuvant radiotherapy. NCCN guidelines favor clinical trial or neoadjuvant chemoradiation for patients who are not locally resectable. Lymph node dissection includes levels VI and VII.

Surgical Management of Rare Thyroid Cancers

Lymphoma

Symptomatic airway obstruction is a frequent indication for surgery in patients with thyroid lymphoma [88]. Rapid enlargement of a thyroid lesion heightens suspicion for lymphoma, especially in the setting of Hashimoto's thyroiditis. The surgical goals are symptom resolution, airway patency, and sufficient tissue for immunohistochemistry to determine the type of lymphoma. Cytoreduction is unnecessary as adjuvant therapies are sufficient for treatment.

Squamous Cell Carcinoma

The development of primary squamous cell carcinoma of the thyroid is rare and positive biopsy results should initiate a thorough search for a primary tumor. The natural history and prognosis of primary thyroid carcinoma is similar to that of anaplastic carcinoma, e.g., advanced stage at diagnosis, rapidly progressive, and high 12-month mortality. Early macroscopically negative surgery followed by radiation therapy seems to provide the best opportunity for increased longevity [89].

Sarcoma

Just as histologic features of primary sarcomas are similar to undifferentiated thyroid cancers such as anaplastic carcinoma, likewise treatment approach is also remarkably similar. Both primary and metastatic sarcomas are very rare but their appearance is often quite dramatic, recurrence is frequent, and prognosis is poor. As in primary squamous cell carcinoma, macroscopic cytoreduction, neck dissection, as well as adjuvant radiation therapy provide the best opportunity for longevity. Overall a 5-year survival is 50% [90], which is better than both anaplastic and squamous cell carcinomas.

Metastasis to Thyroid

Detectable metastatic disease to the thyroid usually portends a poor prognosis [91]. Thyroid metastasis is found in 1.2–24% of patients with widespread malignancy in post-mortem studies [92, 93]. In similar studies, breast (26%), lung (25%), and malignant melanoma (11%) were the most common primary sites [88]. Clinically, there are more opportunities to address metastasis from the kidney (33%) in addition to the lung (16%), breast (16%), and esophagus (9%). In the setting of source control and in the absence of uncontrollable extrathyroidal metastasis, metastectomy may provide a survival benefit. Depending on the responsiveness of the primary tumor type, preoperative chemoradiation may improve resectability and/or postoperative adjuvant therapy may underscore the survival benefit.

Reoperative Surgery

Recurrent disease may occur anywhere in the central compartment – including the remnant thyroid, structures adjacent to the thyroid, and lymph node basin – or lateral compartment. Overall recurrence following surgical therapy for PTMC is 6.2%. Independent risk factors included surgery less than near-total thyroidectomy and lymph node metastasis. Less than near-total thyroidectomy (NTT) was associated with greater recurrence rates when compared to total thyroidectomy or NTT (18 versus 4%, $p=0.01$). When the authors reviewed all patients who did not receive RAI, they noted that the multifocal group was more likely to experience recurrence than the unifocal group (7% versus 2%, $p=0.02$). Nevertheless, in patients whose disease was either multifocal or metastatic to the lymph nodes, RAI administration was not protective against recurrence [94].

When recurrences occur, the risks of reoperative surgery are higher, especially in less experienced hands. The reasons are related to scarring around the RLN and other structures, uncertainty about the status of parathyroid glands, and at times lack of information on the prior procedure(s). Concern about complications following reoperative surgery of the central compartment – including thyroid bed and lymph node basin – encourages prophylactic CLND at the time of initial thyroid surgery. Although inadvertent parathyroidectomy occurs in 31% of secondary lymphadenectomies, glandular loss is not associated with clinically evident changes in calcium homeostasis [95] due to presence of contralateral or other ipsilateral parathyroid glands. There are studies that indicate that reoperative central compartment surgery is not associated with a significant increase in temporary hypocalcemia, permanent hypoparathyroidism, temporary vocal cord dysfunction, wound infection, or hematoma [59].

Rates of permanent RLN injury are increased following reoperative surgery to rates of 1–12% versus < 1% following primary surgery [96]. Surgeon experience level and volume likely affect these rates.

Persistent or new elevation in serum thyroglobulin in patients undergoing postoperative surveillance leads to surgical referral. Locating recurrent or persistent disease detected by elevated thyroglobulin alone may be challenging. Imaging modalities such as ultrasound, PET, CT, or MRI are usually diagnostic. Sonographic biopsy follows identification of the lesion. If the lesion evades conventional imaging, scintigraphy with iodine-131 is effective guidance in iodine-avid lesions. In non-iodine-avid lesions, preoperative injection of alternative radioisotope, such as Technetium 99m-labeled methoxyisobutylisonitrile (99mTc-MIBI) or Technetium 99m sulfur colloid (Sn-99mTc), is an option in combination with intraoperative localization with a gamma probe. In the face of laboratory evidence suggesting that residual or recurrent disease is present, every effort must be made in the preoperative setting to localize the lesion. It is usually ill-advised to proceed to the operating room without localization of the suspected recurrent disease. For tumors which have dedifferentiated to the extent that they no longer produce thyroglobulin, detection will not occur until they are either palpable or visible on imaging.

Once recurrence is detected, recognition of risk factors coupled with adequate treatment is essential to avoid additional treatment failures. Clinical risk factors for multiple recurrences include male gender, stage III or IV primary tumor, primary tumor size, and primary extrathyroidal extension [97]. Multiple recurrences diminish disease-specific actuarial survival at 20 years from 100% in patients with no recurrence, 94% with one recurrence, and 60% with multiple recurrences [97].

Complications of Thyroid Surgery

During the last 150 years, thanks to significant improvements in surgical techniques and training, better understanding of surgical anatomy and progress in anesthesia and intraoperative monitoring, outcomes of thyroid surgery have improved tremendously. Prior to 1850, operative mortality in thyroid surgery was around 50% rendering thyroid surgery a dangerous undertaking both for the patient and the surgeon. Nobel laureate Theodor Kocher is credited for pioneering technical advancements, including meticulous effort in preserving laryngeal nerves and parathyroid glands. His advancements drove his own operative mortality from 13% to less than 0.5% [36, 98]. In the era of modern thyroid surgery, the reported perioperative mortality is in the 0.1–0.2% range [36, 99].

Thyroid surgery in twenty-first century is considered a routine, safe, and effective surgical procedure and should be accomplished with minimal complication and morbidity in the hands of well-trained surgeons [4, 100]. With strict adherence to meticulous surgical technique and with thorough knowledge of surgical anatomy and physiology, morbidity and complication rates are minimized. While prevention of complications is always the best strategy and in most cases complications are preventable, nevertheless, like in all other surgical procedures, complications do occur in the hands of best thyroid surgeons. Recognition of such complications and their timely and appropriate management are of utmost importance in achieving favorable outcomes.

The extent and type of thyroid surgery directly correlate with the rate of complications and the outcome. While in standard thyroid surgery complication rates overall occur in 1–2% range, in revision thyroid surgery incidence of complications may be significantly higher [101]. When completion thyroidectomy is compared to initial total thyroidectomy, there is no significant difference in rate of complications except for increased length of hospitalization [102]. Moreover, the timing of completion thyroidectomy, in and by itself, does not impact rate of complications [103]. In one study, the complication rate of thyroidectomy in patients with radiation-induced thyroid neoplasm was similar to complication rate in patients without history of radiation exposure [104]. With increasing age of the population in general, and increasing need for thyroid surgery in elderly patients, several studies have found no significant difference in rate of complications in the geriatric population based on the patients' age alone independent of other factors [105, 106]. Well-defined and compartment-oriented prophylactic and therapeutic central compartment nodal dissections, whether done concurrently with the thyroidectomy or secondarily, as a separate procedure after diagnosis of malignancy, have resulted in fewer cases of recurrence in the central compartment. The extent of the procedure (unilateral versus bilateral), however, has been subject of much controversy primarily due to balancing its therapeutic benefits against the potentially higher complications revolving around inadvertent removal or devitalization of parathyroid glands and higher need for autotransplantation of devitalized glands and, to a lesser extent, due to potentially higher incidence of temporary or permanent RLN paralysis [51, 53, 59, 107]. Substernal thyroidectomy and mediastinal dissection have been associated with somewhat higher rates of morbidity and mortality when compared to cervical thyroidectomy without need for mediastinal dissection [108, 109]. On the technological front, intraoperative real time vocal nerve monitoring and low current nerve stimulation, in the hands of many surgeons, has proven to be quite effective in identification and safeguarding of the RLNs in revision operations in scarred operative fields and in complex oncologic or substernal cases where the nerves are at higher risk of injury due to increased exposure [110]. Refinements in surgical instrumentation technology have allowed use of ultrasonic Harmonic Scalpels and LigaSure which allow the

surgeon to perform suture-less surgery with improved operative time and with minimal access in selected cases reducing postoperative pain, scarring, and healing time. In addition, use of these instruments has not resulted in added perioperative complications such as postoperative bleeding, RLN paralysis, or hypocalcemia [111–113]. The added cost of using such instruments in thyroid surgery may be compensated by allowing shorter operative time and improved outcomes in the hands of experienced surgeons [111, 114].

In the following sections we will review the most common and significant complications associated with thyroid surgery which includes vocal dysfunction, hypoparathyroidism, airway obstruction, bleeding, hematoma, seroma, and wound infection.

Voice Changes After Thyroid Surgery

Alteration of voice and quality of phonation, with no visible evidence of RLN or SLN injury on fiberoptic laryngoscopy, occurs in a large population of patients after thyroid surgery with an incidence as high as 87% [115]. While most of such changes improve and resolve over time, even transient alterations may have significant adverse impact on the singing and speaking professional voice [116]. These changes in voice quality as well as their subsequent improvement are not only perceived by the patient, but can also be objectively measured by videolaryngostroboscopy as well as through comparison of functional and acoustic voice assessment both before and after surgery [115, 116]. Possible causes are multifactorial and complex. Depending on surgical technique and tumor extent, strap muscles are subject to surgical trauma (transection or retraction) as well as formation of adhesion to the laryngotracheal complex. The result is alteration in external skeletal support of the phonatory apparatus [115, 116]. Intubation may contribute to laryngotracheal edema and/or injury as well as intraoperative traction of laryngotracheal complex, both of which may significantly contribute to postthyroidectomy dysphonia [117]. Use of single intravenous dose of dexamethasone prior to thyroidectomy has resulted in significant reductions in postoperative dysphonia (presumably due to decreased vocal cord or RLN edema) as well as nausea, vomiting, and pain [118]. The informed consent process should include a thorough discussion of the high probability of such voice changes, particularly when transient or even subtle changes will impact the patient's profession. The most common cause of significant dysphonia after thyroid surgery, however, is iatrogenic injury to any combination of the RLN or SLN.

Recurrent Laryngeal Nerve Injury

The incidence of RLN palsy after thyroid surgery, as reported in the literature, varies widely from 0% to 30% [4, 37, 100]. There are several reasons for this degree of relatively large variation in reported ranges by different authors including (1) the extent and type of thyroid surgery, and whether the surgery was performed for malignant or benign disease; (2) the surgeons' level of experience; and (3) the degree to which such complication is accurately sought and detected in the postoperative period. In addition, physiologic presentation of RLN paralysis postoperatively may vary a great deal from asymptomatic and clinically inevident injury based on perceived voice quality alone to severe dysphonia, dysphagia, and aspiration which may worsen over time after the surgery [4, 37, 100, 119]. The degree of lateralization of the paralyzed vocal cord (whether in median or paramedian position) and the extent of compensation offered by the opposite mobile cord determine the degree and severity of the dysphonia. While the generally expected rate of permanent RLN paralysis in the hands of experienced thyroid surgeons is approximately 1%, some authors report much higher incidence with substernal and reoperative thyroidectomy. Higher incidence may also be reported in cases wherein thyroidectomy is performed for malignancy and requires extensive paratracheal or mediastinal tumor or nodal dissection placing the nerve at higher risk of injury by avulsion, traction, or transection. Direct invasion by neoplasm and known paralysis of the nerve prior to surgery might be an indication for intentional sacrifice and en bloc resection of the RLN

for oncologic reasons. Bilateral RLN injury is a rare but devastating complication of thyroid surgery which may result in airway compromise in the immediate postoperative period. In most cases, bilateral RLN injury will require urgent reintubation and possibly tracheostomy to secure the patient's airway.

The incidence of RLN paralysis is significantly reduced by identification, careful dissection and maintaining nerve visualization during thyroidectomy, CLND, as well as mediastinal dissection. Thorough knowledge of expected anatomical variations helps the surgeon anticipate the location of the RLN. Laryngeal nerve "nonrecurrence" is a variant that occurs more commonly on the right side in about 1% of cases [36]. Extralaryngeal branching patterns of the RLN as well as its relationship with the posterior capsule of the thyroid gland, inferior thyroid artery, as well as the posterior suspensory ligament (Berry's Ligament) are essential to the prevention of inadvertent injury to RLN. The most consistent surgical landmark for identification of the RLN is the cricothyroid joint, which is the point of entry of RLN into the larynx. The nerve can also be sought and identified in the thoracic inlet below the inferior border of the thyroid lobe, between the carotid artery and the trachea [37]. Proper handling of the nerve, including gentle and meticulous dissection, avoidance of excessive traction, and protection it from trauma – mechanical, thermal, or electrical – will minimize iatrogenic injury to the RLN. Intraoperative RLNM and low current (<1.0 milliamp) nerve stimulator probes may assist the surgeon in both identification and safeguarding of the nerve during dissection in all thyroid surgical procedures. Both methods may be particularly helpful in complex and reoperative thyroid procedures where the surgeon anticipates difficult surgical dissection due to tumor involvement, heavy inflammation, or scarring in the vicinity of the RLN.

Unilateral RLN Injury

Prompt recognition of RLN injury followed by timely intervention with a treatment plan based on the patient's level of symptoms is of utmost significance in achieving satisfactory outcomes

[119]. Asymptomatic or minimally symptomatic patients may be observed and later benefit from speech therapy alone. At the other end of the spectrum, patients with severe dysphonia or aspiration will require immediate intervention with vocal cord or arytenoid medialization. Knowledge of the prognosis of recovery by the surgeon is critical to outlining the appropriate plan of intervention. If the severance of the nerve is evident intraoperatively, end-to-end repair or grafting of the nerve is indicated. Although full return of abductor and adductor function may not be achieved by such repair, injury-related dysphonia may improve significantly by prevention of vocalis muscular atrophy [4, 36, 119]. Laryngeal reinnervation techniques with neuromuscular pedicled flaps have been attempted but have not resulted in consistently favorable results in restoring vocal cord function. Likewise, laryngeal electrical pacing is currently considered experimental and not a standard therapeutic modality [119]. Detection of RLN injury intraoperatively is frequently difficult. Nevertheless, if it is suspected postoperatively and confirmed by bedside fiberoptic evaluation of the larynx, the patient should be returned to the operating room for re-exploration of the nerve, confirmation of its structural continuity, as well as removal of any sutures or clips in the proximity of the nerve. In symptomatic patients who have a potential for spontaneous recovery within 12 months postoperatively, vocal cord injection with a variety of absorbable and inert materials may be utilized. Injection materials such as Gelfoam, collagen, autologous fat, and decellularized human dermal tissue have various properties and half-lives.

If prognosis for spontaneous recovery is poor or vocal cord motion is not restored at 12 months after surgery, permanent medialization techniques such as medialization laryngoplasty (Isshiki type I thyroplasty) may be employed utilizing a variety of materials (Silicone, Gore-Tex or Hydroxyappetite) with excellent results and chance of subsequent revision or removal of the implant if necessary [120]. Teflon initially revolutionized vocal cord medialization in unilateral RLN paralysis in 1960s but later fell out of favor due to undesirable migration of Teflon. This migration later caused vocal cord fibrosis, stiffness, and intense foreign body reaction ("Teflon granuloma") in many cases. Recently, Hydroxyappetite paste was developed as a permanent vocal cord medializing agent replacing Teflon and other older permanent substances. Injection medialization laryngoplasty may be performed under local or general anesthesia, endoscopically, or percutaneously depending on both experience and preference of the surgeon [119, 120]. In addition, arytenoid adduction can be combined with medialization laryngoplasty to reduce the posterior glottal gap, to improve dysphagia, as well as to further restore voice quality.

Bilateral RLN Injury

Management of bilateral vocal cord paralysis requires a different treatment strategy often focused on managing an airway emergency. In the immediate postoperative phase, if the patient has airway compromise evident by stridor, labored breathing, and desaturation, the highest priority is securing the patient's airway. To that end, urgent reintubation is performed in the operating room or postanesthesia care unit (PACU). Vocal cord function is then assessed postoperatively with fiberoptic laryngoscopy. If the absence of function confirmed by bedside fiberoptic laryngoscopy persists after a few days, a tracheostomy is then performed. The appropriate tracheostomy procedure will provide the patient with a long-term secure airway. Persistent symptoms beyond 9–12 months after surgery are addressed by a variety of vocal cord lateralization procedures if the following criteria are met:

1. There is no spontaneous recovery
2. Laryngeal electromyography (EMG) confirms denervation bilaterally
3. The patient desires decannulation

Vocal cord lateralization procedure options include external arytenoidectomy, endoscopic arytenoidectomy, endoscopic laser cordotomy, or endoscopic cordectomy. The most important factor in achieving optimum results is to obtain an adequate airway to allow decannulation, without compromising voice quality or aspiration-free swallowing.

Superior Laryngeal Nerve Injury

SLN originates at nodose ganglion of Vagus nerve and courses caudally posterior to the carotid artery. The larger internal branch (IBSLN), carrying afferent sensory and secretory fibers, pierces the thyrohyoid membrane to supply sensation to the larynx and hypopharynx and is rarely at risk of injury in thyroid surgery due to its superior location prior to entering the larynx. The smaller external branch (EBSLN) carries motor fibers and travels in close proximity and usually medial to the superior thyroid vascular pedicle and lateral to inferior constrictor muscles, innervating it and terminating in the cricothyroid muscle, the tensor of true vocal cords. Due to its close proximity to the superior pole the EBSLN of the thyroid gland and variability in its anatomic relationship to the vascular pedicle and the cricothyroid muscle in the vicinity of the superior pole the EBSLN is at relatively high risk of injury during thyroidectomy [36, 37, 119]. The reported incidence of EBSLN injury in thyroid surgery ranges from 0% to 20%, with most studies reporting less than 5% incidence. The true incidence of this complication is often underestimated and under-reported due to its subtle presentation for the normal speaking voice. Since in approximately 20% of cases the nerve still remains intertwined with the superior thyroid artery at the point of entry into the superior pole capsule, en masse and indiscriminate ligation of the superior vascular pedicle may result in severance of the nerve. In 20–25% of cases, the EBSLN cannot be visualized due to its anatomic location. Unlike the RLN, identification of EBSLN during thyroidectomy is not standard practice. However, by conscious attempt at its identification, if possible, during the dissection of the superior pole, by maintaining the dissection and ligation of the vessels low and close to the capsule of the superior pole, and by gentle inferior and lateral retraction applied to the superior pole during ligation of the superior vascular pedicle, chances of injury to this nerve can be reduced [37, 119, 121].

Unilateral injury to EBSLN results in denervation of the ipsilateral cricothyroid muscle which lengthens and tenses the true vocal cord while in contraction. As such, with paralysis of the crico-thyroid muscle, the ipsilateral vocal cord assumes a shorter, lower, and more bowed position compared to the unaffected normal counterpart. EBSLN injury may result in subtle changes in normal speaking voice and may go undetected by surgeon and patient due to subtleties of the presenting symptoms. However, its injury may prove to be quite detrimental to professional voice as was the case for the famous soprano opera singer Amelita Galli-Curci who sustained such injury after thyroidectomy for toxic multinodular thyroid in 1935 ending her singing career [36]. Unilateral injury to EBSLN results in loss of high pitch, easy fatigability of voice, and tilting of the larynx to the normal side due to unopposed contraction of the normal cricothyroid muscle. Bilateral injury to the EBSLN may result in weak, low pitch, and breathy voice with symmetrical appearance of larynx on fiberoptic laryngoscopy, though the vocal cords will assume symmetrically bowed and shortened position during phonatory effort allowing tilting of the epiglottis anteriorly. Mainstay rehabilitation method of choice for dysphonia resulting from unilateral or bilateral EBSLN injury is voice and speech therapy to allow the intralaryngeal adductors and tensors of vocal cords to compensate for the loss sustained from paralysis of cricothyroid muscles.

Hypocalcemia (Hypoparathyroidism)

Among all complications associated with thyroid surgery, postoperative hypocalcemia is the most common in incidence and the most likely cause of prolonged length of stay in the hospital. Although the reported incidence of transient hypocalcemia ranges from 0% to 50%, permanent hypocalcemia, lasting more than 6 months, is less common in the range of 0% to 13% [4, 36, 37, 100, 119]. While the reported incidence in older literature is much higher, and in the days of Bilroth and Kocher accounted for significant cause of morbidity and mortality, the currently acceptable combined rate of permanent hypocalcemia should be less than 5%. Extent and type of surgery (lobectomy versus total thyroidectomy or completion thyroidectomy), indication for surgery (benign versus malignant disease), need for central compartment nodal and mediastinal dissection, surgeons' experience and volume, reoperative thyroid surgery, and surgery for Graves' disease are among important factors that correlate with incidence of postoperative hypocalcemia [4, 36, 37, 100, 101, 119, 122, 123].

The exact causation of hypoparathyroidism after thyroidectomy is unknown and most likely is multifactorial. Although multiple factors including intraoperative hemodilution via non-specific release of ADH or excessive perioperative hydration by the anesthesiologist, parathyroid gland manipulation, and excessive release of calcitonin during thyroid manipulation have been named as possible etiologies [1, 9], the most plausible etiology of postoperative hypocalcemia is ischemia, devascularization, or inadvertent removal of parathyroid glands during thyroid surgery, leaving inadequate parathyroid glandular function to maintain the calcium metabolism. Incidental removal of a single parathyroid gland or unilateral lobectomy, however, seldom leads to clinically significant hypocalcemia [4, 36, 119]. Immediate intramuscular autotransplantation of biopsy-proven devascularized parathyroid tissue removed unintentionally during thyroidectomy or central compartment nodal dissection; an occurrence with an incidence of 10–15%, as well as autotransplantation of devascularized and dusky parathyroid glands identified during surgery, has shown to be successful in restoring parathyroid hormone levels and maintaining normocalcemia, though with delay of few weeks to months after surgery.

Thorough knowledge of anatomic relationship of the parathyroid glands to the thyroid capsule, their expected locations, and their variable blood supply from inferior or superior thyroid arteries is essential in preserving the integrity of the parathyroid glands during thyroid surgery as previously discussed. Thus, careful visual identification of the glands, atraumatic dissection and preservation of their blood supply with gentle microsurgical techniques, and ligature of the terminal branches of the inferior and superior thyroid arteries as close as possible to the thyroid capsule will optimize the viability of the parathyroid glands postoperatively.

Inadvertent parathyroidectomy rates range between 11% and 18% [124–126]. When compared to thyroidectomy for benign disease, thyroid malignancy is associated with similar [124] or decreased [127] rates of inadvertent parathyroidectomy. Type of surgery does not increase the risk, usually only 1–2 glands are removed, and any hypocalcemia is almost always transient. Nevertheless, to avoid inadvertent parathyroidectomy, the thyroidectomy specimen should be carefully inspected intraoperatively.

In the modern era of cost containment, reducing the length of stay after thyroidectomy has been subject of significant attention, not only by employing the routine practice of same day surgery but also by a strong trend toward outpatient thyroid surgery in selected cases. To this end, establishing reliable clinical criteria for effective management of postoperative calcium levels for early and safe discharge of patients is highly desirable and has been subject of several studies. Both early serum intact PTH measured 6–8 h postoperatively and serum calcium measurements within 8–14 h after surgery can be reliably used with high degree of sensitivity and specificity to predict the feasibility of discharge of those patients who are at no or low risk of hypocalcemia. In addition, same indicators are helpful in determining the need for replacement with calcium and/or vitamin D (Calcitrol) for those patients who are symptomatic or are at high risk of developing hypocalcemia. Postoperative PTH levels <10 pg/ml or negative slope of calcium levels with calcium <8.0 mg/dl are predictors of need for replacement and observation of the patient in the hospital. On the other hand, PTH levels of >15 pg/ml and positive slope of serial postoperative calcium levels with calcium >8.5 mg/dl may allow for safe discharge [100, 128–132].

In symptomatic or high-risk patients, in addition to adequate replacement of calcium orally or intravenously and supplementation of vitamin D for improved absorption of dietary calcium, correction of hyperphosphatemia and hypomagnesaemia is also important in maintaining adequate calcium levels. The calcium levels, their positive or negative trend, as well as serum phosphate and magnesium levels need to be monitored closely to determine the need for replacement therapy and corrective measures. Symptomatic patients or those who have required intravenous calcium supplementation should not be discharged from the hospital until their calcium levels have been stabilized and the clinical symptoms have resolved. All patients undergoing thyroid surgery should receive clear and thorough discharge instructions for recognition and immediate management of symptoms of hypocalcemia. Though symptomatic, iatrogenic hypercalcemia and vitamin D toxicosis are quite rare, the continued need for calcium and vitamin D supplementation should be reassessed on a regular basis, weekly or every other week. Regular assessment concludes when either the patient is weaned from the supplements, the appropriate level of supplementation to achieve asymptomatic normocalcemia is obtained, the patient is deemed to have permanent hypoparathyroidism, or 6 months after thyroid surgery.

Airway Obstruction and Injury

Airway management is of particular concern in substernal thyroidectomy and when there is significant compression, distortion, or direct invasion of the trachea and the larynx. Predictors of airway complications after thyroidectomy include large and compressive substernal thyroid tumors with airway compression visible on preoperative imaging studies, advanced age of the patient, presence of tracheomalacia, and direct involvement or penetration of the trachea by the tumor requiring resection and reconstructive procedures on the airway [36, 37, 108, 109]. Close communication and cooperation between the surgeon and the anesthesiologist and adequate preparation for atraumatic and endoscopically guided intubation may avoid serious airway complications at the time of induction. Intraoperative finding of tracheal invasion and tracheomalacia, though rare, should alert the surgeon as to possibility of airway compromise postoperatively. After thyroidectomy, hematoma, postoperative

bleeding, and bilateral RLN paralysis may result in stridor, dyspnea, and immediate need for reintubation in the early postoperative period to secure the airway. In the case of hematoma and bleeding, the skin and subcutaneous sutures should be released immediately at the bedside to decompress the airway and the patient should be returned to the operating room urgently for wound exploration and control of the hemorrhage. To avoid contamination of the "clean" thyroidectomy surgical field, reintubation is the preferred method of airway management. Tracheostomy is best to be avoided during thyroid surgery unless absolutely necessary as dictated by the intraoperative circumstances. For further and long-term management of airway obstruction resulting from bilateral RLN injury, tracheostomy and other corrective laryngeal surgeries may be necessary if the patient fails successful extubation within a few days of the thyroid surgery.

Wound Complications

Hemorrhage and hematoma formation may occur intraoperatively in less than 1% of thyroidectomy cases [37] immediately at the time of extubation concurrent with straining and coughing or in a delayed fashion postoperatively. Most significant bleeders become evident within the first 8 h after surgery [100]. The general incidence of postoperative bleeding is approximately 1% or less and is usually arterial in origin. The presence of drains or compressive wound dressings has not reduced the incidence of hematoma formation. Substernal thyroid surgery is associated with higher incidence of bleeding. Meticulous hemostasis at the time of surgery is the single most effective modality in prevention of postoperative bleeding and hematoma.

Seroma can occur after thyroid surgery with reported incidence of 0–6% [37]. Seromas occur more likely when the surgery includes extensive substernal dissection, bilateral surgery, and subtotal thyroidectomy or when there is a substantial surgical "dead space" created from the resection. Wound drains and compressive dressings have not shown to reduce the incidence of seroma formation. Needle aspiration drainage or placement of active or passive drains for recurrent seromas may be necessary for the management of seromas.

Wound infections in thyroid surgery are quite uncommon with overall reported incidence of less than 2% [37] and more acceptable range of 0.1–0.3% [100]. Thyroid surgery, unless associated with violation of the airway (larynx and trachea) or upper gastrointestinal tract (esophagus), is considered a "clean" surgical procedure with very low expected incidence of infection, and as such, with no indication for prophylactic antibiotics. Strict adherence to the sterile surgical technique throughout the procedure, absolute avoidance of retained foreign body in the surgical wound (drains, sponge gauze etc.), and meticulous postoperative wound care would maintain the infection rate low. Mild wound cellulitis will, in most cases, respond to broad spectrum antibiotics active against common skin pathogens, Staphylococcus and Streptococcus species. Abscess formation is more commonly associated with violation and penetration of trachea or esophagus, formation of fistula, as well as infected large cavity hematomas or seromas and will require incision, drainage, and evacuation of the abscess cavity in addition to instituting antibiotic therapy.

Pneumothorax and hemothorax are uncommon in routine thyroid surgery unless significant and difficult mediastinal and subclavicular dissection is performed concurrently with thyroidectomy. Perforation of airway (trachea) and pleura may result in pneumothorax or pneumomediastinum which, if significant, will become clinically apparent in the early postoperative phase evidenced with poor oxygenation, ventilation, and decreased breath sounds on the involved hemithorax. This complication may require placement of chest tube for management. Since incidence of this complication is quite low, routine postoperative chest radiography is not indicated unless there is a high suspicion for possibility of such problem based on intraoperative circumstances and extent of surgical dissection.

Chyle leaks are uncommon in thyroid surgery alone with increased incidence to about 1% when neck dissection or thoracic inlet dissection is performed in conjunction with thyroidectomy plac-ing the thoracic duct at risk of injury. Low-output leaks can be managed conservatively and expectantly with low fat diet, closed drainage system, and pressure dressing. High-output and refractory cases need operative intervention, exploration, and ligation of leaking lymphatic vessels.

Unsightly scars, often the signature of old thyroid surgeries many decades ago, has, by and large, been replaced with cosmetically acceptable small scars in the era of "minimally invasive" and "minimal access" surgery. Attention to details and gentle handling of tissues as well as careful layered and anatomical closure of the wound results in highly acceptable scars in thyroid and neck surgery. Keloid formation may occur in susceptible individuals based on personal history of propensity for formation of keloids from previous surgical scars and can be reduced in incidence by intraoperative injection of dilute steroid in the skin at the time of closure of the wound.

Postoperative Care

Immediate Postoperative Period

The progress of postoperative care is brisk and focused on early discharge. Uncomplicated thyroidectomy patients are usually discharged within 24 h and lobectomy patients are discharged the same day. Evaluation begins in the postanesthesia care unit with observation for signs necessitating an emergent bedside procedure and returns to the operating room (Table 12.6). As soon as the patient is alert, signs of nerve dysfunction are sought. In particular, RLN nerve dysfunction is sought in all patients and cranial nerve dysfunction is sought after lateral neck dissection. Postanesthesia care unit (PACU) assessment for adequate pain control is an important responsibility shared with the anesthesiologist. Achieving adequate control is rarely a postoperative challenge. Finally, signs of hypocalcemia are sought. Either serial calcium levels are trended or PTH levels provide an indirect assessment of calcium homeostasis. Fortunately, most cases of postoperative hypocalcemia are transient.

Table 12.6 Signs and symptoms of complications

Complication	Signs and symptoms	Management
PACU signs and symptoms of complications		
Active bleeding	Rapidly expanding neck mass	Open wound at bedside Return to OR for hemostasis
Changes in voice quality: • Unilateral RLN injury • Intubation-related vocal cord edema	Hoarseness Hot potato voice Early voice fatigue at high pitch	Prevent with single preoperative dose of steroids Observation
Respiratory compromise → bilateral RLN injury	In absence of expanding neck mass: • Stridor • Dyspnea • Oxygen desaturation	Intubation, vocal cord assessment, possible tracheostomy
Respiratory compromise following mediastinal dissection → pneumothorax	• Shortness of breath • Absent breath sounds • Oxygen desaturation	Needle thoracostomy followed by tube thoracostomy and CXR
Parathyroid devitalization or resection causing hypocalcemia	Chvostek's sign, carpopedal spasm	Calcium and vitamin D supplementation
Cranial nerve dysfunction	Unable to shrug shoulders	Observation
Delayed signs and symptoms of complications		
Surgical site infection	Erythema, localized swelling, tenderness, purulent drainage from wound, fever	Minimally open wound to drain; antibiotics
Seroma or chylous collection	Localized swelling without infectious sign	Aspiration; surgical repair may be required if chylous leak persists

PACU post anesthesia care unit, *OR* operating room, *RLN* recurrent laryngeal nerve, *CXR* chest radiograph

Surgical Drains and Perioperative Antibiotics

The placement of surgical drains following thyroidectomy is controversial and is usually guided by surgeon's preference. A recent meta-analysis of RCTs failed to demonstrate definitive evidence that supports routine use of drains following thyroidectomy and suggested that use may significantly increase hospital length of stay [133]. Further, there is a tendency to provide perioperative antibiotic prophylaxis to patients who emerge from the operating room with a surgical drain. Again, this practice was not supported by the data reported in a recent double-blind RCT evaluating perioperative prophylactic antibiotic use in 500 thyroidectomy patients [134]. High-quality studies demonstrate that there is no clinically significant decrease in the incidence of collections that require aspiration between drained and nondrained groups [133]. Nevertheless, if surgical drains are placed, it appears that removal on postoperative day 1 may safely occur in over 90%.

Outpatient Follow-Up

In uncomplicated cases, postoperative follow-up is often more related to the nature of the cancer. Postoperatively, the patient will follow up primarily with the endocrinologist and/or oncologist for adjuvant therapy, physiologic optimization, and surveillance for recurrent disease. Usually, there are no sutures or drains to remove and the surgical dressing may be removed during endocrinology or medical oncology visits. The uncommon instance of a drain retention following hospital discharge requires outpatient care and maintenance by the surgeon. Patients experiencing intraoperative complications should be followed closely by the surgeon for the first 30 days. Once complications resolve or stabilize, the necessity of surgical follow-up is diminished.

References

1. DuBose J, Barnett R, Ragsdale T. Honest and sensible surgeons: the history of thyroid surgery. Curr Surg. 2004;61:213–9.
2. Hegner CF. A history of thyroid surgery. Ann Surg. 1932;95:481–92.
3. Rogers-Stevane J, Kauffman GL. A historical perspective on surgery of the thyroid and parathyroid glands. Otolaryngol Clin North Am. 2008;41:1059.
4. Summers G. Thyroid and parathyroid surgery. In: Krespi Y, Ossoff R, editors. Complications in head and neck surgery. Philadelphia: W.B. Saunders; 1993.
5. Werner JA, Davis RK. Metastases in head and neck cancer. Berlin: Springer; 2004. 233.
6. Heimgartner S, Zbaeren P. Thyroid carcinoma presenting as a metastasis to the parapharyngeal space. Otolaryngol Head Neck Surg. 2009;140:435–6.
7. Sundram F. Clinical use of PET/CT in thyroid cancer diagnosis and management. Biomed Imag Interv J. 2006;2:1–5.
8. Shaha AR, Shah JP, Loree TR. Risk group stratification and prognostic factors in papillary carcinoma of thyroid. Ann Surg Oncol. 1996;3:534–8.
9. Podnos YD, Smith D, Wagman LD, Ellenhorn JD. The implication of lymph node metastasis on survival in patients with well-differentiated thyroid cancer. Am Surg. 2005;71:731–4.
10. Shaha AR, Shah JP, Loree TR. Low-risk differentiated thyroid cancer: the need for selective treatment. Ann Surg Oncol. 1997;4:328–33.
11. Hay ID, McConahey WM, Goellner JR. Managing patients with papillary thyroid carcinoma: insights gained from the Mayo Clinic's experience of treating 2,512 consecutive patients during 1940 through 2000. Trans Am Clin Climatol Assoc. 2002;113:241–60.
12. Bilimoria KY, Bentrem DJ, Linn JG, et al. Utilization of total thyroidectomy for papillary thyroid cancer in the United States. Surgery. 2007;142:906–13. discussion 913.e901-902.
13. Suliburk J, Delbridge L. Surgical management of well-differentiated thyroid cancer: state of the art. Surg Clin North Am. 2009;89:1171.
14. Cooper DS, Doherty GM, Haugen BR, et al. Revised American Thyroid Association Management guidelines for patients with thyroid nodules and differentiated thyroid cancer. Thyroid. 2009;19:1167–214.
15. Haymart MR, Cayo M, Chen H. Papillary thyroid microcarcinomas: big decisions for a small tumor. Ann Surg Oncol. 2009;16:3132–9.
16. Sugitani I, Toda K, Yamada K, Yamamoto N, Ikenaga M, Fujimoto Y. Three distinctly different kinds of papillary thyroid microcarcinoma should be recognized: our treatment strategies and outcomes. World J Surg. 2010;12:12.
17. Kloos RT, Amer Thyroid A. Medullary thyroid cancer: management guidelines of the American Thyroid Association (vol 19, pg 565, 2009). Thyroid. 2009;19:1295–5.
18. Terris DJ, Seybt MW, Gourin CG, Chin E. Ultrasonic technology facilitates minimal access thyroid surgery. Laryngoscope. 2006;116:851–4.
19. Koutsoumanis K, Koutras AS, Drimousis PG, et al. The use of a harmonic scalpel in thyroid surgery: report of a 3-year experience. Am J Surg. 2007;193:693–6.
20. Shimizu K, Akira S, Jasmi AY, et al. Video-assisted neck surgery: endoscopic resection of thyroid tumors with a very minimal neck wound. J Am Coll Surg. 1999;188:697–703.
21. Miccoli P, Berti P, Conte M, Bendinelli C, Marcocci C. Minimally invasive surgery for thyroid small nodules: preliminary report. J Endocrinol Invest. 1999;22:849–51.
22. Del Rio P, Sommaruga L, Cataldo S, Robuschi G, Arcuri MF, Sianesi M. Minimally invasive video-assisted thyroidectomy: the learning curve. Eur Surg Resarch. 2008;41:33–6.
23. Miccoli P, Berti P, Frustaci GL, Ambrosini CE, Materazzi G. Video-assisted thyroidectomy: indications and results. Langenbecks Arch Surg. 2006;391:68–71.
24. Lombardi CP, Raffaelli M, Princi P, et al. Safety of video-assisted thyroidectomy versus conventional surgery. Head Neck. 2005;27:58–64.
25. Tabaqchali MA, Hanson JM, Proud G. Drains for thyroidectomy/parathyroidectomy: fact or fiction? Ann R Coll Surg Engl. 1999;81:302–5.
26. Terris DJ, Anderson SK, Watts TL, Chin E. Laryngeal nerve monitoring and minimally invasive thyroid surgery. Arch Otolaryngol Head Neck Surg. 2007;133:1254–7.
27. Miccoli P, Elisei R, Materazzi G, et al. Minimally invasive video-assisted thyroidectomy for papillary carcinoma: a prospective study of its completeness. Surgery. 2002;132:1070–3. discussion 1073–1074.
28. Terris DJ, Angelos P, Steward DL, Simental AA. Minimally invasive video-assisted thyroidectomy – a multi-institutional North American experience. Arch Otolaryngol Head Neck Surg. 2008;134:81–4.
29. Lewis CM, Chung WY, Holsinger FC. Feasibility and surgical approach of transaxillary robotic thyroidectomy without CO2 insufflation. Head Neck. 2010;32:121–6.
30. Kang SW, Lee SC, Lee SH, et al. Robotic thyroid surgery using a gasless, transaxillary approach and the da Vinci S system: the operative outcomes of 338 consecutive patients. Surgery. 2009;146:1048–55.
31. Lahey FH, Hoover WB. Injuries to the recurrent laryngeal nerve in thyroid operations: their management and avoidance. Ann Surg. 1938;108:545–62.
32. Thomusch O, Machens A, Sekulla C, et al. Multivariate analysis of risk factors for postoperative complications in benign goiter surgery: prospective multicenter study in Germany. World J Surg. 2000;24:1335–41.
33. Myssiorek D. Recurrent laryngeal nerve paralysis: anatomy and etiology. Otolaryngol Clin North Am. 2004;37:25–44.
34. Dralle H, Sekulla C, Haerting J, et al. Risk factors of paralysis and functional outcome after recurrent

laryngeal nerve monitoring in thyroid surgery. Surgery. 2004;136:1310–22.

35. Donnellan KA, Pitman KT, Cannon CR, Replogle WH, Simmons JD. Intraoperative laryngeal nerve monitoring during thyroidectomy. Arch Otolaryngol Head Neck Surg. 2009;135:1196–8.

36. Zarnegar R, Brunaud L, Clark OH. Prevention, evaluation, and management of complications following thyroidectomy for thyroid carcinoma. Endocrinol Metab Clin North Am. 2003;32:483–502.

37. Gourin CG, Johnson JT. Postoperative complications. In: RG W, editor. Surgery of thyroid and parathyroid glands. Philadelphia: Saunders (Elsevier Science); 2003. p. 433–43.

38. Wingert DJ, Friesen SR, Iliopoulos JI, Pierce GE, Thomas JH, Hermreck AS. Post-thyroidectomy hypocalcemia. Incidence and risk factors. Am J Surg. 1986;152:606–10.

39. Rimpl I, Wahl RA. Surgery of nodular goiter: postoperative hypocalcemia in relation to extent of resection and manipulation of the parathyroid glands. Langenbecks Arch Chir Suppl Kongressbd. 1998;115:1063–6.

40. Sosa JA, Bowman HM, Tielsch JM, Powe NR, Gordon TA, Udelsman R. The importance of surgeon experience for clinical and economic outcomes from thyroidectomy. Ann Surg. 1998;228:320–30.

41. Kihara M, Yokomise H, Miyauchi A, Matsusaka K. Recovery of parathyroid function after total thyroidectomy. Surg Today. 2000;30:333–8.

42. Zedenius J, Wadstrom C, Delbridge L. Routine autotransplantation of at least one parathyroid gland during total thyroidectomy may reduce permanent hypoparathyroidism to zero. Aust N Z J Surg. 1999;69:794–7.

43. El-Sharaky MI, Kahalil MR, Sharaky O, et al. Assessment of parathyroid autotransplantation for preservation of parathyroid function after total thyroidectomy. Head Neck. 2003;25:799–807.

44. Lo C, Lam K. Routine parathyroid autotransplantation during thyroidectomy. Surgery. 2001;129:318–23.

45. Higgins KM, Mandell DL, Govindaraj S, et al. The role of intraoperative rapid parathyroid hormone monitoring for predicting thyroidectomy-related hypocalcemia. Arch Otolaryngol Head Neck Surg. 2004;130:63–7.

46. Attie JN, Khafif RA, Steckler RM. Elective neck dissection in papillary carcinoma of the thyroid. Am J Surg. 1971;122:464–71.

47. Machens A, Holzhausen HJ, Dralle H. The prognostic value of primary tumor size in papillary and follicular thyroid carcinoma. Cancer. 2005;103:2269–73.

48. Frankenthaler RA, Sellin RV, Cangir A, Goepfert H. Lymph node metastasis from papillary-follicular thyroid carcinoma in young patients. Am J Surg. 1990;160:341–3.

49. Lee SH, Lee SS, Jin SM, Kim JH, Rho YS. Predictive factors for central compartment lymph node metastasis in thyroid papillary microcarcinoma. Laryngoscope. 2008;118:659–62.

50. Wada N, Duh QY, Sugino K, et al. Lymph node metastasis from 259 papillary thyroid microcarcinomas: frequency, pattern of occurrence and recurrence, and optimal strategy for neck dissection. Ann Surg. 2003;237:399–407.

51. Pereira J, Jimeno J, Miquel J, et al. Nodal yield, morbidity, and recurrence after central neck dissection for papillary thyroid carcinoma. Surgery. 2005;138:1095–100.

52. Noguchi S, Noguchi A, Murakami N. Papillary carcinoma of the thyroid. II. Value of prophylactic lymph node excision. Cancer. 1970;26:1061–4.

53. Carty SE, Cooper DS, Doherty GM, et al. Consensus statement on the terminology and classification of central neck dissection for thyroid cancer. Thyroid. 2009;19:1153–8.

54. Bardet S, Malville E, Rame JP, et al. Macroscopic lymph-node involvement and neck dissection predict lymph-node recurrence in papillary thyroid carcinoma. Eur J Endocrinol. 2008;158:551–60.

55. White ML, Gauger PG, Doherty GM. Central lymph node dissection in differentiated thyroid cancer. World J Surg. 2007;31:895–904.

56. Sippel RS, Chen H. Controversies in the surgical management of newly diagnosed and recurrent/residual thyroid cancer. Thyroid. 2009;19:1373–80.

57. Shen WT, Ogawa L, Ruan D, et al. Central neck lymph node dissection for papillary thyroid cancer comparison of complication and recurrence rates in 295 initial dissections and reoperations. Arch Surg. 2010;145:272–5.

58. Pederson LC, Shapiro SE, Fritsche HAJ, et al. Potential role for intraoperative gamma probe identification of normal parathyroid glands. Am J Surg. 2003;186:711–7.

59. Alvarado R, Sywak MS, Delbridge L, Sidhu SB. Central lymph node dissection as a secondary procedure for papillary thyroid cancer: Is there added morbidity? Surgery. 2009;145:514–8.

60. Wada N, Suganuma N, Nakayama H, et al. Microscopic regional lymph node status in papillary thyroid carcinoma with and without lymphadenopathy and its relation to outcomes. Langenbecks Arch Surg. 2007;392:417–22.

61. Mirallie E, Visset J, Sagan C, Hamy AL, Bodic MF, Paineau J. Localization of cervical node metastasis of papillary thyroid carcinoma. World J Surg. 1999;23:970–3. discussion 973–974.

62. Takeyama H, Tabei I, Uchida K, Morikawa T. Sentinel node biopsy for follicular tumours of the thyroid gland. Br J Surg. 2009;96:490–5.

63. Carcoforo P, Feggi L, Trasforini G, et al. Use of preoperative lymphoscintigraphy and intraoperative gamma-probe detection for identification of the sentinel lymph node in patients with papillary thyroid carcinoma. Eur J Surg Oncol. 2007;33:1075–80. Epub 2007 Mar 1076.

64. Rettenbacher L, Sungler P, Gmeiner D, Kassmann H, Galvan G. Detecting the sentinel lymph node in

patients with differentiated thyroid carcinoma. Eur J Nucl Med. 2000;27:1399–401.

65. Catarci M, Zaraca F, Angeloni R, et al. Preoperative lymphoscintigraphy and sentinel lymph node biopsy in papillary thyroid cancer. A pilot study. J Surg Oncol. 2001;77:21–4. discussion 25.

66. Carcoforo P, Sortini D, Soliani G, Basaglia E, Feggi L, Liboni A. Accuracy and reliability of sentinel node biopsy in patients with breast cancer. Single centre study with long term follow-up. Breast Cancer Res Treat. 2006;95:111–6.

67. Ferlito A, Silver CE, Pelizzo MR, Rinaldo A, Toniato A, Owen RP. Surgical management of the neck in thyroid cancer. ORL J Otorhinolaryngol Relat Spec. 2001;63:63–5.

68. Dzodic R, Markovic I, Inic M, et al. Sentinel lymph node biopsy may be used to support the decision to perform modified radical neck dissection in differentiated thyroid carcinoma. World J Surg. 2006;30:841–6.

69. Fukui Y, Yamakawa T, Taniki T, Numoto S, Miki H, Monden Y. Sentinel lymph node biopsy in patients with papillary thyroid carcinoma. Cancer. 2001;92:2868–74.

70. Chow TL, Lim BH, Kwok SP. Sentinel lymph node dissection in papillary thyroid carcinoma. ANZ J Surg. 2004;74:10–2.

71. Arch-Ferrer J, Velazquez D, Fajardo R, Gamboa-Dominguez A, Herrera MF. Accuracy of sentinel lymph node in papillary thyroid carcinoma. Surgery. 2001;130:907–13.

72. Kelemen PR, Van Herle AJ, Giuliano AE. Sentinel lymphadenectomy in thyroid malignant neoplasms. Arch Surg. 1998;133:288–92.

73. Dixon E, McKinnon JG, Pasieka JL. Feasibility of sentinel lymph node biopsy and lymphatic mapping in nodular thyroid neoplasms. World J Surg. 2000;24:1396–401.

74. Lee SK, Choi JH, Lim HI, et al. Sentinel lymph node biopsy in papillary thyroid cancer: comparison study of blue dye method and combined radioisotope and blue dye method in papillary thyroid cancer. Eur J Surg Oncol. 2009;35:974–9.

75. Silliphant WM, Klinck GH, Levitin MS. Thyroid carcinoma and death. A clinicopathological study of 193 autopsies. Cancer. 1964;17:513–25.

76. McConahey WM, Hay ID, Woolner LB, van Heerden JA, Taylor WF. Papillary thyroid cancer treated at the Mayo Clinic, 1946 through 1970: initial manifestations, pathologic findings, therapy, and outcome. Mayo Clin Proc. 1986;61:978–96.

77. McCaffrey JC. Aerodigestive tract invasion by well-differentiated thyroid carcinoma: diagnosis, management, prognosis, and biology. Laryngoscope. 2006;116:1–11.

78. Tuttle RM, Leboeuf R, Martorella AJ. Papillary thyroid cancer: Monitoring and therapy. Endocrinol Metab Clin N Am. 2007;36:753.

79. Al-Dhahri SF, Al-Amro AS, Al-Shakwer W, Terkawi AS. Cerebellar mass as a primary presentation of papillary thyroid carcinoma: case report and literature review. Head Neck Oncol. 2009;1:23.

80. Lee J, Soh EY. Differentiated thyroid carcinoma presenting with distant metastasis at initial diagnosis clinical outcomes and prognostic factors. Ann Surg. 2010;251:114–9.

81. Shaha AR, Ferlito A, Rinaldo A. Distant metastases from thyroid and parathyroid cancer. ORL J Otorhinolaryngol Relat Spec. 2001;63:243–9.

82. Mihailovic J, Stefanovic L, Malesevic M, Markoski B. The importance of age over radioiodine avidity as a prognostic factor in differentiated thyroid carcinoma with distant metastases. Thyroid. 2009;19:227–32.

83. Worm AM, Holten I, Taaning E. Nuclear imaging of pulmonary metastases in thyroid carcinoma. Acta Radiol Oncol. 1980;19:401–3.

84. Fonseca P. Thyroid lung metastasis diagnosed 47 years after thyroidectomy. Ann Thorac Surg. 1999;67:856–7.

85. Brignardello E, Gallo M, Baldi I, et al. Anaplastic thyroid carcinoma: clinical outcome of 30 consecutive patients referred to a single institution in the past 5 years. Eur J Endocrinol. 2007;156:425–30.

86. Chen J, Tward JD, Shrieve DC, Hitchcock YJ. Surgery and radiotherapy improves survival in patients with anaplastic thyroid carcinoma: analysis of the surveillance, epidemiology, and end results 1983–2002. Am J Clin Oncol. 2008;31:460–4.

87. Yau T, Lo CY, Epstein RJ, Lam AKY, Wan KY, Lang BH. Treatment outcomes in anaplastic thyroid carcinoma: survival improvement in young patients with localized disease treated by combination of surgery and radiotherapy. Ann Surg Oncol. 2008;15:2500–5.

88. Haq MS, Harmer C. Rare thyroid cancers. In: Mazzaferri EL, Harmer C, Mallick UK, Kendall-Taylor P, editors. Practical management of thyroid cancer. London: Springer; 2006.

89. Harmer C, Bidmead M, Shepherd S, Sharpe A, Vini L. Radiotherapy planning techniques for thyroid cancer. Br J Radiol. 1998;71:1069–75.

90. Eeles RA, Fisher C, A'Hern RP, et al. Head and neck sarcomas: prognostic factors and implications for treatment. Br J Cancer. 1993;68:201–7.

91. Chen H, Nicol TL, Udelsman R. Clinically significant, isolated metastatic disease to the thyroid gland. World J Surg. 1999;23:177–80. discussion 181.

92. Shimaoka K, Sokal JE, Pickren JW. Metastatic neoplasms in the thyroid gland. Pathological and clinical findings. Cancer. 1962;15:557–65.

93. Silverberg SG, Vidone RA. Carcinoma of the thyroid in surgical and postmortem material. Analysis of 300 cases at autopsy and literature review. Ann Surg. 1966;164:291–9.

94. Ross DS, Litofsky D, Ain KB, et al. Recurrence after treatment of micropapillary thyroid cancer. Thyroid. 2009;19:1043–U1043.

95. Ondik MP, McGinn J, Ruggiero F, Goldenberg D. Unintentional parathyroidectomy and hypoparathyroidism in secondary central compartment surgery for thyroid cancer. Head Neck. 2009;24:24.

96. Kim MK, Mandel SH, Baloch Z, et al. Morbidity following central compartment reoperation for recurrent or persistent thyroid cancer. Arch Otolaryngol Head Neck Surg. 2004;130:1214–6.

97. Palme CE, Waseem Z, Raza SN, Eski S, Walfish P, Freeman JL. Management and outcome of recurrent well-differentiated thyroid carcinoma. Arch Otolaryngol Head Neck Surg. 2004;130:819–24.

98. Becker WF. Presidential address: pioneers in thyroid surgery. Ann Surg. 1977;185:493–504.

99. Bhattacharyya N, Fried MP. Assessment of the morbidity and complications of total thyroidectomy. Arch Otolaryngol Head Neck Surg. 2002;128:389–92.

100. Jameson MJ, Levine PA. Complications of thyroid surgery. In: TD J, GC G, editors. Thyroid and parathyroid diseases, Medical and surgical management. New York: Theime; 2009. p. 247–52.

101. Shaha AR. Revision thyroid surgery – technical considerations. Otolaryngol Clin North Am. 2008; 41:1169.

102. Rafferty MA, Goldstein DP, Rotstein L, et al. Completion thyroidectomy versus total thyroidectomy: Is there a difference in complication rates? An analysis of 350 patients. J Am Coll Surg. 2007;205: 602–7.

103. Tan M, Agarwal G, Reeve T, Barraclough B, Delbridge L. Impact of timing on completion thyroidectomy for thyroid cancer. Br J Surg. 2002;89:802–4.

104. Kikuchi S, Perrier N, Cheah W, Siperstein A, Duh Q, Clark O. Complication of thyroidectomy in patients with radiation-induced thyroid neoplasms. Arch Surg. 2004;139:1185–8.

105. Seybt MW, Khichi S, Terris DJ. Geriatric thyroidectomy safety of thyroid surgery in an aging population. Arch Otolaryngol Head Neck Surg. 2009;135:1041–4.

106. Mekel M, Stephen AE, Gaz RD, Perry ZH, Hodin RA, Parangi S. Thyroid surgery in octogenarians is associated with higher complication rates. Surgery. 2009;146:913–21.

107. Moo TAS, Umunna B, Kato M, et al. Ipsilateral versus bilateral central neck lymph node dissection in papillary thyroid carcinoma. Ann Surg. 2009;250:403–8.

108. Pieracci FM, Fahey TJ. Substernal thyroidectomy is associated with increased morbidity and mortality as compared with conventional cervical thyroidectomy. J Am Coll Surg. 2007;205:1–7.

109. Shen WT, Kebebew E, Duh QY, Clark OH. Predictors of airway complications after thyroidectomy for substernal goiter. Arch Surg. 2004;139:656–9. discussion 659–660.

110. Ulmer C, Koch KP, Seimer A, et al. Real-time monitoring of the recurrent laryngeal nerve: an observational clinical trial. Surgery. 2008;143:359–65.

111. Miccoli P, Berti P, Dionigi G, D'Agostino J, Orlandini C, Donatini G. Randomized controlled trial of harmonic scalpel use during thyroidectomy. Arch Otolaryngol Head Neck Surg. 2006;132:1069–73.

112. Siperstein AE, Berber E, Morkoyun E. The use of the harmonic scalpel vs conventional knot tying for vessel ligation in thyroid surgery. Arch Surg. 2002;137:137–42.

113. Koh YW, Park JH, Lee SW, Choi EC. The harmonic scalpel technique without supplementary, ligation in total thyroidectomy with central neck dissection – a prospective randomized study. Ann Surg. 2008;247:945–9.

114. Saint Marc O, Cogliandolo A, Piquard A, Fama F, Pidoto RR. LigaSure vs clamp-and-tie technique to achieve hemostasis in total thyroidectomy for benign multinodular goiter – a prospective randomized study. Arch Surg. 2007;142:150–6.

115. Sinagra D, Montesinos M, Tacchi V, et al. Voice changes after thyroidectomy without recurrent laryngeal nerve injury. J Am Coll Surg. 2004;199:556–60.

116. Musholt TJ, Musholt PB, Garm J, Napiontek U, Keilmann A. Changes of the speaking and singing voice after thyroid or parathyroid surgery. Surgery. 2006;140:978–88. discussion 988–979.

117. Maurer CA. Laryngeal complications after thyroidectomy: is it always the surgeon? (vol 144, pg 149, 2009). Arch Surg. 2009;144:595–5.

118. Worni M, Schudel HH, Seifert E, et al. Randomized controlled trial on single dose steroid before thyroidectomy for benign disease to improve postoperative nausea, pain, and vocal function. Ann Surg. 2008;248: 1060–6.

119. Fewins J, Simpson C, Miller F. Complications of thyroid and parathyroid surgery. Otolaryngol Clin North Am. 2003;36:189–206.

120. Hartl DM, Travagli JP, Leboulleux S, Baudin E, Brasnu DF, Schlumberger M. Clinical review: current concepts in the management of unilateral recurrent laryngeal nerve paralysis after thyroid surgery. J Clin Endocrinol Metab. 2005;90:3084–8.

121. Bellantone R, Boscherini M, Lombardi CP, et al. Is the identification of the external branch of the superior laryngeal nerve mandatory in thyroid operation? Results of a prospective randomized study. Surgery. 2001;130:1055–9.

122. Stavrakis AI, Ituarte PHG, Ko CY, Yeh MW. Surgeon volume as a predictor of outcomes in inpatient and outpatient endocrine surgery. Surgery. 2007;142:887–94.

123. McHenry CR. Patient volumes and complications in thyroid surgery. Br J Surg. 2002;89:821–3.

124. Abboud B, Sleilaty G, Braidy C, et al. Careful examination of thyroid specimen intraoperatively to reduce incidence of inadvertent parathyroidectomy during thyroid surgery. Arch Otolaryngol Head Neck Surg. 2007;133:1105–10.

125. Sasson AR, Pingpank JFJ, Wetherington RW, Hanlon AL, Ridge JA. Incidental parathyroidectomy during thyroid surgery does not cause transient symptomatic hypocalcemia. Arch Otolaryngol Head Neck Surg. 2001;127:304–8.

126. Sakorafas GH, Stafyla V, Bramis C, Kotsifopoulos N, Kolettis T, Kassaras G. Incidental parathyroidectomy during thyroid surgery: an underappreciated complication of thyroidectomy. World J Surg. 2005;29:1539–43.

127. Gourgiotis S, Moustafellos P, Dimopoulos N, Papaxoinis G, Baratsis S, Hadjiyannakis E. Inadvertent parathyroidectomy during thyroid surgery: the incidence of a complication of thyroidectomy. Langenbecks Arch Surg. 2006;391:557–60.
128. Lam A, Kerr PD. Parathyroid hormone: an early predictor of postthyroidectomy hypocalcemia. Laryngoscope. 2003;113:2196–200.
129. Vescan A, Witterick I, Freeman J. Parathyroid hormone as a predictor of hypocalcemia after thyroidectomy. Laryngoscope. 2005;115:2105–8.
130. Luu Q, Andersen PE, Adams J, Wax MK, Cohen JI. The predictive value of perioperative calcium levels after thyroid/parathyroid surgery. Head Neck. 2002;24:63–7.
131. Gulluoglu BM, Manukyan MN, Cingi A, Yegen C, Yalin R, Aktan AO. Early prediction of normocalcemia after thyroid surgery. World J Surg. 2005; 29:1288–93.
132. Payne RJ, Hier MP, Tamilia M, Mac Namara E, Young J, Black MJ. Same-day discharge after total thyroidectomy: the value of 6-hour serum parathyroid hormone and calcium levels. Head Neck. 2005; 27:1–7.
133. Samraj K, Gurusamy KS. Wound drains following thyroid surgery. Cochrane Database Syst Rev. 2007;4:CD006099.
134. Avenia N, Sanguinetti A, Cirocchi R, et al. Antibiotic prophylaxis in thyroid surgery: a preliminary multicentric Italian experience. Ann Surg Innov Res. 2009;3:10.
135. Elaraj D, Sturgeon C. Papillary thyroid carcinoma. In: Morita S, Dackiw A, Zeiger M, editors. Endocrine surgery. New York: McGraw-Hill; 2009. p. 47–64.
136. McCaffrey JC. Evaluation and treatment of aerodigestive tract invasion by well- differentiated thyroid carcinoma. Cancer Control. 2000;7(3):246–52.

Radioactive Iodine Therapy

13

Wendy Sacks and Alan D. Waxman

Introduction

Radioactive iodine (RAI; ^{131}I) has been used to destroy thyroid carcinoma tissue postoperatively in patients with and without known residual disease since the mid-twentieth century [1]. By eliminating remaining normal thyroid tissue, RAI ablation facilitates monitoring for persistent or recurrent thyroid carcinoma with thyroglobulin levels and iodine scans. Furthermore, for those patients with invasive cancers, extensive locoregional or distant metastases, many studies demonstrate that RAI treatment improves cause-specific and disease-free survival [2, 3], but there are many challenges in the thyroid cancer literature to evaluating the benefits of RAI remnant ablation. There is a lack of prospective randomized controlled trials to identify effectiveness of RAI [4]. Moreover, the use of as many as 16 staging systems, pooling of histological subtypes that respond differently to iodine, and lack of agreement of definitions for "low risk" versus "high risk" make it difficult to compare the outcomes for different stages/risks from across studies [5–7]. In addition, the majority of analyses do not account for ethnic and geographic differences in total incidence and incidence of different histological types of differentiated thyroid cancer (DTC). Furthermore, since recurrence and death from thyroid cancer can be seen many years after the initial diagnosis, attaining significant outcome data depends upon the duration of a study which is, oftentimes, too short to provide meaningful data. Lastly, recent studies use newer methods for detecting recurrence of disease such as with more sensitive thyroglobulin assays and high-resolution ultrasound, making it difficult to compare outcomes from older studies where less sensitive whole-body scanning was performed [8, 9].

Whom to Treat

Over the past several decades, there has been an increase in DTC primarily due to small tumors with the largest rate of growth in those tumors 1 cm or less in size [10]. The mortality rate has remained the same, while the use of RAI for remnant ablation in this group of patients has decreased. The effectiveness of RAI for improving outcomes of patients with DTC has been challenged [2, 11] and the Mayo Clinic and other centers have been more selective in their use of RAI for remnant ablation, especially in patients with small tumors confined to the thyroid without lymph node involvement [11]. Retrospective reviews have demonstrated similar excellent outcomes in this subset of patients whether RAI

W. Sacks (✉)
Division of Endocrinology, Diabetes, and Metabolism, Department of Medicine, Cedars-Sinai Medical Center, 8700 Beverly Boulevard, Becker Room 130, Los Angeles, CA 90048, USA
e-mail: wendy.sacks@cshs.org

A.D. Waxman
Department of Imaging, Cedars-Sinai Medical Center, Los Angeles, CA, USA

G.D. Braunstein (ed.), *Thyroid Cancer*, Endocrine Updates 30,
DOI 10.1007/978-1-4614-0875-8_13, © Springer Science+Business Media, LLC 2012

was administered or not [2, 11]. Subsequent studies have also called into question the effectiveness of RAI for patients with stage I disease is defined by AJCC 6th ed (TNM) and MACIS staging systems [12, 13]. Therefore, despite the widespread use of RAI for all stages of DTC, its use in low-risk patients who have an excellent prognosis has become controversial. The revised 2009 American Thyroid Association (ATA) guidelines reflect this in their recommendation against RAI for the very low risk population of patients with small tumors (<1 cm, microscopic, uni- or multifocal). The guidelines advocate for selective use for low-risk patients with tumors between 1 and 4 cm. The reason for these recommandations is due to the fact that the data are conflicting whether RAI will improve recurrence and it has not been shown to improve survival in this group [14]. Furthermore, Hay and colleagues demonstrated that young low-risk patients (MACIS < 6) with central compartment lymph node involvement had the same recurrence rate whether treated with RAI or not (19.6%, P = NS). While RAI therapy does facilitate staging and follow-up, trends in thyroglobulin levels and high-resolution ultrasound are still useful to monitor for recurrent or persistent disease for those who go untreated.

The 2009 ATA guidelines for management of DTC recommend postoperative radioiodine ablation for American Joint Committee on Cancer (AJCC, Sixth Edition) stages III/IV disease, stage II disease in patients younger than age 45 years (and selected patients 45 years or older), and select cases of stage I disease, especially for those patients with multifocal disease, nodal metastases, extrathyroidal or vascular invasion, and/or more aggressive histologies [14]. The 2006 European consensus guideline risk-stratifies patients into very-low-risk, low-risk, or high-risk groups according to the AJCC TNM staging system and recommends RAI for patients in the high-risk group, including stage III/IV disease, stage II disease in patients younger than age 45, or those with incomplete tumor resection. They also recommend RAI for select cases in the low-risk group, including patients with stage I or stage II disease (in those over age 45) who did not have a complete surgery or lymph node dissection, age under 18 years, or tumor size between 1 and 4 cm

with no metastases [15]. A systematic review examining the effects of RAI remnant ablation on the risk of thyroid cancer-related mortality and disease recurrence in early stage DTC published by Sawka and colleagues also found a lack of benefit of RAI remnant ablation in decreasing cause-specific mortality or recurrence for low-risk patients; however, remnant ablation was associated with a decrease in risk of distant metastatic recurrence with a risk difference of −2% (P = 0.005) [16]. Furthermore, a systematic analysis of the peer-reviewed literature from 1966 through 2008 did not find a recurrence or survival benefit to using RAI for patients under age 45 with very-low-risk (MACIS <6; TNM stage I; T0–T2, N0, and M0) or low-risk (MACIS <6; TNM stage I; T0–T2, N0–N1a, and M0) disease [17]. High-risk patients under age 45 (TNM stage 2 disease or MACIS >6) do benefit from RAI treatment. It is unclear whether those patients who fall in the moderate risk category due to extensive lymph node involvement, extrathyroidal extension, and aggressive histologic variants of papillary thyroid carcinoma (PTC) have survival or recurrence benefit from RAI ablation and, therefore, these authors suggest clinical judgment be used for selective use in this category of patients.

With a growing body of evidence on RAI side effects, including secondary malignancies (see section on "Side Effects of Radioactive Iodine") [18, 19], judicious use of RAI should be considered for those patients with a low risk for recurrence and otherwise excellent cause-specific survival. For those patients with a high risk for recurrence and higher stage disease conferring a poorer prognosis, RAI benefits outweigh the risks. In conclusion, the use of RAI should be individualized based on each patient's overall risk for recurrence and survival.

Radioiodine Dose for Remnant Ablation

The most effective ^{131}I dose for thyroid remnant ablation is controversial. It was believed for a long time that the higher the treatment dose, the more effective the ablation. However, some retrospective studies have shown successful results with doses ≤30 mCi when compared to higher doses such as 100–200 mCi [20–22]. In 1983, a study by Maxon and colleagues found that for 70 patients treated for remnant ablation, best results occurred when a dose of ^{131}I was administered such that the patient received 30,000 rad or 45 mCi. There was no apparent gain using progressively increasing doses above 45 mCi [23].

A prospective randomized clinical trial published by Bal et al. in 1996, sought to determine the optimal dose of ^{131}I required for successful ablation in patients without evidence of extrathyroidal or distant metastases. Of the 149 patients [58.4% with PTC and 41.6% with follicular thyroid cancer (FTC)], with a mean age of 39, 27 patients were empirically assigned a single dose of ^{131}I ranging from 25 to 34 mCi, 54 given 35–64 mCi, 38 were given 65–119 mCi, and 30 were given 120–200 mCi. Criteria for complete ablation included no scintigraphic visualization of radiotracer concentration at the thyroid bed or extrathyroidal sites by a standard 5 mCi ^{131}I whole-body scan, uptake of less than 0.2% at 48 h post-treatment, and thyroglobulin less than 10 ng/mL off l-thyroxine. As per these criteria, successful ablation was achieved in 63% of 25–35-mCi group, 77.8% of the 35–64-mCi group, 73.7% of the 65–119-mCi group, and 76.7% of the 120–200-mCi group [24]. Their results seemed to demonstrate no additional benefit in uptake in the higher dose groups. Some limitations to their study include: total thyroidectomy was not performed in the majority of cases (many fewer than in comparative studies in the US), hence uptake should be >5%, resulting in less effect; there were a high number of FTCs which do not take up iodine as readily as PTCs; lastly, the 5 mCi pretreatment dose to assess for metastases may have affected the uptake of iodine after the treatment dose (see section on stunning). In a randomized study, complete ablation was achieved in 86% of patients who received 60 mCi, superior results compared to those treated with 30 mCi [25]. In a subsequent study, Bal et al. randomized 509 patients into eight groups receiving between 15 and 50 mCi ^{131}I for remnant ablation. Patients who received less than 25 mCi were not as effectively ablated (61.8%) versus those who received 25–50 mCi (81.6%) [26]. This large-scale study suggests that lower doses are equally effective. A contributing factor to the efficacy of low and high doses for remnant ablation is the amount of remnant tissue left behind after surgery. Rosario et al. looked at cervical uptake and ablation efficacy with low- and high-dose [131]I. Postoperative cervical uptake was measured 24 h after administration of 300 μCi [131]I. When the uptake was <2%, there was no difference in efficacy of ablation in those who received 30 mCi ($N=30$) versus those who received 100 mCi ($N=40$). However, larger doses of ^{131}I were needed for those with >5% of uptake on pretreatment scan in that success rates were 46.6% for patients treated with 30 mCi and 70% for patients treated with 100 mCi ($N=20$) ($p=0.16$) [27]. One of the main limitations to all of the studies evaluating the best dose for remnant ablation is that the literature lacks data on long-term follow-up of recurrence for patients treated with low doses of [131]I.

A 2007 systematic review of all relevant retrospective studies and prospective cohorts evaluating rates of successful ^{131}I ablation with high- and low-dose ^{131}I found a paucity of robust evidence regarding the lowest activity that can be used for ablation [28]. Variability in the reported rates of ablation resulted from the lack of a significant number of randomized trials, large variability in the definition of successful ablation, and differences in the method of TSH stimulation, extent of surgery, whether a low-iodine diet was recommended, use of preablative ^{131}I scan, and length of time from treatment to follow-up. Overall, they found that studies confirmed the use of 100 mCi for successful ablation in approximately 80% of cases. When looking at the observational studies, the success rate was lower for 30 mCi than 100 mCi (51 vs. 79%) [28], but a meta-analysis of the risk ratios indicated only a modest effect (a 10% reduction). The results of the meta-analysis based on the randomized trials included in their review ($N=6$) were equivocal and the authors suggest that there is a need for further appropriately powered randomized trials with ablation success and recurrence rates as outcome measures. The 2009 American Thyroid Association guidelines state that ^{131}I doses between 30 and

100 mCi generally show similarly successful ablation rates, although higher activities may be better [14]. The recommendation is to use the "minimum activity necessary to achieve successful remnant ablation" [14].

The proponents of higher initial doses of RAI argue that larger doses will not only ablate the remnant tissue but also ablate possible micrometastases resulting in improved recurrence rates [29]. However, Mazzaferri and Jhiang found no difference in the long-term tumor recurrence rate (7% vs. 9%; $P=$NS) following low-dose (29–50 mCi) and high-dose (51–200 mCi) [131]I treatment in their large cohort of patients ($N=1,355$) [30]. For patients with known locoregional or distant metastases and a high risk for recurrence, activity ≥ 100 mCi is generally recommended.

Patient Preparation for Remnant Ablation in Patients with Differentiated Thyroid Cancer

Treatment for patients with DTC often includes a total thyroidectomy or near-total thyroidectomy. This is most often followed by ablation of the remnant tissue with [131]I. For some patients, total thyroidectomy coupled with ^{131}I treatment results in a lower recurrence rate of thyroid cancer. In patients with moderate to high risk of recurrent disease, it has been demonstrated that the administration of radioiodine coupled with total thyroidectomy results in lower incidence of disease recurrence, especially in patients with higher initial staging of their thyroid cancer [3, 30–48]. Ablation also is useful in allowing the patient to be followed by the serum tumor marker thyroglobulin (Tg) as well as subsequent radioiodine whole-body scan when necessary. Having a remnant of thyroid tissue present does not allow for a meaningful and accurate follow-up since the remaining remnant may produce thyroglobulin and will result in a positive diagnostic ^{131}I scan. However, one can follow the thyroglobulin trend and use ultrasound of the neck to identify recurrent disease. Thyroid hormone replacement and

suppression of TSH are generally recommended to reduce recurrence.

RAI remnant ablation is performed to optimize follow-up of patients who have undergone total thyroidectomy, while it is also used as adjunctive therapy for those with residual thyroid cancer in the neck postoperatively. A 6-week period following surgery generally is recommended for purposes of healing prior to giving the high-dose ^{131}I therapy. To prepare patients for optimal treatment with radioactive iodine, the TSH must be elevated to enhance the uptake of iodine into remnant thyroid tissue as well as residual thyroid cancer. The most prevalent method for stimulating residual iodine-avid tissue is to employ a withdrawal method in which the patient is taken off thyroid hormone replacement. Many regimens have been proposed for withdrawing thyroid hormone, but all require sufficient time for thyroid hormone levels to fall significantly, resulting in an adequate rise in TSH secretion. Thyroxine (T4) has a half-life in the blood of approximately 1 week, while the shorter-acting liothyronine (T3) has a half-life of approximately 1 day. The target goal for TSH is generally accepted to be approximately 25–40 mIU/L for RAI treatment preparation [49–51].

In order to prepare patients for ^{131}I ablative therapy, or for maximizing stimulation of iodine-avid tissue for diagnostic testing, it is critical to determine the optimum regimen for achieving a target goal of TSH which is felt to be necessary for achieving successful stimulation and adequate ^{131}I for therapeutic purposes [49–52]. Some groups recommend T4 withdrawal alone, whereas others recommend T3 withdrawal to achieve a TSH greater than 30 mIU/L [52, 53].

Goldman et al. studied 27 patients after 2 weeks of T3 withdrawal and again after 4 weeks of T3 withdrawal. They visually assessed scans and whole-body retention 48 h post-^{131}I administration as well as whole-body results at 72 and 96 h. They demonstrated that the 2-week scans were subjectively equal or better than the 4-week scan and concluded that a 2-week period off T3 was all that was necessary for achieving appropriate TSH stimulation [52]. Other studies suggest that T4 withdrawal alone is simpler and sufficient to achieve a goal TSH greater than 30 mIu/L needed for ^{131}I remnant ablation [49–51]. One study of 13 consecutive patients with DTC on suppressive doses of levothyroxine demonstrated that a mean withdrawal interval of 17 days was required to reach the target TSH concentration of 30 mIU/L [49]. Serhal et al. obtained similar results demonstrating that serum TSH concentrations reached more than 30 mIU/L 18.1 days after T4 withdrawal [50]. They suggested T3 preparation did not add benefit in achieving a rapid rise in TSH over a T4 withdrawal strategy.

While this approach for withdrawal is effective, the majority of patients have significant side effects from overt hypothyroidism and, therefore, Guimaras and DeGroot suggest a reduced thyroxin dose of half the usual amount for 5 weeks which they demonstrated achieved a TSH level 25–30 mIU/L and advantageously reduced symptoms of hypothyroidism [54].

The Society of Nuclear Medicine's recommended protocol for preparation of postoperative remnant ablation and that which is employed in our Center is for the patient to be placed on replacement doses of T3 for 3 weeks after surgery or, for the first three weeks after discontinuing l-thyroxine and then discontinued 2 weeks prior to RAI treatment [53]. Unless a significant thyroid remnant has been left in the neck, we have had success in achieving adequate TSH levels in our patients. Occasionally, patients with failure to achieve a target TSH level have been found to have pituitary failure or rarely other causes, especially in elderly patients.

The T3 withdrawal regimen has resulted in a shorter duration of symptomatic hypothyroidism than if the patient were not given replacement T3 and allowed to achieve a hypothyroid status sooner. The same withdrawal regimen is used to prepare patients for follow-up diagnostic scans to assess for recurrent thyroid cancer. Prior to a diagnostic 4-millicurie (mCi) dose of ^{131}I, thyroxine is replaced with T3 for a period of 3–4 weeks followed by a 2-week period of withdrawal to achieve optimal TSH levels.

The Use of Human Recombinant TSH

To minimize the side effects and discomfort during the hypothyroid period prior to radioiodine treatment or scans, human recombinant TSH (rhTSH) has been developed and approved for use as an alternative to the endogenous withdrawal protocol. Studies by Haugen et al. and Robbins et al. have demonstrated that the sensitivity and specificity for whole-body radioiodine imaging for detection of residual iodine-avid tissue are nearly identical whether one uses the withdrawal technique to increase endogenous production of TSH or if one uses the rhTSH stimulation technique [55, 56].

While these techniques are similar, it is important to recognize that the diagnostic whole-body scan for detecting radioiodine-avid tissue is relatively insensitive for small residual volumes. Nevertheless, the use of rhTSH has nearly equal sensitivity for detecting thyroid cancer metastasis as the withdrawal method and therefore its use has been substantiated for therapeutic purposes. In a retrospective analysis, Robbins et al. found that 84% of patients who were prepared using rhTSH and 81% of patients prepared by hormone withdrawal had complete resolution of visible thyroid remnant. Additional studies have published comparable results in some cases reducing serum thyroglobulin to undetectable levels and demonstrating complete ablation of the normal thyroid remnant using whole-body radioiodine follow-up scans [57–61].

Data from 394 consecutive thyroid cancer patients published by investigators at Sloan-Kettering demonstrated that rhTSH-prepared patients achieved short-term clinical recurrence rates similar to patients who underwent the traditional hormone withdrawal protocols with a median follow-up of 2.5 years after remnant ablation [62]. Using a definition of no clinical evidence of disease, including suppressed thyroglobulin levels of less than 1 ng/mL and a stimulated thyroglobulin level of less than 2 ng/mL, the rhTSH ablation protocol was associated with significantly higher rates of no clinical evidence of disease (74%) versus 55% who were treated with hormone withdrawal. The study also demonstrated a significant lower rate of persistent disease using rhTSH. The authors concluded that rhTSH-assisted iodine ablation is associated with rates of clinically evident disease recurrence and persistent uptake in the thyroid bed that are similar to those treated with the conventional method of thyroid hormone withdrawal [62].

There are multiple factors that contribute to successful ablation of iodine-avid tissue after total thyroidectomy in patients with thyroid cancer, the majority of which relates to the ability to deliver high concentrations of ^{131}I to residual iodine-avid tissue. Factors such as the initial dose, the amount of radioiodine concentration in the thyroid remnant, and volume of residual neoplastic iodine-avid tissue are critical in achieving successful ablation [31–46]. In order to maximize ^{131}I concentration within iodine-avid tissue in the neck, it is desirable to reduce the nonradioactive iodine in order for ^{131}I to enter thyroid tissue without competition.

The accepted method for reducing iodine within the body is to restrict iodine intake. The normal dietary intake in the United States is approximately 1,000 μg of iodine with iodine-fortified bread and rolls responsible for the majority of iodine intake. Effective therapy with rigid low-iodine diets will generally provide 30–50 μg/day dietary iodine, which has been shown to result in increased ^{131}I tumor dose (Gy per 100 mCi) in patients with DTC [63–66]. The dosimetric increase has been found to be 2–3 times that in patients who have been on a regular diet. Maruca et al. found a 146% increase in tumor retention, and also demonstrated decreased ^{131}I clearance and an increase in the total body ^{131}I dose of 68% after low-iodine diet for 5 days [67].

While some centers recommend patients adhere to a strict low-iodine diet, others recommend simply avoiding high-iodine-containing food such as kelp, iodized salt, multivitamin, or mineral preparations that contain iodine and seafood including sushi, shellfish, and other fish for 10–14 days prior to ^{131}I treatment. Morris et al. demonstrated that despite the observed reduction in urinary iodine with a low-iodine diet when compared to patients on a regular diet, simply avoiding high-iodine-containing foods resulted in ablation outcomes that were equivalent [68]. Following high-dose ^{131}I therapy, patients were assessed for residual iodine-avid tissue within the neck using the endogenous TSH stimulation protocol. The success of ablation was determined using a 3–6-mCi ^{131}I scan ranging from 4 to 42 months post-ablative ^{131}I therapy (mean 11.8 months). The patient was considered ablated if the scan was visually interpreted as negative with no activity remaining in the thyroid bed. Ablation rates were calculated for both groups and found not to be statistically significantly different. There was a definite trend, however, in which the patients who were on the strict low-iodine diet tended to have a better ablation rate following 100 or 150 mCi of ^{131}I. The ablation rate after 100 mCi in those patients who followed a strict low-iodine diet was 60%, whereas for patients continuing a regular diet the rate was 50%. However, since there were only 24 patients in this group, statistical significance was not achieved ($p=0.51$). A similar finding was noted for the 150-mCi therapy group in which 30 patients were included. Ablation rate for 150 mCi was 76.9% for the low-iodine-diet group and 66.7% for the regular-diet subgroup. Statistical significance was not reached ($p=0.50$). The findings suggest that a strict low-iodine diet generated numerically, but not statistically, greater ablation rates in thyroid cancer patients. The authors discussed several potential mechanisms that may explain why they did not obtain greater outcomes in the low-iodine group versus the regular-diet group including that it was possible that the limited restrictions in the regular diet were enough to significantly reduce the iodine pool. However, since a trend was observed for improved efficacy of ^{131}I ablation with adherence to a strict low-iodine diet, the authors suggested that perhaps larger studies are need to demonstrate statistical significance [68]. Even though this study suggests that a regular diet limiting foods with high-iodine content may be sufficient in preparation for ^{131}I treatment, our center recommends a strict low-iodine diet as seen on http://www.thyca.org.

Pre-therapy Diagnostic Iodine Imaging

There is ongoing controversy as to whether a diagnostic ^{131}I scan should be performed prior to high-dose ^{131}I therapy. A pre-therapy diagnostic scan can provide important information that may alter the treatment a patient would receive. Arguments for a pre-therapy ^{131}I scan include avoidance of ^{131}I therapy in patients with a negative diagnostic scan; ability to adjust the therapeutic dose if distant metastases are detected; identification of possible brain or spinal cord metastasis which may cause a serious adverse event if high-dose therapy were given; and ability to identify a large thyroid remnant which would require a lower treatment dose to avoid painful radiation thyroiditis.

While a pre-therapy scan may be beneficial in some cases, there are also significant downsides. Arguments against a pre-therapy scan include the rare incidence of a negative pre-therapy diagnostic scan and treatment benefit for occult disease; the possibility of a stunning effect of the diagnostic ^{131}I dose on uptake by the subsequent therapeutic dose (see section on "Stunning" for further details); additional cost for the diagnostic study; and lack of management changes based on the diagnostic study.

Although the Society of Nuclear Medicine Procedure Guidelines favors pre-therapy scans [53], others found that the diagnostic study was not justified [69]. The most recent guidelines from the American Thyroid Association (ATA) do not recommend pre-therapy diagnostic studies following total thyroidectomy prior to ^{131}I therapy [14].

Comparison of ^{123}I and ^{131}I as the Radiopharmaceutical of Choice for Performance of Diagnostic Iodine Scans in Patients Following Total Thyroidectomy

Siddiqui et al. advocated the use of ^{123}I plus thyroglobulin (Tg) levels rather than ^{131}I imaging for patients needing evaluation of recurrent or persistent thyroid cancer [70]. They found that for those patients ($N = 12$) treated with ^{131}I who had detectable serum Tg levels, a 5-mCi ^{123}I diagnostic uptake pattern was concordant with that of a 150-mCi ^{131}I treatment whole-body scan. Mandel et al. visualized more foci in the thyroid bed on 13 patients' diagnostic scans using ^{123}I than [131]I (91% concordance) [71]. Sarkar et al., however, found a lower sensitivity for ^{123}I in detecting iodine-avid tissue when compared to [131]I [72]. Gerard et al. compared ^{123}I diagnostic scans using 3–5 mCi of ^{123}I with the post-therapy ^{131}I scans [73] and found a sensitivity of 87% when compared to the gold standard of ^{131}I post-therapy results. They also found that some of the lesions increased in target-to-background activity ratios between 6 and 24 h and again between 24 and 48 h. This suggests that the target-to-background ratio will increase over time. The relatively short half-life of ^{123}I when compared to ^{131}I may limit the target-to-background ratios as the shorter half-life of ^{123}I prevents the optimization of differential kinetics. This tends to reduce the sensitivity of detecting metastases when ^{123}I is used as compared to [131]I. We have discontinued routine iodine scanning prior to therapy in patients who have recently undergone total thyroidectomy as recommended by the ATA Guidelines [14]. [123]I is more expensive, less sensitive, was found to be less accurate in most studies, and has a half-life which allows delayed imaging only up to 36 h even when high doses of ^{123}I are given (5–20 mCi), all reasons which make it not ideal for diagnostic use.

Stunning

Thyroid stunning is defined as a temporary impairment of thyroid tissue uptake of ^{131}I after a diagnostic ^{131}I scan, which decreases the final absorbed dose following subsequent ablative therapy. Thyroid stunning was first described by Rawson et al. in 1951 [74]. Since the initial observations, there have been many studies attempting to determine if stunning is a significant clinical concern in that it is implied that stunning diminishes the effectiveness of the ablative dose to an extent that causes lower ablation rates in patients who are given diagnostic scans prior to therapy [70, 74–93].

Pre-therapeutic diagnostic radioiodine scans for many years have utilized ^{131}I as the diagnostic radiopharmaceutical. More recently, ^{123}I has been advocated for pre-therapeutic diagnostic scans in order to avoid the stunning affect. Pre-therapeutic diagnostic radioiodine scans after thyroidectomy had been advocated to determine the amount of residual tissue remaining, the iodine avidity of residual tissue, safety factors with respect to potential brain and/or spinal cord-related damage, and the appropriate ^{131}I dose to be given.

Those who believe in stunning advocate using 2 mCi of ^{131}I or less as the diagnostic scanning dose or the use of [123]I. The negative aspect of this practice revolves around the fact that low-dose [131]I (2 mCi) is less sensitive in detection of iodine-avid residual tissue than 10 mCi [94]. The value of ^{123}I or small diagnostic doses of ^{131}I is controversial as several studies indicate that patients who have had no thyroid tumor seen with low-dose ^{131}I or ^{123}I may have high-dose post-therapeutic scans (30–100 mCi) which yield markedly positive scans despite the negative diagnostic scans [94–98].

The issue of whether stunning actually exists continues to be controversial in the literature. Many investigators have concluded stunning is not a real phenomenon, while others have insisted that it is real and will definitely impact ablation rates in patients who are treated with therapeutic doses of ^{131}I after the diagnostic scan. The large numbers of studies published on stunning have differing protocols with respect to the scanning doses, treatment doses, and time from the administration of the diagnostic scan to time of administering the therapeutic [131]I. The time from the treatment of the patient with high-dose ^{131}I to time of scan may have considerable importance. The definition of ablation can be extremely variable, especially with many confounding variables affecting results. Reports favoring a stunning effect were reported by Park et al. and Huic et al., who published manuscripts in which post-diagnostic scans were compared with post-therapy scans performed 24–72 h post-therapy dose administration [76, 78, 79].

It has been demonstrated that the iodine-avid tissue-to-background ratio in assessing iodine-avid tissue is extremely low when scans are performed within 72 h following therapy due to high background activity [99]. For this reason, procedure guidelines now recommend performing the whole-body scans 7–10 days post-administration of the ^{131}I treatment dose [14, 53]. Thus, if a diagnostic dose is performed with 4 mCi of ^{131}I and the scans on the diagnostic dose are performed at 48–72 h, the tissue-to-background ratio may be higher than the post-therapy scans performed 24–72 h post-administration due to the high body background. Figure 13.5 is an example of perceived stunning. A diagnostic scan is compared with post-^{131}I therapy (100 mCi) scans performed at 2 and 7 days post-therapy.

Other researchers find no evidence for a stunning effect. Cholewinski et al. could find no evidence for stunning after giving a diagnostic dose of 5 mCi followed by a 150-mCi therapeutic dose [85]. The post-therapy scans were read at 72 h. Studies by Park and Huic et al. were incorrectly interpreted as evidence for stunning simply based upon the visual assessment within a relatively short period of time (less than 3 days) post-therapy diagnostic scan.

Another variable needing further study is the impact of the time lapse between the performance of a diagnostic scan and the subsequent delivery of a larger therapeutic dose. Bajen et al. found that stunning occurred in 26.5% of patients using visual assessment [72]. The time between the diagnostic and therapeutic scans ranges from 7 to 112 days with a mean of 50 days [88]. The long lag time between diagnostic and therapeutic dose administration may have played a role in the apparent decrease in the therapy scan as compared to the diagnostic scan. Cholewinski et al., on the other hand, delivered the therapeutic dose the same day the diagnostic scan was done. Of the 104 patients in Cholewinski's study who required therapy, there were no patients who were felt to have a stunning effect [85]. Kao et al. found a stunning effect in 73.5% of patients but did not deliver a therapy dose for 7–30 days following the diagnostic dose [83].

Diagnostic doses are not generally thought of as having therapeutic effects. It is likely however, that, over time, treatment doses of 2–10 mCi are large enough to be considered therapeutic as these doses are used in patients who have hyperthyroidism. McDougall et al. observed stunning in only 2 of 147 patients using a 2-mCi diagnostic dose [81]. Time between diagnostic scan and therapy was less than 4 days (21% were on same day) [81]. The variability of results using the same diagnostic doses appears to demonstrate that other factors are playing an essential role in post-radioiodine effect on thyroid tissue.

If stunning is of a concern and a real phenomenon, choosing the appropriate diagnostic dose of ^{131}I is important. One must consider the effects of stunning with the effectiveness of discovering radioiodine-avid tissue using lower doses. Many of the stunning studies recommend the use of small (less than 3 mCi) diagnostic doses of ^{131}I or ^{123}I but do not thoroughly discuss or consider the lack of ability to visualize thyroid remnants and metastases with these lower doses. In a study of follow-up scans (6–8 months after initial therapy) to assess for residual iodine-avid tissue, Waxman et al. reported a 400% increase in sensitivity in visualizing thyroid remnant or metastasis using a 10-mCi dose of ^{131}I compared with the 2-mCi ^{131}I dose in the same patient [94]. Forty-three percent of the patients in this study had a negative 2-mCi ^{131}I scan but had a positive 10-mCi ^{131}I diagnostic scan. This study also demonstrated a positive correlation between uptake in residual iodine-avid tissue and increasing ^{131}I dose in iodine-avid tissue visualization in patients given 10 mCi followed by 30 mCi of ^{131}I as well as in those given 10 mCi followed by 100 mCi of ^{131}I [94].

Shlumberger et al. and Nemec et al. both demonstrated that a 2-mCi diagnostic dose missed metastasis to the lung in nearly 20–50% of patients whose disease was identified after a subsequent therapeutic dose of 80–120 mCi [95, 96]. Lastly, Pacini et al. reported on patients with elevated thyroglobulin levels who had previously received high-dose radioiodine therapy (50–150 mCi) [97]. All of the patients in this series had a negative 5-mCi ^{131}I scan but positive post-therapy scans in 94% of patients studied. The findings of markedly improved detection of iodine-avid tissue with therapeutic doses question the value of a diagnostic scan in patients following total thyroidectomy. Scans performed with therapeutic doses of ^{131}I along with a delayed scan (7–10 days) appear to benefit from advantages of increasing photon flux due to the higher initial dose and the differential washout rates between normal and iodine-avid tissue.

Quantitative Measurements of Iodine Uptake Following a Diagnostic Dose of ^{131}I

Quantitative studies of thyroid stunning have compared percent uptake of radioiodine after a diagnostic dose compared to uptake following therapeutic doses. This has therapeutic implications as successful treatment is related to maximizing tumor radiation since improved outcomes of radioiodine therapy for thyroid cancer is directly related to effective radiation dose to the area to be ablated [23]. Huic et al. demonstrated that quantitative measurements of biologic and effective half-life of post-diagnostic versus post-therapeutic uptake were influenced by the effective half-life of radioisotope uptake in the tumor [78]. Patients with tumors, especially with long effective half-life (greater than 40 h), demonstrated significantly greater reductions in uptake between the diagnostic and the therapeutic whole-body scans when compared to tumors with shorter half-life. This is presumed to be due to the effective radiation of the tumor which depends upon initial dose to the tumor as well as residence time of the iodine ^{131}I within the tumor. They found that patients with a 24-h uptake greater than 2% of ^{131}I had significantly reduced uptake on the therapeutic scans compared to patients with less than 2% 24-h accumulation of ^{131}I. The reductions in uptake between diagnostic and therapeutic scans range from 6.8 to 73.4%, indicating that individual biologic responses to radioiodine were considerable [78].

Sabri et al. evaluated patients with benign thyroid disease (Graves' disease or diffuse toxic multinodular goiter) who were given a 0.05-mCi diagnostic dose of ^{131}I and a therapy dose of 5–17 mCi of [131]I 4 days later [92]. They observed reduction in uptake of nearly 32% between the diagnostic and therapeutic doses. This was attributed directly to the effect of the absorbed energy dose of the diagnostic [131]I. Jeevanram et al. evaluated radioiodine uptake in patients with DTC following initial diagnostic doses (0.1–5 mCi) compared to a second dose. The radioiodine uptake decreased by 40–75% between the two doses in six of seven patients who received a second 4.5-mCi dose. It should be noted that there was a significant time lapse between 10 and 40 days between the initial diagnostic dose and the second dose [75].

Medvedec et al. measured absorbed dose after administration of 2 mCi of ^{131}I as a diagnostic dose to 41 patients [86]. They used the uptake value to predict the therapeutic absorbed dose. The higher the diagnostic absorbed dose, the greater the percent reduction of the diagnostically predicted therapeutic absorbed dose. The cut-off level for the significance of stunning effects in this study was 10 Gy, prompting the authors to recommend a dose of 1 mCi or less for diagnostic scanning prior to ^{131}I therapy. However, outcome measures by follow-up scintigraphy demonstrated an 88% ablation rate which is considerably higher than that reported in the majority of outcome studies [76, 80, 84, 85, 87]. Park et al. is the only group to date that reported stunning in patients treated immediately after receiving the diagnostic scan [76]. This group attempted to interpret the post-therapy scan 24–48 h following the therapeutic dose. Performing a total-body scan within 48 h following a therapeutic dose will result in an extremely high background and, therefore, falsely reduce the target-to-background ratio in iodine-avid tissue. Optimal time for interpreting the therapeutic scan appears to be 5–10 days post-therapy. Therefore, the reports of stunning based upon comparing a diagnostic scan with 5 mCi performed 48 h post-diagnostic dose may not be readily compared with scans performed at 48 h using a therapeutic dose of 100 mCi or greater.

It is becoming more evident that the time elapsed between diagnostic and treatment dose administration as well as the time between the therapeutic dose and post-therapeutic scans are important factors that may impact perceptions of stunning.

Impact of Stunning on Clinical Outcomes

Due to the conflicting nature of multiple reports with respect to whether stunning is present using quantitative or visual ^{131}I studies to determine the presence of reduced activity between the diagnostic and therapeutic scans, multiple investigators have simply attempted to assess successful ablation by comparing groups of patients who did and did not receive diagnostic radioiodine studies. Morris et al. summarized multiple reports on outcomes of patients given diagnostic doses of ^{131}I ranging from no diagnostic scan to 10 mCi of [131]I. While the definition of ablation was extremely variable ranging from low-dose scans at 4 months up to higher-dose scans at 1 year, they found only one study which demonstrated that stunning had an impact on outcomes. Overall, they reported little or no impact of stunning on ablation from ^{131}I therapy [80].

Other factors such as method of stimulation (rh TSH or endogenous stimulation) are also inconsistent between studies. Size of the iodine pool (iodine-restricted diet), TSH levels at the time of diagnostic dose administration, and type of instrumentation used in performing the diagnostic scan are additional variables which may impact the perception of successful ablation. Outcomes may also be impacted by the quantity of residual thyroid tissue remaining after surgery and the dose of iodine ^{131}I used for therapy.

Using ^{131}I or ^{123}I as the diagnostic scan prior to ^{131}I high-dose ablation did not appear to influence therapeutic outcomes. Silberstein evaluated 50 patients with nonmetastatic PTC or FTC who have received total thyroidectomy [100]. These patients underwent thyroid hormone withdrawal to achieve serum TSH levels above 30 μIU/mL. They were divided prospectively into two separate groups. One group had a diagnostic imaging with 0.4 mCi of ^{123}I followed by thyroid remnant ablation with 100 mCi of [131]I. The other group had empiric ablation with 100-mCi ^{131}I but the preceding diagnostic scan was performed using 2 mCi of [131]I. Post-ablation outcomes were evaluated by both the groups. Successful ablation required a negative follow-up ^{131}I diagnostic scan 6–8 months after ablation and also an undetectable serum thyroglobulin level in the absence of anti-thyroglobulin antibodies. There was no significant difference between the two groups with respect to ablation rates. Silberstein concluded that if indeed thyroid remnant stunning was present due to 2-mCi ^{131}I used as a diagnostic agent before ^{131}I ablation, there was no significant clinical correlation between the use of ^{131}I or ^{123}I since the ablation rates were identical whether ^{123}I or ^{131}I was used as the pre-therapy diagnostic agent [100].

Given all of the confounding variables in the use of ^{131}I to treat thyroid cancer, it is difficult to determine not only if stunning exists but also the magnitude of the stunning effect. A radiation effect may be insignificant if an extremely limited time exists following the diagnostic scan. A partial therapeutic effect may account for reports of stunning, especially when many days or weeks separate the diagnostic dose from the therapeutic dose.

Side Effects of Radioactive Iodine

Side effects of ^{131}I can be categorized by their time and occurrence after therapy [101] and fall into three categories, early (first 10 days after treatment), intermediate (10 days until 1 year), and late effects (over 1 year) (Table 13.1), based on the time periods in which patients are observed after treatment.

While the most common side effects from ^{131}I treatment are gastrointestinal in nature, including nausea and vomiting occurring in up to 67% of patients, the symptoms are limited and can usually be well managed by preventative measures with antinausea medications given 30 min prior to taking the ^{131}I pill [102]. Nausea is related to the dose of ^{131}I administered. Higher doses (>150 mCi) are associated with increased nausea and vomiting, while only 5.35% of patients were

Table 13.1 Early, intermediate and late side effects of ^{131}I therapy (modified from Von Nostrand. Thyroid; December 2009:1381–1391. Used with permission)

Early (day of therapy ~10 days after therapy)
Acute sialoadenitis
Xerostomia
Ageusia
Stomatitis and/or ulcers
Abnormalities in smell
Epistaxis
Thyroiditis
Gastoenteritis
Nausea
Vomiting
Intermediate (~10 days after therapy to 1 year)
Xerophthalmia
Chronic sialoadenitis
Salivary duct obstruction
Ageusia
Abnormalities in smell
Epiphoria
Conjunctivitis
Recurrent laryngeal nerve injury (very rare)
Hypoparathyroidism (very rare)
Acute radiation pneumonitis (very rare when guidelines followed)
Pulmonary fibrosis (very rare when guidelines followed)
Transient decreased ovarian or testicular function
Neutropenia; Thrombocytopenia; Anemia
Late (≥1 year after therapy)
Xerophthalmia
Chronic sialoadenitis
Salivary duct obstruction
Epiphoria
Conjunctivitis
Infertility; azoospermia; premature menopause
Pulmonary fibrosis
Bone marrow aplasia
Second primary malignancies?

symptomatic with low doses (30 mCi) of [131]I [102–104].

Another side effect of ^{131}I that is fairly common in the short term and can have persistent residual effects in the long term is sialoadenitis or inflammation of the salivary glands. Radioiodine can be taken up by the salivary glands and in large doses can cause inflammation (sialoadenitis), xerostomia (dry mouth), salivary duct obstruction, and, possibly, even malignancy of the salivary glands [105]. The incidence of sialoadenitis ranges from 10 to 67% and the course and severity have been shown to be dose dependent [102, 106, 107]. Even though most patients who have long-term sequelae of sialoadenitis, such as xerostomia, do not experience acute sialoadenitis, others have symptoms including pain, swelling, and tenderness of the parotid, submandibular, or lingual glands. These symptoms can last anywhere from a few days to many years after treatment. To treat the symptoms, hydration and anti-inflammatory medications, in addition to analgesics, may be necessary. Many studies suggest that frequent hydration and the use of saliva-producing products (sialogogs) such as sour candies and lemon juice, in addition to massage and cessation of anti-cholinergic use, which decrease salivation prior to ^{131}I treatment, can all decrease the risk for sialoadenitis [107].

Uptake of ^{131}I by the lacrimal glands can result in xerophthalmia [101, 107, 108] which was reported in 25% of cases in one study of 79 patients receiving 50–500-mCi ^{131}I [108]. The sicca symptoms in the majority of these patients disappeared by 1 year; however, a small number continued to have persistent symptoms for more than 3 years [108].

Taste dysfunction occurs after ^{131}I treatment because of its effect on the serous Ebner's glands that facilitate the ability of food's chemicals to get to the taste buds [107]. Transient loss of taste occurred in 27% of patients ($N = 203$) in one study after treatment with over 200 mCi ^{131}I, while 58% of patients were affected in a second study [106, 109]. Occasionally, loss of taste can persist for more than a few weeks or months, particularly with higher cumulative doses of ^{131}I [107].

While not a common complication of radioiodine treatment, Levinson reported two cases of transient facial nerve paralysis following ^{131}I therapy [110]. The mechanism is thought to be due to sialoadenitis of the parotid gland through which the facial nerve traverses, resulting in compression and subsequent paralysis of the facial nerve. Resolution seems to occur over time due to decreased inflammation.

Radiation thyroiditis is commonly seen in patients who have had a suboptimal surgery with a significant amount of residual thyroid tissue left behind or if there is significant bulky neck disease that is unobtainable via surgery. Symptoms include dysphagia or painful swallowing, neck and ear pain, and swelling in the thyroid bed, and rarely results in airway compromise requiring intubation [102].

In patients with pulmonary metastases, a high uptake of ^{131}I can result in acute radiation pneumonitis and subsequent pulmonary fibrosis, which is a rare, but severe and potentially fatal complication of ^{131}I therapy [102]. A case report by Rall et al. describes two patients with pulmonary metastases who developed radiation pneumonitis and subsequent fibrosis [111]. These patients presented 60 and 61 days after RAI treatment with fairly nonspecific symptoms including shortness of breath, fatigue, substernal pressure during exertion, and mild cough. Death occurred within 2 months after presenting symptoms. Despite the fact that radiation pneumonitis is a rare entity, we learn from Rall's patients that even if initial symptoms may appear to be minor and nonspecific, they should not be dismissed since early treatment with steroids may help prevent progressive respiratory failure [102]. To decrease the risk for radiation pneumonitis and its sequelae, Benua et al. first introduced the dosimetric approach to administering RAI. Their technique used blood and urine measurements to calculate activity levels in areas of interest such as bone marrow and lungs which they then used to limit the patient's whole-body retention of ^{131}I to less than 80 mCi, a dose thought to be safe [32]. Subsequently, a review of the literature by Van Nostrand and Freitas [102] demonstrated in a pooled analysis of patients treated with a dosimetry protocol a frequency of observed radiation pneumonitis of 2%, pulmonary fibrosis 3%, and death due to radiation effects on the lung 2% [102]. Significant improvements have been made to dosimetric techniques since Benua first introduced his method in 1962. Many centers either have adopted the Benua dosimetry method or use an empiric formula to decrease the whole-body uptake of ^{131}I in patients with pulmonary metastases at risk for radiation pneumonitis and its sequelae.

Female and male fertility are transiently affected by high doses of [131]I. Vini et al. assessed the prognosis of ovarian function and fertility in almost 500 women receiving one or more doses of [131]I (>81 mCi). Amenorrhea occurred between 1 and 3 months after RAI in 20% of patients, and, in those patients, there was a transient increase in FSH and LH indicating transient ovarian failure ($N=83$). Only one patient who desired to conceive 1 year after treatment was unable to conceive. Menstrual disturbances were associated with greater cumulative radiation doses [112]. A study by Bal and colleagues evaluated the genetic risk to offspring of mothers who received ^{131}I after 1990 by assessing pregnancy outcomes and health status of children of female patients. Forty women who desired pregnancy were able to conceive a minimum of 12 months after ^{131}I treatment and 47 babies were born of 50 pregnancies with a miscarriage rate of 6%, within range for the general population. Three of the babies had complications that were deemed to be unrelated to RAI treatment, concluding that high-dose RAI was not associated with a genetic risk to offspring [113]. The male gonadal effects of ^{131}I also seem to have a limited course. Studies have reported transient elevations in FSH, which is a sensitive marker of testicular failure and suggests azoospermia; however, FSH levels normalize by 12–18 months after treatment and the risk of infertility is minimal [114–116]. Fertility in men after multiple administrations of ^{131}I for those with recurrent thyroid carcinoma has not been well studied as the numbers are small.

The brain is a rare site for metastatic thyroid carcinoma occurring in approximately 1% of patients [117]. Several case reports have described complications such as seizures, cerebral edema, and hemorrhage causing focal neurologic deficits after treatment with ^{131}I in patients with brain metastases. [118–120]. The MD Anderson experience demonstrated that radioactive iodine uptake by brain metastases occurred infrequently in 17% of patients ($N=18$) [117]. Corticosteroids begun 48–72 h prior to ^{131}I treatment have been used to reduce the risk for peritumor cerebral edema [117, 119].

A concern for any patient receiving ionizing radiation is the risk of development of second primary malignancies. The data are challenging because factors such as timing of detection of cancer, insufficient time for follow-up, and confounding factors such as additional treatments including external beam radiation may alone increase one's risk for malignancy. In 2003, Rubino et al. published the results of a pooled analysis of patients with DTC from Swedish, Italian, and French cohorts ($N=6841$) where they found a 27% increased risk for cancer compared to the general population in patients treated with a minimum of 100 mCi (3.7 GBq). After adjusting for external beam radiation therapy, the relative risk of second primary malignancy occurrence in relation to ^{131}I administration was increased for salivary gland, bone, and soft-tissue cancers (RR=4), cancers of female genital organs (RR=2.2), central nervous system cancers (RR=2.2), and leukemia (RR=2.5) [121]. From the SEER Database of over 29,000 thyroid cancer patients, Chuang et al. did not note an overall increase in the risk of second primary malignancies relative to therapeutic radiation exposure, but there was a significant association between upper gastrointestinal malignancies and myeloid leukemias [122]. It is likely that those patients with more advanced disease received radiation therapy which may overestimate the rate of related second primary malignancies.

In 2007, after a careful systematic review of the literature, Sawka and colleagues published a meta-analysis looking at second primary malignancies in thyroid cancer patients treated with RAI versus the general population. They found an increased risk of second primary malignancies in thyroid cancer patients with a standardized incidence ratio of 1.2% compared to the general population [123]. A study by Brown and colleagues sought to determine the risk factors and characteristics of patients who develop second primary malignancies [18]. The study population came from the SEER registry ($N=30,278$).

They found that patients receiving RAI from 1973 to 2002 were at a slightly increased risk of developing second primary cancers over the general population as well as nonirradiated survivors; however, when they isolated the analysis period from 1988 to 2002, increased risk was observed in both those who were and were not treated with RAI. There was an increased incidence of breast cancer for women aged 25–75 at diagnosis and only within 10 years of the thyroid cancer diagnosis and an increase in prostate cancers. The reason for this increase is not understood and may be due to genetic or environmental factors in addition to surveillance bias. There was also an increased risk of kidney cancer in both those who were and were not irradiated, while only those treated with RAI had significantly increased stomach cancer. Salivary gland cancers were increased in those not irradiated, and the reason for this is difficult to explain. As demonstrated in prior studies, the frequency of leukemia was increased in patients receiving radioisotope compared with those who were not irradiated [18].

Although the above data demonstrate an increased risk of secondary malignancies in the thyroid cancer population when compared with the general population, it is not clear that this is due to ^{131}I treatment. The Sawka group subsequently queried whether there would be an increase in second primary malignancies in thyroid cancer patients treated with ^{131}I versus thyroid cancer patients not treated with [131]I. A meta-analysis published in 2009 included only two multi-center studies (Europe and North America) that compared second primary malignancies in thyroid cancer patients treated with RAI and not treated with RAI. The results demonstrated an increased relative risk of second primary malignancies at 1.19 ($P=0.010$) relative to thyroid cancer survivors not treated with RAI ($N=16,502$). These data seem to suggest the possibility that perhaps the factors that induce thyroid cancer or the genetics of patients with thyroid cancer may make them more susceptible to second primary malignancies; whether, RAI therapy alone does or dose to increase the risk is unclear [19].

Other Imaging Modalities

^{18}F-FluoroDeoxyGlucose (FDG) Positron Emission Tomography (PET) with Computerized Tomography (CT) in the Assessment of Patients with Thyroid Cancer

Significance of Incidentalomas in the Thyroid on FDG-PET Scanning

FDG-PET and FDG-PET/CT have been extensively utilized and published in the oncology literature. FDG is a glucose analog that is transported across the cell membrane by the cell membrane transporter GLUT-1. The FDG is phosphorylated by hexokinase and cannot enter the glycolytic pathway nor can it leave the cell. Since tumors utilize more glucose than the surrounding tissue, high target-to-background ratios have been achieved using FDG-PET, allowing the detection of subcentimeter tumors. This technique has achieved significant importance in the evaluation of thyroid cancer (Fig. 13.1).

FDG uptake in malignancies is dependent on the high activity of the glucose transport protein GLUT-1 which is highly expressed in many tumor cells. Immunostaining for GLUT-1 has been frequently detected in differentiated and

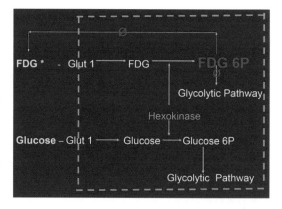

Fig. 13.1 Diagram of mechanism of FDG concentration in malignant cell. Note the GLUT-1 transporter which is upregulated in thyroid cancer cell. Phosphorylation of FDG by hexokinase prevents FDG from leaving the cell while FDG cannot enter the glycolytic pathway. This results in high concentration of FDG in less well-differentiated thyroid cancer

Fig. 13.2 (**a**) Incidental
FDG focus (incidentaloma)
in the right thyroid lobe on
FDG-PET in patient being
staged for lymphoma.
Pathology demonstrated
7 mm papillary cancer
(*broken arrow*) with
positive cervical lymph
node (*solid arrow*).
(**b**) FDG-PET/CT in same
patient. Note the intense
FDG activity correspond-
ing to a low-density
abnormality in the right
thyroid lobe

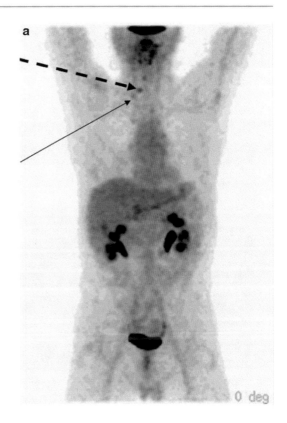

anaplastic thyroid cancers but not benign nodules or normal thyroid. Lazar et al. demonstrated 1 of 24 adenomas to have high GLUT-1 mRNA levels and 8 of 43 thyroid carcinomas had elevated GLUT-1 mRNA levels [124].

There are several reports indicating that focal FDG increases in the thyroid gland may represent a neoplastic process [125–137].

Cancer metastases to the thyroid gland are uncommon and account for less than 1% of all thyroid malignancies [125]. Results from autopsy series, however, report higher incidence ranging between 2 and 26%. Most of the metastases in the series originate from lung cancer and to a lesser extent breast cancer [125–128].

Multiple reports indicate that focal uptake of FDG in the thyroid may be due to primary malignancy of the thyroid [129–138]. The incidence of malignancy in the published "incidentaloma" group ranges from 14 up to 50% [129–136]. Choi et al. demonstrated an incidence of focal FDG activity in the thyroid of 4% with a malignancy rate of approximately 37% [136]. Standardized uptake values (SUVs) in this and other series have shown a correlation between

SUV and malignancy with SUV above 3.0 more likely to be malignant [129, 131–133, 135]. Others have found no correlation [134, 137]. Kim et al. suggested that a cytologic diagnosis is needed regardless of SUV, since too much overlap of SUV values exists between benign and malignant thyroid nodules [135]. Eloy et al. found a 28% incidence of well-differentiated thyroid cancer in "incidentalomas" with no statistical difference in SUV between benign and malignant thyroid nodules [138]. Eloy recommends thyroid ultrasound and fine needle aspiration biopsy or surgery in patients with focal thyroid uptake on FDG-PET with nonsuppressed TSH regardless of SUV [138]. Further imaging with high-resolution ultrasound and ultrasound-guided FNA is now the recommended standard of practice for thyroid nodules detected by FDG uptake on a PET scan [14]. One must be aware that false-positive results may occur in patients with focal or diffuse increases of FDG within the thyroid. Follicular adenomas may cause a focal increase, while diffuse bilateral FDG activity in the thyroid is often associated with thyroiditis [139]. Figure 13.2 is an FDG-PET scan in a

Fig. 13.2 (continued)

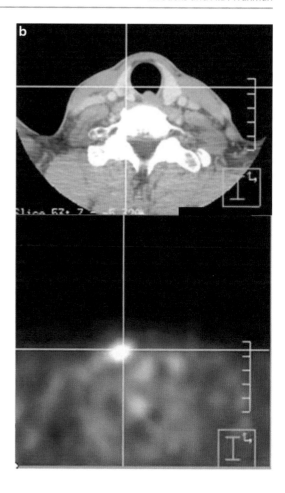

patient being staged for lymphoma. Focal increase in the thyroid (incidentaloma) was found to be a papillary thyroid cancer.

Most DTCs will accumulate iodine; therefore, the primary staging modality has been the use of whole-body radioiodine scans. This test has been shown to have an approximately 99% specificity but a relatively low sensitivity ranging between 50 and 70%. It is estimated that 75% or fewer DTCs will be detected using radioiodine whole-body scans. In addition, the low sensitivity is dose dependent. Most guidelines for ^{131}I therapy now utilize a post-high-dose therapy scan in order to maximize the detection of metastatic disease since low-dose (2–5 mCi) diagnostic scans have a lower sensitivity than post-therapy high-dose scans. Figure 13.3 is a comparison of a pre-therapy 3-mCi ^{131}I scan compared to a post-therapy 150-mCi ^{131}I scan.

A significant number of patients being followed up for possible recurrence of DTC will present with elevated thyroglobulin serum levels, but a negative diagnostic whole-body scan, suggesting that the tumor no longer has the ability to take up iodine, or the disease is too small to show up after a diagnostic dose. For these patients, PET–CT scanning is often helpful for localization of disease recurrence. It has been demonstrated that the greater the FDG activity in patients with residual or metastatic DTC, the greater the degree of de-differentiation has occurred in the tumor [140–142]. Generally, these patients do not benefit from additional radioiodine therapy but may have benefit from surgery or radiation therapy [143, 144]. Figure 13.4 is an FDG-PET scan in a patient with elevated Tg and negative ^{131}I study. Note the extensive pulmonary disease detected only by FDG-PET indicating a de-differ-

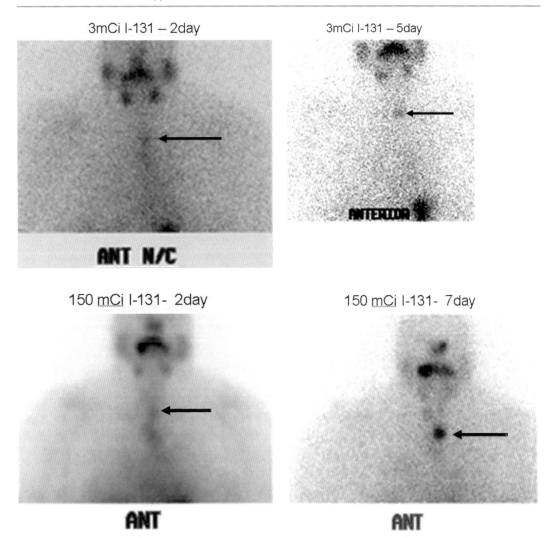

3mCi I-131 – 2day

3mCi I-131 – 5day

ANT N/C

ANTERIOR

150 mCi I-131- 2day

150 mCi I-131- 7day

ANT

ANT

Fig. 13.3 (a) 3-mCi [131]I 2-day pre-therapy scan. (b) 3-mCi [131]I 5-day pre-therapy scan (note: increased target /background ratio compared to 2-day scan). (c) 150-mCi [131]I 2-day post therapy scan. (d) 150-mCi [131]I 7-day post therapy scan [note: marked increase in target/background ratio (T/B) compared to 2-day 150-mCi as well as 2- and 5-day 3-mCi scan]. If a 3-mCi ^{131}I scan is compared to 2-day post-therapy scan, a false assumption of stunning may occur. A 7-day ^{131}I post Rx allows background to clear which improves T/B ratios

entiated tumor to be present. Multiple studies have demonstrated the success of FDG PET–CT in localizing DTC including iodine-negative tumors with sensitivities of 70–94% [140–142, 145–167]. Small tumor burden such as microscopic nodal deposits as well as miliary disease in the lungs is difficult for FDG-PET to detect because of resolution limitations. The use of FDG-PET in patients with elevated thyroglobulin levels and negative radioiodine levels is well established and reimbursed by the majority of insurance carriers including Medicare.

With the advent of PET–CT, localization of recurrent thyroid cancer has been made simpler and has improved patient management. Chung et al. demonstrated superiority of both sensitivity (94% vs. 55%) and specificity (95% vs. 76%) of FDG-PET over thyroglobulin for detecting metastases in 33 patients with known tumor metastasis and in 21 patients who were in clinical remission

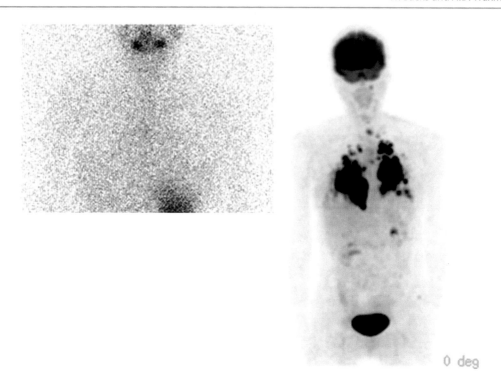

Fig. 13.4 (**a**) 5-mCi ^{131}I diagnostic scan in a patient with papillary thyroid cancer and rising thyroglobulin levels. (**b**) FDG-PET scan in same patient. Note the negative ^{131}I study and markedly positive FDG pulmonary uptake in patient with pulmonary metastasis

[153]. Additionally, FDG-PET was positive in 14 of 15 patients with metastatic cancer and normal thyroglobulin levels. FDG-PET detected cervical lymph node metastasis in 88% of patients with negative ^{131}I scans. Lung metastasis was detected in 27% and mediastinal metastasis in 33% along with bone metastasis in 9%. Chung also compared the effectiveness of ^{131}I scans with PET–CT scans in detecting metastatic thyroid cancer. Of the 117 patients, ^{131}I scans were superior in detecting metastasis especially in cervical nodes and lung; however, FDG-PET scans localized metastatic sites in ^{131}I scan negative thyroid cancer with a high degree of accuracy. For patients with negative ^{131}I scans who had locoregional or distant metastasis, FDG-PET scans were superior to ^{131}I whole-body studies and serum thyroglobulin measurements in detecting metastasis to cervical lymph nodes. Furthermore, FDG-PET is useful for determining subsequent surgical management [153].

FDG-PET results may be influenced by increasing TSH levels by endogenous stimulation or by exogenous rhTSH administration [168–173]. Leboulleux et al. found an increased sensitivity for lesion detection using rhTSH compared to basal PET (95% vs. 79%), but they did not find an increased sensitivity on a per-patient basis [172]. Petrich using rhTSH found a sensitivity of 87% versus 53% for basal PET [171]. Other investigators found no significant difference between TSH stimulation and basal FDG-PET [149, 154].

At our institution, we have successfully employed a combined 5-day protocol where intramuscular injections of 0.9 mg rhTSH are given on Monday and Tuesday (days 1 and 2) with FDG-PET scan performed on Wednesday (day 3). Immediately following the FDG-PET, a 4-mCi capsule of ^{131}I is given, and on Friday (day #5), a whole-body ^{131}I scan is performed. Additionally, serum thyroglobulin is tested on days 1 and 5. In 1 week, with one sequence of rhTSH injections, the patient is assessed with respect to the amount of iodine-avid tissue as well as the amount of FDG-avid tissue. This may have prognostic significance as it has been demonstrated that FDG-positive subjects have a poorer prognosis than subjects with mainly iodine avidity and no or minimal FDG activity (157, 158).

A relationship between thyroglobulin levels and FDG activity of recurrent or metastatic thyroid cancer has been reported [174, 175]. Bertagna et al. found a statistically significant positive correlation between FDG-PET/CT and Tg levels with positive imaging scans compared with negative scans [175] and the highest accuracy was achieved with Tg levels greater than 21 ng/mL. Iagaru et al. found FDG-PET/CT had a sensitivity of 88.6% and specificity of 89.3% for detection of recurrent or metastatic thyroid cancer [174]. The mean Tg level in positive studies was 1203 ng/mL and 9.72 ng/mL in negative studies. The authors concluded FDG-PET/CT has excellent sensitivity and specificity for recurrent or metastatic disease.

FDG-PET in Hurthle Cell Cancer of the Thyroid

Since Hurthle cell carcinomas typically have low avidity for iodine, attempts to localize sites of tumor recurrence have included other types of labeled scans including [201]Thallium chloride, 99mTc sestamibi, anti-carcinoembryonic antigen antibodies, and [111]Indium-labeled pentatreotide [140, 141, 146, 176–180]. The success in localizing is often superior to ^{131}I but sensitivity and specificity are still marginal. FDG-PET use for Hurthle cell carcinoma of the thyroid has been studied and found to be superior to other molecular imaging techniques including ^{131}I scanning [181–184]. Pryma et al. found in 50% of Hurthle cell cancer patients with positive ^{131}I studies, the iodine scans underestimated disease extent [184]. Of the 44 patients, 10 with positive FDG-PET had negative ^{131}I scans. The authors concluded FDG-

PET was superior to CT and ^{131}I studies in localizing Hurthle cell cancers and intense uptake on FDG-PET was associated with worse outcomes [184]. Figure 13.5 demonstrates an ^{131}I scan for restaging compared to an FDG-PET scan in a patient with Hurthle cell-dominant thyroid neoplasm. Note the discordant neck foci.

FDG-PET in Medullary Thyroid Cancer

Medullary thyroid cancer (MTC) accounts for 3–10% of thyroid neoplasms [185]. At diagnosis, approximately one-third of patients have mediastinal or cervical nodal metastasis [186]. Serum calcitonin is a tumor marker used to detect residual or recurrent tumor [187–190].

Molecular imaging with [99m]Tc(V) dimer captosuccinic acid, ^{111}In pentatreotide, [99m]Tc Sestamibi , ^{201}Tl, and ^{131}I metaiodobenzguanadine have been used to detect disease and stage and restage patients with MTC with limited sensitivity and specificity [191–194].

FDG-PET has added a new dimension in evaluating MTC for staging and restaging [195–202]. Ong et al. found a relationship of FDG activity to serum calcitonin levels. FDG-PET detected residual, recurrent, or metastatic MTC with a sensitivity of 78% with calcitonin levels >1,000 pg/mL but could not detect tumor when calcitonin was less than 506 pg/mL [200]. Lastly, F18-DOPA has been shown to be effective in the detection of MTC [202]; however, studies are limited and the radiopharmaceutical is not readily available.

[124]I PET Imaging

[124]I is a positron-emitting isotope with potential for imaging residual, recurrent, or metastatic thyroid cancer. Due to limited availability and purity considerations, most applications have been limited to dosimetry calculations for ^{131}I thyroid cancer therapy [203–207]. Eventually, [124]I PET may become a widely used isotope for imaging residual, recurrent, or metastatic cancer.

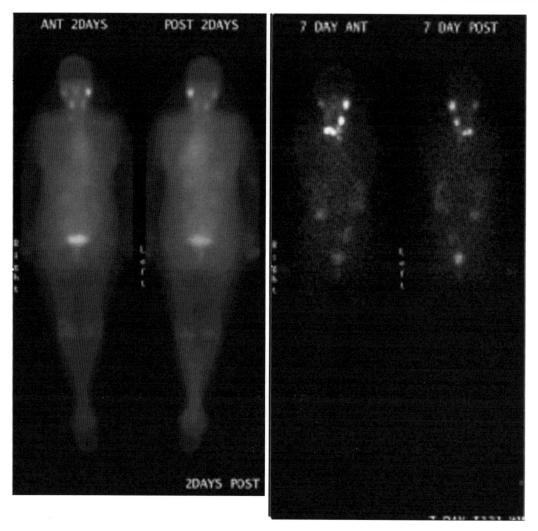

Fig. 13.5 (**a**) 100-mCi ^{131}I scan 2 days post-^{131}I Rx 8 weeks following total thyroidectomy in patient with Stage III papillary cancer with Hurthle cell features. (**b**) Same patient 7 days post-^{131}I Rx. Note marked increase in iodine-avid foci detected. (**c**) FDG-PET same patient 8 weeks following ^{131}I Rx. Note regions of high ^{131}I T/B ratio to have low FDG activity, while areas of low ^{131}I T/B ratio to have high FDG activity (*solid arrows*). High FDG activity correlates with less well-differentiated tumor. Hurthle cell tumors have high avidity for FDG

Summary

Radioactive iodine ablation is used successfully for postoperative remnant ablation as well as adjuvant therapy for patients with residual thyroid cancer remaining after surgery. While there are many controversies in the literature surrounding the use of RAI such as whom to treat, the optimal ^{131}I dose for long-term benefit, whether stunning exists, and the usefulness of pre-therapy diagnostic scans, RAI is a unique treatment in the management of thyroid cancer and disease-free and cause-specific survival can be improved with its use in certain patients. Further prospective studies are needed to clarify some of the discrepancies in management.

Fig. 13.5 (continued)

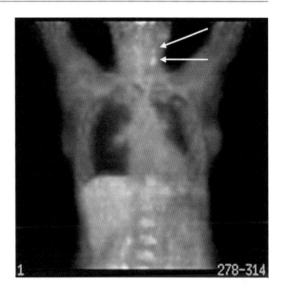

References

1. Seidlin SM, Marinelli LD, Oshry E. Radioactive iodine therapy: effect on functioning metastases of adenocarcinoma of the thyroid. CA Cancer J Clin. 1990;40:299–317.
2. Jonklaas J, Sarlis NJ, Litofsky D, Ain KB, Bigos ST, Brierley JD, et al. Outcomes of patients with differentiated thyroid carcinoma following initial therapy. Thyroid. 2006;16(12):1229–42.
3. Sawka AM, Thabane L, Browman G, Gerstein HC. A systematic review and meta-analysis of the effectiveness of radioactive iodine remnant ablation for well-differentiated thyroid cancer. J Clin Endocrinol Metab. 2004;89:3668–76.
4. Mazzaferri E. A randomized trial of remnant ablation – in search of an impossible dream? J Clin Endocrinol Metab. 2004;89:3662–4.
5. Lang BH, Lo CY, Chan WF, Lam KY, Wan KY. Staging systems for papillary thyroid carcinoma: a review and comparison. Ann Surg. 2007;245:366–78.
6. Chow SM, Law SC, Mendenhall WMAuSK, Chan PT, Leung TW, Tong CC, et al. Papillary thyroid carcinoma: prognostic factors and the role of radioiodine and external radiotherapy. Int J Radiat Oncol Biol Phys. 2002;52:784–95.
7. Lal G, O'Dorisio T, McDougall R, Weigel RJ. Cancer of the head and neck. In: Abeloff MD, Armitage JO, Niederhuber JE, Kastan MB, McKenna WG, editors. Abeloff's clinical oncology. Philadelphia, PA: Churchill Livingstone Elsevier; 2008. p. 148.
8. Pacini F, Molinaro E, Castagna MG, Agate L, Elisei R, Ceccarelli C, et al. Recombinant human thyrotropin-stimulated serum thyroglobulin combined with neck ultrasonography has the highest sensitivity in monitoring differentiated thyroid carcinoma. J Clin Endocrinol Metab. 2003;88:3668–73.
9. Torlontano M, Attard M, Crocetti U, Tumino S, Bruno R, Costante G, et al. Follow-up of low risk patients with papillary thyroid cancer: role of neck ultrasonography in detecting lymph node metastases. J Clin Endocrinol Metab. 2004;89:3402–7.
10. Davies L, Welch G. Increasing Incidence of thyroid cancer in the United States, 1973–2002. JAMA. 2006;295(18):2164–7.
11. Hay ID, Thompson GB, Grant CS, Bergstralh EJ, Dvorak CE, Gorman CA, et al. Papillary thyroid carcinoma managed at the Mayo Clinic during six decades (1940–1999): temporal trends in initial therapy and long-term outcome in 2444 consecutively treated patients. World J Surg. 2002;26:879–85.
12. Shaha AR. TNM classification of thyroid carcinoma. World J Surg. 2007;31:879–87.
13. Hay ID, Bergstralh EJ, Goellner JR, Ebersold JR, Grant CS. Predicting outcome in papillary thyroid carcinoma: development of a reliable prognostic scoring system in a cohort of 1779 patients surgically treated at one institution during 1940 through 1989. Surgery. 1993;114:1050–8.
14. Cooper DS, Doherty GM, Haugen BR, Kloos RT, Lee SL, Mandel SJ, et al. American Thyroid Association (ATA) guidelines taskforce on thyroid nodules and differentiated thyroid cancer. Thyroid. 2009;19:1167–214.
15. Pacini F, Schlumberger M, Dralle H, Elisei R, Smit J, Wiersinga W, et al. European consensus for the management of patients with differentiated thyroid carcinoma of the follicular epithelium. Eur J Endocrinol. 2006;154:787–803.
16. Sawka AM, Brierley JD, Tsang RW, Thabane L, Rotstein L, Gafni A, et al. An updated systematic review and commentary examining the effectiveness of radioactive iodine remnant ablation in well-differentiated thyroid cancer. Endocrinol Metab Clin N Am. 2008;37:457–80.

17. Sacks WL, Fung CH, Chang JT, Waxman A, Braunstein GD. The effectiveness of radioactive iodine for treatment of low-risk thyroid cancer: a systematic analysis of the peer-reviewed literature from 1966 to April 2008. Thyroid. 2010;20(11):1235–45.

18. Brown AP, Chen J, Hitchcock YJ, Szabo A, Shrieve DC, Tward JD. The risk of second primary malignancies up to three decades after the treatment of differentiated thyroid cancer. J Clin Endocrinol Metab. 2008;93:504–15.

19. Sawka AM, Thabane L, Parlea L, Ibrahim-Zada I, Tsang RW, Brierley JD, et al. Second primary malignancy risk after radioactive iodine treatment for thyroid cancer: a systematic review and meta-analysis. Thyroid. 2009;19(5):451–7.

20. McCowen KD, Adler RA, Ghaed N, Verdon T, Hofeldt FD. Low dose radioiodine thyroid ablation in post surgical patients with thyroid cancer. Am J Med. 1976;61:52–8.

21. Ramacciotti C, Pretorius HT, Line BR, Goldman JM, Robbins J. Ablation of non-malignant thyroid remnants with low doses of radioactive iodine: concise communication. J Nucl Med. 1982;23:483–9.

22. DeGroot LJ, Reilly M. Comparison of 30 and 50 mCi doses of I-131 for thyroid ablation. Ann Intern Med. 1982;96:51–3.

23. Maxon HR, Thomas SR, Thomas SR, Hertzberg VS, Kereiakes JG, Chen I-W, et al. Relation between effective radiation dose and outcome of radioiodine therapy for thyroid cancer. N Engl J Med. 1983; 309(16):937–41.

24. Bal C, Padhy AK, Jana S, Pant GS, Basu AK. Prospective randomized clinical trial to evaluate the optimal dose of 131-I for remnant ablation in patients with differentiated thyroid carcinoma. Cancer. 1996; 77(12):2574–80.

25. Gawkowska-Suwinska M, Turska M, Roskosz J, Puch Z, Jurecka-Tuleja B, Handkiewicz-Junak D, et al. Early evaluation of treatment effectiveness using 131 iodine radiotherapy in patients with differentiated thyroid cancer. Wiad Lek. 2001;54:278–88.

26. Bal CS, Kumar A, Pant GS. Radioiodine dose for remnant ablation in differentiated thyroid cancer: a randomized clinical trial in 509 patients. J Clin Endocrinol Metab. 2004;89:1666–73.

27. Rosario PWS, Reis JS, Barroso AL, Rezende LL, Padrao EL, Fagundes TA. Efficacy of low and high 131-I doses for thyroid remnant ablation in patients with differentiated thyroid carcinoma based on postoperative cervical uptake. Nucl Med Commun. 2004;25(11):1077–81.

28. Hackshaw A, Harmer C, Mallick Ujjal, Haq M, Franklyn JA. 131I activity for remnant ablation in patients with differentiated thyroid cancer: a systematic review. J Clin Endocrinol Metab. 2007;92:28–38.

29. Beierwaltes WH, Rabbani R, Dmuchowski C, Lloyd RV, Eyre P, Mallette S. An analysis of "ablation of thyroid remnants" with I-131 in 511 patients from 1947–1984: experience at University of Michigan. J Nucl Med. 1984;25:1287–93.

30. Mazzaferri EL, Jhiang SM. Long-term impact of initial surgical and medical therapy on papillary and follicular thyroid cancer. Am J Med. 1994;97:418–28.

31. Seidlin S, Marinelli L, Oshry E. Radioactive iodine therapy effect on functioning metastases of adenocarcinoma of the thyroid. JAMA. 1946;132:838–47.

32. Benua RS, Cicale NR, Sonenberg M, Rawson RW. The relation of radioiodine dosimetry to results and complications in the treatment of metastatic thyroid cancer. Am J Roentgenol Radium Ther Nucl Med. 1962;87:171–82.

33. Thomas SR, Maxon HR, Kereiakes JG. In vivo quantitation of lesion radioactivity using external counting methods. Med Phys. 1976;03:253–5.

34. Krishnamurthy GT, Blahd WH. Radioiodine I-131 therapy in the management of thyroid cancer: a prospective study. Cancer. 1977;40:195–202.

35. Beierwaltes WH. The treatment of thyroid carcinoma with radioactive iodine. Semin Nucl Med. 1978;8: 79–94.

36. Ruegemer JJ, Hay ID, Bergstralh EJ, Ryan JJ, Offord KP, Gorman CA. Distant metastases in differentiated thyroid carcinoma: a multivariate analysis of prognostic variables. J Clin Endocrinol Metab. 1988;67:501–8.

37. Simpson WJ, Panzarella T, Carruthers JS, Gospodarowicz MK, Sutcliffe SB. Papillary and follicular thyroid cancer: impact of treatment in 1578 patients. Int J Radiat Oncol Biol Phys. 1988;14:1063–75.

38. Maxon HR, Smith HS. Radioiodine I-131 in the diagnosis and treatment of metastatic well differentiated thyroid cancer. Endocrinol Metab Clin North Am. 1990;19:685–718.

39. DeGroot LJ, Kaplan EL, McCormick M, Straus FH. Natural history, treatment, and course of papillary thyroid carcinoma. J Clin Endocrinol Metab. 1990; 71:414–24.

40. Robbins J, Merino MJ, Boice JD, et al. Thyroid cancer: a lethal endocrine neoplasm. Ann Intern Med. 1991;115:133–47.

41. Samaan NA, Schultz PN, Hickey RC, et al. The results of various modalities of treatment of well-differentiated thyroid carcinoma: a retrospective review of 1599 patients. J Clin Endocrinol Metab. 1992;75:714–20.

42. Dulgeroff AJ, Hershman JM. Medical therapy for differentiated thyroid carcinoma. Endocrinol Rev. 1994; 15:500–15.

43. Menzel C, Grunwald F, Schomburg A, et al. "High dose" radioiodine therapy in advanced differentiated thyroid carcinoma. J Nucl Med. 1996;37:1496–503.

44. Sisson JC. Practical dosimetry of I-131 in patients with thyroid carcinoma. Cancer Biother Radiopharm. 2002;17:101–5.

45. Van Nostrand D, Atkins F, Yeganeh F, Acio E, Bursaw R, Wartofsky L. Dosimetrically determined doses of radioiodine for the treatment of metastatic thyroid carcinoma. Thyroid. 2002;12:121–34.

46. Sgouros G, Kolbert KS, Sheikh A, et al. Patient specific dosimetry for I-131 thyroid cancer therapy using I-124 PET and 3 dimensional internal dosimetry 3D-ID) software. J Nucl Med. 2004;45:1366–72.

47. Doi, Suhail AE, Woodhouse NJ, Thalib L, Onitilo A. Ablation of the thyroid remnant and I-131 dose in differentiated thyroid cancer: a meta analysis revisited. Clin Med Res. 2007;5(2):87–90.

48. Verberg FA, de Keizer D, Lips CJ, Zelissen PM, de Kierk JM. Prognostic significance of successful ablation with radioiodine of differentiated thyroid cancer patients. Eur J Endocrinol. 2005;152(1):33–7.

49. Liel Y. Preparation for radioactive iodine administration in differentiated thyroid cancer patients. Clin Endocrinol. 2002;57(4):523–7.

50. Serhal DI, Nasrallah MP, Arafah BM. Rapid rise in serum thyrotropin concentrations after thyroidectomy or withdrawal of suppressive thyroxine therapy in preparation for radioactive iodine administration to patients with differentiated thyroid cancer. J Clin Endocrinol Metab. 2004;89(7):3285–9.

51. Leboeuf R, Perro P, Carpentier AC, Verreault J, Langlois MF. Preparation for whole body scintigraphy: a randomized controlled trial. Clin Endocrinol (Oxf). 2007;7(6):839–44.

52. Goldman JM, Line BR, Aarmodt RL, Robbins J. Influence of triiodothyronine withdrawal time on I-131 uptake postthyroidectomy for thyroid cancer. J Clin Endocrinol Metab. 1980;50(4):734–9.

53. Silberstein EB, Alavi A, Balon HR, Becker D, Charkes ND, Clarke SEM, Divgi CR, Donohoe KJ, Delbeke D, Goldsmith SJ, Meier DA, Sarkar SD, Waxman AD. Society of nuclear medicine procedure guideline for scintigraphy for differentiated papillary and follicular thyroid cancer. September 5, 2006. http://interactive.snm.org/docs/Scintigraphy%20for%20Differentiated%20Thyroid%20Cancer%20V3%200%20(9-25-06).pdf.

54. Guimaraes V, DeGroot LJ. Moderate hypothyroidism in preparation for whole body I-131 scintiscans and thyroglobulin testing. Thyroid. 1996;6(2):69–73.

55. Haugen B, Pacini F, Reiners C, et al. A comparison of recombinant human thyrotropin and thyroid hormone withdrawal for the detection of thyroid remnant or cancer. J Clin Endocrinol Metab. 1999;84:3877–85.

56. Robbins RJ, Tuttle RM, Sharaf RN, et al. Preparation by recombinant human thyrotropin or thyroid hormone withdrawal are comparable for the detection of residual differentiated thyroid carcinoma. J Clin Endocrinol Metab. 2001;86:619–25.

57. Luster M, Lippi F, Jarzab B, et al. rhTSH-aided radioiodine ablation and treatment of differentiated thyroid carcinoma: a comprehensive review. Endocr Relat Cancer. 2005;12:49–64.

58. Robbins RJ, Larson SM, Sinha N, et al. A retrospective review of the effectiveness of recombinant human TSH as a preparation for radioiodine thyroid remnant ablation. J Nucl Med. 2002;43:1482–8.

59. Pacini F, Ladenson PW, Schlumberger M, et al. Radioiodine ablation of thyroid remnants after preparation with recombinant human thyrotropin in differentiated thyroid carcinoma: results of an international, randomized controlled study. J Clin Endocrinol Metab. 2006;91:926–32.

60. Barbaro D, Boni G, Meucci G, et al. Radioiodine treatment with 30mCi after recombinant human thyrotropin stimulation in thyroid cancer: effectiveness for postsurgical remnants ablation and possible role of iodine content in l-thyroxine in the outcome of ablation. J Clin Endocrinol Metab. 2003;88:4110–5.

61. Pacini F, Molinaro E, Castagna MG, Lippi F, Ceccarelli C, Agate L, et al. Ablation of thyroid residues with 30 mCi I-131: a comparison in thyroid cancer patients prepared with recombinant human TSH or thyroid hormone withdrawal. J Clin Endocrinol Metab. 2002;87:4063–8.

62. Tuttle RM, Brokhin M, Omry G, Martorella AJ, Larson SM, Grewal RK, et al. Recombinant human TSH-assisted radioactive iodine remnant ablation achieves short-term clinical recurrence rates similar to those of traditional thyroid hormone withdrawal. J Nucl Med. 2008;49(5):764–70.

63. Maxon HR, Thomas SR, Boehringer A, Drilling J, Sperling MI, Sparks JC, et al. Low iodine diet in I-131 ablation of thyroid remnants. Clin Nucl Med. 1983; 8:123–6.

64. Goslings BM. Effect of a low iodine diet on I-131 therapy in follicular thyroid carcinoma. J Endocrinol. 1975;64:30P.

65. Lakshmanan M, Schaffer A, Robbins J, Reynolds J, Norton J. A simplified low iodine diet in I-131 scanning and therapy of thyroid cancer. Clin Nucl Med. 1988;13:866–8.

66. Pluijmen MJ, Eustatia-Rutten C, Goslings BM, Stokkel MP, Arias AM, Diamant M, et al. Effects of low-iodine diet on postsurgical radioiodide ablation therapy in patients with differentiated thyroid carcinoma. Clin Endocrinol (Oxf). 2003;58(4):428–35.

67. Maruca J, Santner S, Miller K, Santen RJ. Prolonged iodine clearance with a depletion regimen for thyroid carcinoma: concise communication. J Nucl Med. 1984;25(10):1089–93.

68. Morris LF, Wilder MS, Waxman AD, Braunstein GD. Reevaluation of the impact of a stringent low-iodine diet on ablation rates in radioiodine treatment of thyroid carcinoma. Thyroid. 2001;11:749–55.

69. Cailleux AF, Baudin E, Travagli JP, Ricard M, Schlumberger M. Is diagnostic iodine-131 scanning useful after total thyroid ablation for differentiated thyroid cancer? J Clin Endocrinol Metab. 2000;85: 175–8.

70. Siddiqui AR, Foley RR, Britton KE, Sibtain A, Plowman N, Grossman AB, et al. The role of I-123 diagnostic imaging in the follow-up of patients with differentiated thyroid carcinoma as compared to I-131 scanning: avoidance of negative therapeutic uptake due to stunning. Clin Endocrinol. 2001;55: 515–21.

71. Mandel SJ, Shankar LK, Benard F, Yamamoto A, Alavi A. Superiority if iodine-123 compared with iodine-131 scanning for thyroid remnants in patients with differentiated thyroid cancer. Clin Nucl Med. 2001;26:6–9.

72. Sarkar SD, Kalapparambath TP, Palestro CJ. Comparison of I-123 and I-131 for whole body imaging in thyroid cancer. J Nucl Med. 2002;43:632–4.

73. Gerard SK, Cavalieri RR. I-123 diagnostic thyroid tumor whole body scanning with imaging at 6, 24, and 48 hours. Clin Nucl Med. 2002;27:1–8.

74. Rawson RW, Rall JE, Peacock W. Limitations and indications in the treatment of cancer of the thyroid with radioactive iodine. J Clin Endocrinol. 1951;11:1128–42.

75. Jeevanram RK, Shah DH, Sharma SM, Ganatra RD. Influence of initial large dose on subsequent uptake of therapeutic radioiodine in thyroid cancer patients. Int J Rad Appl Instrum B. 1986;13:277–9.

76. Park H, Perkins OW, Edmondson JW, Schnute RB, Manutunga M. Influence of diagnostic radioiodines on the uptake of ablative dose of iodine-131. Thyroid. 1994;4:49–54.

77. Chopra S, Wastie ML, Cha S, Vincent RM, Rezeslak A, Perkins AC, et al. Assessment of completeness of thyroid ablation by estimation of neck uptake of I-131 on whole-body scans: comparison of quantification and visual assessment of thyroid bed uptake. Nucl Med Commun. 1996;17:687–91.

78. Huic D, Medvedec M, Dodig D, Popovic S, Ivancevic D, Pavlinovic Z, et al. Radioiodine uptake in thyroid cancer patients after diagnostic application of low-dose I-131. Nucl Med Commun. 1996;17:839–42.

79. Park H, Park Y, Zhou X. Detection of thyroid remnant/metastasis without stunning: an ongoing dilemma. Thyroid. 1997;7:277–80.

80. Morris LF, Waxman AD, Braunstein GD. The nonimpact of thyroid stunning: remnant ablation rates in I-131 scanned and nonscanned individuals. J Clin Endocrinol Metab. 2001;86:3507–11.

81. McDougall IR. 74 MBq radioiodine I-131 does not prevent uptake on therapeutic doses of I-131 (i.e. it does not cause stunning) in differentiated thyroid cancer. Nucl Med Commun. 1997;18:505–12.

82. Leger FA, Izembart M, Dagousset F, Barritault L, Baillet G, Chevalier A, et al. Decreased uptake of therapeutic doses of iodine-131 after 185-MBq iodine-131 diagnostic imaging for thyroid remnants in differentiated thyroid carcinoma. Eur J Nucl Med. 1998;25:242–6.

83. Kao CH, Yen TC. Stunning effects after a diagnostic dose of iodine-131. Nuklearmedizin. 1998;37:23–5.

84. Muratet JP, Daver A, Minier JF, Larra F. Influence of scanning doses of iodine-131 on subsequent first ablative treatment outcome in patients operated on for differentiated thyroid carcinoma. J Nucl Med. 1998;39:1546–50.

85. Cholewinski SP, Yoo KS, Klieger PS, O'Mara RE. Absence of thyroid stunning after diagnostic whole-body scanning with 185 MBq I-131. J Nucl Med. 2000;41:1198–202.

86. Medvedec M, Grosev D, Loncarix S, Pavlinovic Z, Dodig D. Thyroid stunning: full quantitative explanation based on radiation absorbed dose analysis [abstract]. Eur J Nucl Med. 2000;27:923.

87. Comtosis R, Theriault C, Vecchio P. Assessment of the efficacy of iodine-131 for thyroid ablation. J Nucl Med. 1993;34:1927–30.

88. Bajen T, Mane S, Munoz A, Garcia JR. Effect of a diagnostic dose of 185 MBq I-131 on postsurgical thyroid remnants. J Nucl Med. 2000;41:2038–42.

89. Medvedec M. Seeking a radiobiological explanation for thyroid stunning [letter]. Eur J Nucl Med. 2001;28:393–4.

90. McMenemin RM, Hilditch TE, Dempsey MF, Reed NS. Thyroid stunning after I-131 diagnostic whole body scanning [letter]. J Nucl Med. 2001;42:986–7.

91. Postgard P, Himmelman J, Lindencrona U, Bhogal N, Wilberg D, Berg G, et al. Stunning of iodide transport by [131]-I irradiation in cultured thyroid epithelial cells. J Nucl Med. 2002;43:828–34.

92. Sabri O, Zimmy M, Schreckenberger M, Meyer-Oelmann A, Reinartz P, Buell U. Does thyroid stunning exist? A model with benign thyroid disease. Eur J Nucl Med. 2002;27:1591–7.

93. Gerard SK, Dam HQ. Stunning with I-131 diagnostic whole-body imaging of patients with thyroid cancer. Radiology. 2005;234(3):972–4.

94. Waxman AD, Ramanna L, Chapman N, Brachman M, Tanasescu DE, Berman D, et al. The significance of I-131 scan dose in patients with thyroid cancer: determination of ablation: concise communication. J Nucl Med. 1981;22:861–5.

95. Schlumberger M, Arcangioli O, Piekerski JD, Tubiana M, Parmentier C. Detection and treatment of lunch metastases of differentiated thyroid carcinoma in patients with normal chest X-rays. J Nucl Med. 1988;29:1790–4.

96. Nemec J, Rohling S, Zamrazil V, Pahunkova D. Comparison of the distribution of diagnostic and thyroablative I-131 in the evaluation of differentiated thyroid cancers. J Nucl Med. 1979;20:92–7.

97. Pacini F, Lippi F, Formica N, Elisei R, Anelli S, Ceccarelli C, et al. Therapeutic doses of iodine-131 reveal undiagnosed metastases in thyroid cancer patients with detectable serum thyroglobulin levels. J Nucl Med. 1987;28:1888–91.

98. Donahue KP, Shah NP, Lee SL, Oates ME. Initial staging of differentiated thyroid carcinoma: continued utility of post therapy 131I whole-body scintigraphy. Radiology. 2008;246(3):887–94.

99. Khan S, Waxman AD, Nagaraj N, Braunstein GD. Optimization of post ablative I-131 scintigraphy: comparison of 2 day vs 7 day post therapy study in patients with differentiated thyroid cancer (DTC). J Nucl Med. 1994;35 Suppl 5:15P.

100. Silberstein EB. Comparison of outcomes after I-123 versus I-131 pre-ablation imaging before radioiodine ablation in differentiated thyroid carcinoma. J Nucl Med. 2007;48(7):1043–6.

101. Van Nostrand D. The benefits and risks of I-131 therapy in patients with well-differentiated thyroid cancer. Thyroid. 2009;19(12):1381–91.

102. Van Nostrand D, Freitas J. Side effects of I-131 for ablation and treatment of well-differentiated thyroid

carcinoma. In: Wartofsky L, Van Nostrand D, editors. Thyroid cancer: a comprehensive guide to clinical management. 2nd ed. Totowa, NJ: Humana Press; 2006. p. 459–80.

103. Schuck A, Biermann M, Pixberg MK, Müller SB, Heinecke A, Schober O, et al. Acute toxicity of adjuvant radiotherapy in locally advanced differentiated thyroid carcinoma. First results of the multicenter study differentiated thyroid carcinoma (MSDS). Strahlenther Onkol. 2003;179:832–9.

104. Kim TH, Yang DS, Jung KY, Kim CY, Choi MS. Value of external irradiation for locally advanced papillary thyroid cancer. Int J Radiat Oncol Biol Phys. 2003;55:1006–12.

105. Klubo-Gwiezdzinska J, Van Nostrand D, Burman KD, Vasko V, Chia S, Deng T, et al. Salivary gland malignancy and radioiodine therapy for thyroid cancer. Thyroid. 2010;20(6):1–5.

106. Alexander C, Bader JB, Schaefer A, Finke C, Kirsch CM. Intermediate and long-term side effects of high-dose radioiodine therapy for thyroid carcinoma. J Nucl Med. 1998;39(9):1551–4.

107. Mandel SJ, Mandel L. Radioactive iodine and the salivary glands. Thyroid. 2003;13(3):265–71.

108. Solans R, Bosch JA, Galofré P, Porta F, Rosselló J, Selva-O'Callagan A, et al. Salivary and lacrimal gland dysfunction (sicca syndrome) after radioiodine therapy. J Nucl Med. 2001;42(5):738–43.

109. Albrecht HH, Creutzig H. Salivary gland scintigraphy after radioiodine therapy. Functional scintigraphy of the salivary gland after high dose radioiodine therapy. Fortschr Rontgenstr. 1976;125(6):546–51.

110. Levenson D, Coulec S, Sonnenberg M, Lai E, Goldsmith SJ, Larson SM. Peripheral facial nerve palsy after high-dose radioiodine therapy in patients with papillary thyroid carcinoma. Ann Intern Med. 1994;120:576–8.

111. Rall JE, Alpers JB, Lewallen CG, Sonenberg M, Berman M, Rawson RW. Radiation pneumonitis and fibrosis: a complication of radioiodine treatment of pulmonary metastases from cancer of the thyroid. J Clin Endocrinol Metab. 1957;17(11):1263–76.

112. Vini L, Hyer S, Al-Saadi A, Pratt B, Harmer C. Prognosis for fertility and ovarian function after treatment with radioiodine for thyroid cancer. Postgrad Med J. 2002;78(916):92–3.

113. Bal C, Kumar A, Tripathi M, Chandrashekar N, Phom H, Murali NR, et al. High-dose radioiodine treatment for differentiated thyroid carcinoma is not associated with change in female fertility or any genetic risk to the offspring. Int J Radiat Oncol Biol Phys. 2005;63(2):449–55.

114. Hyer S, Vini L, O'Connell M, Pratt B, Harmer C. Testicular dose and fertility in men following I-131 therapy for thyroid cancer. Clin Endocrinol. 2002;56:755–8.

115. Wichers M, Benz E, Palmedo H, Biersack HJ, Grunwald F, Klingmuller D. Testicular function after radioiodine therapy for thyroid carcinoma. Eur J Nucl Med. 2000;27:503–7.

116. Pacini F, Gasperi M, Fugazzola L, Ceccarelli C, Lippi F, Centoni R, et al. Testicular function in patients with differentiated thyroid carcinoma treated with radioiodine. J Nucl Med. 1994;35:1418–22.

117. Chiu AC, Delpassand ES, Sherman SI. Prognosis and treatment of brain metastases in thyroid carcinoma. J Clin Endocrinol Metab. 1997;82(11):3637–42.

118. Holmquest DL, Lake P. Sudden hemorrhage in metastatic thyroid carcinoma of the brain during treatment with iodine-131. J Nucl Med. 1976;17(4):307–9.

119. Datz FL. Cerebral edema following iodine-131 therapy for thyroid carcinoma metastatic to the brain. J Nucl Med. 1986;27(5):637–40.

120. Hurley JR, Becker DV. The use of radioiodine in the management of thyroid cancer. In: Freeman LM, Weissmann HS, editors. Nuclear medicine annual. New York: Raven Press; 1983. p. 560–4.

121. Rubino C, de Vathaire F, Dottorini ME, Hall P, Schvartz C, Couette JE, et al. Second primary malignancies in thyroid cancer patients. Br J Cancer. 2003;89:1638–44.

122. Chuang SC, Hashibe M, Yu GP, Le AD, Cao W, Hurwitz EL, et al. Radiotherapy for primary thyroid cancer as a risk factor for second primary cancers. Cancer Lett. 2006;238(1):42–52.

123. Subramanian S, Goldstein DP, Parlea L, Thabane L, Ezzat S, Ibrahim-Zada I, et al. Second primary malignancy risk in thyroid cancer survivors: a systematic review and meta-analysis. Thyroid. 2007;17:1277–88.

124. Lazar V, Bidart J-M, Caillou B, Mahe C, Lacroix L, Filetti S, et al. Expression of the Na$^+$/I$^-$ symporter gene in human thyroid tumors: a comparison study with other thyroid-specific genes. J Clin Endocrinol Metab. 1999;84:3228–34.

125. Fraker DL, Skarulis M, Livolsi V. Thyroid tumors. In: De Vita VT, Jr HS, Rosenberg SA, editors. Cancer principles and practice of oncology. 6th ed. Philadelphia, PA: Lippincott Williams & Wilkins; 2001. p. 1740–63.

126. Nakhjavani MK, Gharib H, Goellner JR, van Heerden JA. Metastasis to the thyroid gland: a report of 43 cases. Cancer. 1997;79:574–8.

127. Lam KY, Lo CY. Metastatic tumors of the thyroid gland: a study of 79 cases in Chinese patients. Arch Pathol Lab Med. 1998;122(1):37–41.

128. Singh R, Lehl SS, Sachdev A, Handa U, D'Cruz S, Bhalla A. Metastasis to thyroid from lung carcinoma. Indian J Chest Dis Allied Sci. 2003;45:203–4.

129. Cohen MS, Arslan N, Dehdashti F, Doherty GM, Lairmore TC, Brunt LM, et al. Risk of malignancy in thyroid incidentalomas identified by fluorodeoxyglucose-positron emission tomography. Surgery. 2001;130:941–6.

130. Ramos CD, Chisin R, Yeung HW, Larson SM, Macapinlac HA. Incidental focal thyroid uptake on FDG positron emission tomographic scans may represent a second primary tumor. Clin Nucl Med. 2001;26:193–7.

131. Kang KW, Kim SK, Kang HS, Lee ES, Sim JS, Lee IG, et al. Prevalence and risk of cancer of focal thyroid

incidentaloma identified by 18F-flurodeoxyglucose positron emission tomography for metastasis evaluation and cancer screening in healthy subjects. J Clin Endocrinol Metab. 2003;88:4100–4.

132. Van den Bruel A, Maes A, De Potter T, Mortelmans L, Drijkoningen M, van Damme B, et al. Clinical relevance of thyroid fluorodeoxyglucose-whole body positron emission tomography incidentaloma. J Clin Endocrinol Metab. 2002;87:1517–20.

133. Chen YK, Ding HJ, Chen KT, Chen YL, Liao AC, Shen YY, et al. Prevalence and risk of cancer of focal thyroid incidentaloma identified by 18-F-fluorodeoxyglucose positron emission tomography for cancer screening in healthy subjects. Anticancer Res. 2005;25(2B):1421–6.

134. Yi JG, Marom EM, Munden RF, Truong MT, Macapinlac HA, Gladish GW, et al. Focal uptake of fluorodeoxyglucose by the thyroid in patients undergoing initial disease staging with combined PET/CT for non-small cell lung cancer. Radiology. 2005; 236:271–5.

135. Kim TY, Kim WB, Ryu JS, Gong G, Hong SJ, Shong YK. 18-F-flurodeoxyglucose uptake in thyroid from positron emission tomogram (PET) for evaluation in cancer patients: high prevalence of malignancy in thyroid PET incidentaloma. Laryngoscope. 2005; 115(6):1074–8.

136. Choi JY, Lee KS, Kim HJ, Shim YM, Kwon OJ, Park K, et al. Focal thyroid lesions incidentally identified by integrated 18-F-FDG-PET/CT: clinical significance and improved characterization. J Nucl Med. 2006;47(4):609–15.

137. Chu Q, Connor MS, Lilien DL, Johnson LW, Turnage RH, Li BD. Positron emission tomography (PET) positive thyroid incidentaloma: the risk of malignancy observed in a tertiary referral center. Am J Surg. 2006;72(3):272–5.

138. Eloy JA, Brett EM, Fatterpekar GM, Kostakoglu L, Som PM, Desai SC, et al. The significance and management of incidental [18F]fluorodeoxyglucose–positron-emission tomography uptake in the thyroid gland in patients with cancer. AJNR Am J Neuroradiol. 2009;30:1431–4.

139. Yasuda S, Shohtsu A, Ide M, Takagi S, Takahashi W, Suzuki Y, et al. Chronic thyroiditis: diffuse uptake of FDG at PET. Radiology. 1998;207(3):775–8.

140. Grunwald F, Menzel C, Bender H, Palmedo H, Wilkomm P, Ruhlmann J, et al. Comparison of [18]-FDG-PET with [131] iodine and ^{99m}Tc-Sestamibi scintigraphy in differentiated thyroid carcinoma. Thyroid. 1997;7:327–35.

141. Fridrich L, Messa C, Landoni C, Lucignani G, Moncayo R, Kendler D, et al. Whole body scintigraphy with ^{99m}Tc-MIBI, [18]-FDG and [131]-I in patients with metastatic thyroid carcinoma. Nucl Med Commun. 1997;18(1):3–9.

142. Altenvoerde G, Lerch H, Kuwert T, Matheja P, Schafers M, Schober O. Positron emission tomography with ^{18}F-fluorodeoxyglucose in patients with differentiated thyroid carcinoma, elevated thyroglobulin

levels and negative iodine scans. Langenbecks Arch Surg. 1998;383:160–3.

143. Helal BO, Merlet P, Toubert ME, Franc B, Schvartz C, Gauthier-Koelesnikov H, et al. Clinical impact of 18-F FDG-PET in thyroid carcinoma patients with elevated thyroglobulin levels and negative (131)I scanning results after therapy. J Nucl Med. 2001; 42(10):1464–9.

144. Khan N, Oriuchi N, Higuchi T, Zhang H, Endo K. PET in the follow-up of differentiated thyroid cancer. Br J Radiol. 2003;76(910):690–5.

145. Yutan E, Clark OH. Hurthle cell carcinoma. Curr Treat Options Oncol. 2001;2(4):331–5.

146. Yen TC, Lin HD, Lee CH, Chang SL, Yeh SH. The role of technetium-99m sestamibi whole body scans in diagnosing metastatic Hurthle cell carcinoma of the thyroid gland after total thyroidectomy: a comparison with iodine-131 and thallium-201 whole body scans. Eur J Nucl Med. 1994;21(9):980–3.

147. Joensuu H, Ahonen A. Imaging of metastases of thyroid carcinoma with fluorine-18 fluorodeoxyglucose. J Nucl Med. 1987;28(5):910–4.

148. Sisson JC, Ackerman RJ, Meyer MA, Wahl RL. Uptake of 18-fluoro-2-deoxy-d-glucose by thyroid cancer: implications for diagnosis and therapy. J Clin Endocrinol Metab. 1993;77:1090–4.

149. Feine U, Leitzenmayer R, Hanke JP, Held J, Wöhrle H, Müller-Schauenburg W. Fluorine-18-FDG and iodine I-131 iodine uptake in thyroid cancer. J Nucl Med. 1996;37(9):1468–72.

150. Dietlein M, Scheidhauer K, Voth E, Theissen P, Schicha H. Fluorine-18 flurodeoxyglucose positron emission tomography and iodine-131 whole body scintigraphy in the follow-up of differentiated thyroid cancer. Eur J Nucl Med. 1997; 24(11):1342–8.

151. Feine U. Fluoro-18-deoxyglucose positron emission tomography in differentiated thyroid carcinoma. Eur J Endocrinol. 1998;138(5):492–6.

152. Grunwald F, Kalicke T, Feine U, et al. Fluorine-18-fluorodeoxyglucose positron emission tomography in thyroid cancer: results of a multicentre study. Eur J Nucl Med. 1999;26:1547–52.

153. Chung JK, So Y, Lee JS, Choi CW, Lim SM, Lee DS, et al. Value of FDG-PET in papillary thyroid carcinoma with negative [131]-I whole body scan. J Nucl Med. 1999;40:986–92.

154. Wang W, Macapinlac H, Larson SM, Yeh SDJ, Akhurst T, Finn RD, et al. ^{18}F-2-fluoro-2-deoxy-d-glucose positron emission tomography localizes residual thyroid cancer in patients with negative diagnostic [131]-I whole body scans and elevated serum thyroglobulin levels. J Clin Endocrinol Metab. 1999; 84:2291–302.

155. Conti PS, Durski JM, Bacqai F, Grafton ST, Singer PA. Imaging of locally recurrent and metastatic thyroid cancer with positron emission tomography. Thyroid. 1999;9(8):797–804.

156. Schirrmeister H, Guhlmann A, Elsner K, et al. Sensitivity in detecting osseous lesions depends on

anatomic localization: planar bone scintigraphy versus F-18 PET. J Nucl Med. 1999;26:1547–52.

157. Wang W, Larson SM, Fazzari M, et al. Prognostic value of ^{18}F-fluorodeoxyglucose positron emission tomographic scanning in patients with thyroid cancer. J Clin Endocrinol Metab. 2000;85:1107–13.

158. Robbins RJ, Wan Q, Grewal RK, et al. Real-time prognosis for metastatic thyroid carcinoma based on 2-F18-fluoro-2-deoxy-d-glucose positron emission tomography scanning. J Clin Endocrinol Metab. 2006;91(2):498–505.

159. Muros MA, Llmas-Elvire JM, Ramirez-Navarro A, et al. Utility of fluorine-18-fluorodeoxyglucose positron emission tomography in differentiated thyroid carcinoma with negative radioiodine scans and elevated serum thyroglobulin levels. Am J Surg. 2000; 179:457–61.

160. Alnafasi NS, Driedger AA, Coates G, Moote DG, Raphael SJ. FDG-PET of recurrent or metastatic I-131 negative papillary thyroid carcinoma. J Nucl Med. 2000;41:1010–5.

161. Schluter B, Bhuslavizki KH, Beyer W, Plotkin M, Buchert R, Clausen M. Impact of FDG-PET on patients with differentiated thyroid cancer who present with elevated thyroglobulin and negative ^{131}I scan. J Nucl Med. 2001;42:71–6.

162. Giammarile F, Hafdi Z, Bournaud C, Janier M, Houzard C, Desuzinges C, et al. Is ^{18}F-2-fluoro-2-deoxy-d-glucose (FDG) scintigraphy with non-dedicated positron emission tomography useful in the diagnostic management of suspected metastatic thyroid carcinoma in patients with no detectable radioiodine uptake? Eur J Endocrinol. 2003;149:293–300.

163. Yeo JS, Chung JK, So Y, et al. ^{18}F-fluorodeoxyglucose positron emission tomography as presurgical evaluation modality for I-131 scan-negative thyroid carcinoma patients with local recurrence in cervical lymph nodes. Head Neck. 2001;23:94–103.

164. Shiga T, Tsukamoto E, Nakada K, et al. Comparison of ^{18}F-FDG, ^{131}I-Na and ^{201}Tl in diagnosis of recurrent or metastatic thyroid carcinoma. J Nucl Med. 2001;42:414–9.

165. Frilling A, Teckenborg K, Gorges R, et al. Preoperative diagnostic value of ^{18}F-fluorodeoxyglucose positron emission tomography in patients with radioiodine negative recurrent well differentiated thyroid carcinoma. Ann Surg. 2001;234:804–11.

166. Helal BO, Merlet P, Toubert ME, et al. Clinical impact of 18-F FDG-PET in thyroid carcinoma patients with elevated thyroglobulin levels and negative I-131 scanning results after therapy. J Nucl Med. 2001;42:1464–9.

167. Larson SM, Robins R. Positron emission tomography in thyroid cancer management. Semin Roentgenol. 2002;37:169–74.

168. Macapinlac HA. Clinical usefulness of FDG-PET in differentiated thyroid cancer. J Nucl Med. 2001; 42(1):77–8.

169. Moog F, Linke R, Manthey N, et al. Influence of thyroid stimulating hormone levels on uptake of FDG in recurrent and metastatic differentiated thyroid carcinoma. J Nucl Med. 2000;41:1989–95.

170. Van Tol KM, Jager PL, Piers DA, et al. Better yield of F18-fluorodeoxyglucose positron emission tomography in patients with metastatic differentiated thyroid carcinoma during thyrotropin stimulation. Thyroid. 2002;12:381–7.

171. Petrich Tl, Borner AR, Otto D, Hoffman M, Knapp WH. Influence of rhTSH on F18-fluorodeoxyglucose uptake by differentiated thyroid carcinoma. Eur J Nucl Med. 2002;29:641–7.

172. Lebouleux S, Schroeder PR, Busaidy NL, et al. Assessment of incremental value of recombinant thyrotropin stimulation before 2-F18-fluoro-2-deoxy-d-glucose positron emission tomography/computed tomography imaging to localize residual differentiated thyroid cancer. J Clin Endocrinol Metab. 2009;94:1310–6.

173. Chin BB, Patel P, Cohade C, Ewertz M, et al. Recombinant human thyrotropin stimulation of fluoro-d-glucose positron emission tomography uptake in well-diffferentiated thyroid carcinoma. J Clin Endocrinol Metab. 2004;89:91–5.

174. Iagaru A, Kalinyak JE, McDougall IR. F-18 FDG-PET/CT in the management of thyroid cancer. Clin Nucl Med. 2007;32:690–5.

175. Bertagna F, Bosio G, Rodella C, et al. F-18 FDG-PET/CT in the evaluation of patients with differentiated thyroid cancer with negative I-131 total body scan and high thyroglobulin level. Clin Nucl Med. 2009;34:756–61.

176. Boi F, Lai ML, Desias C, et al. The usefulness of Tc-99m-sestamibi scan in the diagnostic evaluation of thyroid nodules with oncocytic cytology. Eur J Endocrinol. 2003;149:493–8.

177. Kostoglou-Athanassiou I, Pappas A, Gogou L, et al. Scintigraphy with In-111 octreotide and Tl-201 in a Hurthle cell thyroid carcinoma without detectable radio-iodine uptake. Report of a case and review of the literature. Horm Res. 2003;60:205–8.

178. Christian JA, Cook GJ, Harmer C. Indium-111 labeled octreotide scintigraphy in the diagnosis and management of non-iodine avid metastatic carcinoma of the thyroid. Br J Cancer. 2003;89:258–61.

179. Gulec SA, Serafini AN, Sridhar KS, et al. Somatostatin receptor expression in Hurthle cell cancer of the thyroid. J Nucl Med. 1998;39:243–5.

180. Valili N, Catargi B, Ronci N, et al. Evaluation of indium-111 pentetreotide somatostatin receptor scintigraphy to detect recurrent thyroid carcinoma in patients with negative radioiodine scintigraphy. Thyroid. 1999;9:583–9.

181. Blount CL, Dworkin HJ. F-18-FDG uptake by recurrent Hurthle cell carcinoma of the thyroid using high-energy planar scintigraphy. Clin Nucl Med. 1996;21:831–3.

182. Plotkin M, Hautzel H, Krause BJ, et al. Implication of 2-18-fluoro-2-deoxyglucose positron emission tomography in the follow up of Hurthle cell thyroid cancer. Thyroid. 2002;12:155–61.

183. Lowe VJ, Mullan BP, Hay ID, et al. FDG-PET of patients with Hurthle cell carcinoma. J Nucl Med. 2003;44:1402–6.

184. Pryma DA, Schoder H, Gonen M, Robbins RJ, et al. Diagnostic accuracy and prognostic value of 18-F-FDG PET in Hurthle cell thyroid cancer patients. J Nucl Med. 2006;47:1260–6.

185. Hundahl SA, Fleming ID, Fremgen AM, Menck HR. A National Cancer Data Base report on 53,856 cases of thyroid carcinoma treated in the U.S., 1985–1995. Cancer. 1998;83(12):2638–48.

186. Kloos RT, Eng C, Evans DB, Francis GL, Gagel RF, Gharib H, et al. Medullary thyroid cancer: management guidelines of the American thyroid association. Thyroid. 2009;19(6):565–612.

187. Lairmore TC, Wells Jr SA. Medullary carcinoma of the thyroid: current diagnosis and management. Semin Surg Oncol. 1991;7:92–9.

188. DeLellis RA, Rule AH, Spiler I, Nathanson L, Tashjian Jr AH, et al. Calcitonin and carcinoembryonic antigen as tumor markers in medullary thyroid carcinoma. Am J Clin Pathol. 1978;70:587–94.

189. Busnardo B, Girelli ME, Simioni N, et al. Nonparallel patterns of calcitonin and carcinoembryonic antigen levels in the follow up of medullary thyroid carcinoma. Cancer. 1984;53:278–85.

190. Quayle FJ, Moley JF. Medullary thyroid carcinoma: including MEN 2A and MEN 2B syndromes. J Surg Oncol. 2005;89:122–9.

191. Ugur O, Kostakglu L, Guler N, et al. Comparison of Tc-99m (V)-DMSA, Tl-201, and Tc-99m MIBI imaging in the follow up of patients with medullary carcinoma of the thyroid. Eur J Nucl Med. 1996;23:1367–71.

192. Berna L, Chico A, Matias-Guiu X, et al. Use of somatostatin analogue scintigraphy in the localization of recurrent medullary thyroid carcinoma. Eur J Nucl Med. 1998;25:1482–8.

193. Krausz Y, Rosler A, Guttmann H, et al. Somatostatin receptor scintigraphy for early detection of regional and distant metastases of medullary carcinoma of the thyroid. Clin Nucl Med. 1999;24:256–60.

194. Adalet I, Kocak M, Oguz H, et al. Determination of medullary thyroid carcinoma metastases by Tl-201, Tc-99m (V) DMSA, Tc-99m MIBI and Tc-99m Tetrofosmin. Nucl Med Commun. 1999;20:353–9.

195. Musholt TJ, Musholt PB, Dehdashti F, et al. Evaluation of fluorodeoxyglucose positron emission tomographic scanning and its association with glucose transporter expression in medullary thyroid carcinoma and pheochromocytoma: a clinical and molecular study. Surgery. 1997;122:1049–60.

196. Brandt-Mainz K, Muller SP, Gorges R, et al. The value of fluorine-18-fluorodeoxyglucose PET in patients with medullary thyroid cancer. Eur J Nucl Med. 2000;27:490–6.

197. Diehl M, Risse JH, Brandt-Mainz K, et al. Fluorine-18 fluorodeoxyglucose positron emission tomography in medullary thyroid cancer: results of a multicenter study. Eur J Nucl Med. 2001;28:1671–6.

198. Szakall Jr S, Esik O, Bajzik G, et al. F-18-FDG-PET detection of lymph node metastases in medullary thyroid carcinoma. J Nucl Med. 2002;43:66–71.

199. De Groot JW, Links TP, Jager PL, et al. Impact of F-18-fluorodeoxyglucose positron emission tomography (FDG-PET) in patients with biochemical evidence of recurrent or residual medullary thyroid cancer. Ann Surg Oncol. 2004;11:786–94.

200. Ong SC, Schoder H, Patel SG, Tabangay-Lim IM, et al. Diagnostic accuracy of 18F FDG PET in restaging patients with medullary thyroid carcinoma and elevated calcitonin levels. J Nucl Med. 2007; 48:501–7.

201. Khan N, Oriuchi N, Higuchi T, et al. Review of fluorine 18-2-fluoro-2-deoxyglucose positron emission tomography (FDG-PET) in the follow up of medullary and anaplastic thyroid carcinomas. Cancer Control. 2005;12:254–60.

202. Hoegerle S, Altehoefer C, Ghanem N, Brink I, Moser E, Nitzsche E. F-18 DOPA positron emission tomography for tumour detection in patients with medullary thyroid carcinoma and elevated calcitonin levels. Eur J Nucl Med. 2001;28:64–71.

203. Larson SM, Pentlow KS, Volkow ND, Wolf AP, Finn RD, Lamrecht RM, et al. PET scanning of iodine-124-3-F9 as an approach to tumor dosimetry during treatment planning for radioimmuno-therapy in a child with neuroblastoma. J Nucl Med. 1992;33: 2020–3.

204. Pentlow KS, Graham MC, Lambrecht RM, Cheung NK, Larson SM. Quantitative imaging of I-124 using positron emission tomography with applications to radioimmunodiagnosis and radioimmunotherapy. Med Phys. 1991;18:357–66.

205. Eschmann SM, Reischl G, Bilger K, et al. Evaluations of dosimetry of radioiodine therapy in benign and malignant thyroid disorders by means of iodine-124 and PET. J Nucl Med Mol Imaging. 2002;29: 760–7.

206. Sgouros G, Kolbert KS, Sheikh A, Pentlow KS, et al. Patient-specific dosimetry for I-131 thyroid cancer therapy using I-124 PET and 3-dimensional internal dosimetry (3D-ID) software. J Nucl Med. 2004;45: 1366–72.

207. Erdi YE, Macapinlac HA, Larson SM, et al. Radiation dose assessment for I-131 therapy for thyroid cancer using I-124 PET imaging. Clin Positron Imaging. 1999;2:41–6.

External Beam Radiation Therapy in the Treatment of Differentiated Thyroid Cancers

14

C. Michele Burnison

Introduction

Thyroid cancers include a diffuse group of histologies having intrinsically different biological behaviors and natural histories. Given the location of the thyroid gland in close proximity to major organs, such as the larynx, recurrent laryngeal nerve, trachea, carotid artery, and esophagus, it is well recognized that local control remains itself an important endpoint in the treatment of all these malignancies. With the exception of lymphomas, surgery remains the primary treatment modality. In general, EBRT, as a locoregional treatment, is indicated in situations where surgery or other alternative relatively less toxic therapies, such as ^{131}I or potentially more specifically targeted systemic therapies, are deemed inappropriate or unsuccessful [1, 2].

Radiation Physics and Biology: Basic Principles

Radiation therapy physically directs ionizing radiation to a target, resulting in accumulated hits to account for double-stranded DNA breaks, leading to mitotic cell death at the time of

attempted cell division. Radiobiologically, this is represented by the cell survival curve, depicted by the percentage of cell population surviving plotted against an increasing dose of radiation, with the shoulder representing repair of sublethal damage and the slope representing the efficiency of cell kill. Different normal tissues and tumors have different breadth of shoulders and slope steepness to their cell survival curves, this graphically defining the radiosensitivity for a given microenvironment. The therapeutic ratio, an integral concept as to the efficacy of EBRT, is simply defined as the relative damage to tumor, as compared to normal tissues, for a given radiation dose. It is depicted by the separation of the sigmoid curves between normal tissues and tumors.

A distinction needs to be made of radiosensitivity versus radioresponsiveness. Radiosensitivity refers to cell kill and is a measure of the susceptibility of a specific cell type to damage from ionizing radiation. Radioresponsiveness relates to the observed clinical response of a tumor to EBRT, which is dependent on cell kill, on the rate of cell death, as well as on the rate of clearance, or cell loss, resulting in a corresponding diminution in the volume of measurable disease. Generally, tumors which have slow growth kinetics, such as differentiated thyroid cancer (DTC), also show a slow clinical response to EBRT, accounting for a median time of maximum regression ranging from 6 months to 2 years [3–6] and, if not sterilized, with a correspondingly slow time for repopulation reflected in relatively delayed time to clinical relapse on the order of 5 years for

C.M. Burnison (✉)
Department of Radiation Oncology, Cedars-Sinai Medical Center, 8700 Beverly Blvd #AC-1020, Los Angeles, CA 90048-1865, USA
e-mail: burnisonc@cshs.org

G.D. Braunstein (ed.), *Thyroid Cancer*, Endocrine Updates 30,
DOI 10.1007/978-1-4614-0875-8_14, © Springer Science+Business Media, LLC 2012

microscopic disease. Clinical progression of irradiated bulk disease may take many years with "control" often lasting a lifetime, especially for older patients. On the other extreme, anaplastic thyroid cancer (ATC) may regress quickly; however, sterilization of gross disease is unlikely and with the associated rapid repopulation phenomena, the initial response is not durable, even for a matter of months. For ATC the maximum time to local response is cited often to be at, or near the completion of, a 6 week course of therapy [7, 8].

The interaction of several important radiation parameters, including overall treatment time, total dose, and fractionation schedule (dose per fraction), account for observed clinical responses of both tumor control and toxicities. Additionally, the biological responsiveness to a fractionated course of radiation is abbreviated in the "4 R's" of radiobiology: reoxygenation, reassortment, repopulation, and repair. Fractionation, the delivering integral doses of RT spaced over uniform time periods (Gy/fraction), accounts for observation of repeated shoulders on the cell survival curve and conceptually allows time for accumulated repair of damage. Tumors typically have less sophisticated enzymatic repair mechanisms; hence, result in relatively less efficient repair of radiation damage, as compared to normal tissues. At the same time, fractionation also allows for reoxygenation, improving (tumor) cell kill in an otherwise more radioresistant hypoxic tumor microenvironment. Furthermore, fractionation allows for reassortment, whereby the more rapidly dividing tumor cells (relative to normal tissues) are more likely to be in a radiosensitive portion of their cell cycle. On the other hand, during a protracted course of RT there is also time allowance for accelerated tumor repopulation resulting from cellular mutations and survival of resistant clones, presumably related to growth factors and receptors. Both repopulation and repair represent detrimental effects of fractionation on the efficiency of tumor cell kill. On a clinical basis, different fractionation schedules have been devised in an attempt to overcome the observation of accelerated repopulation [9]. The efficacy of such is strongly contingent on both tumor and normal tissue radiosensitivity and cellular kinetics.

It is observed that for any given tumor and normal tissue, clinical responses vary according to the schedule of radiation. "Standard fractionation (SF)" refers to the delivery of 1.8–2.0 Gy per fraction given on a schedule of one treatment per day, five consecutive days per calendar week. Hyperfractionation and accelerated fractionation refer to multiple (usually two) treatments per day and generally impart greater cell kill of rapidly dividing tissues. However, treatment of rapidly dividing normal tissues, such as the esophageal mucosa, may be dose limiting, and therefore it is important that the time between fractions be sufficient (usually 6 h) to allow for effective repair of normal tissues. In contrast, hypofractionation refers to a daily single fraction of greater than 2 Gy typically given over an abbreviated time course, such as 2–3 weeks. While this schedule may clinically demonstrate similar tumor damage as a more protracted standard fractionation schedule of 4–5 weeks, it is also conceptionally associated with higher risk for late complications.

"Combined modality therapy" entails the concomitant use of EBRT with a chemotherapy agent that has shown to be effective against the specific tumor in question. Ideally, chemo-toxicities should be different from the anticipated radiation toxicities. Possible chemo-sensitizing mechanisms include synergistic DNA damage, inhibition of repair of radiation damage, and inhibition of repopulation. Targeted agents have also been shown to result in radiation sensitization. Cetuximab, a monoclonal antibody against EGFR, has been shown to be an effective radiosensitizer in head and neck cancers, notably with no significant increase in toxicity other than an acneiform rash and infusion reactions [10–12].

One of the most important tenets of radiotherapy is the dose/volume relationship (Fig. 14.1). Generally, for most tumors increasing size of aggregate disease requires increasing dose for sterilization. Using squamous and adenocarcinomas as models, a total dose of 50 Gy over 5 weeks, at standard fractionation should control 95% of subclinical tumors, while 60–65 Gy/SF is required for 2 cm of disease and 70–75 Gy/SF to control a 4 cm tumor [13]. Given that the acceptable tolerant dose for the esophagus is approximately

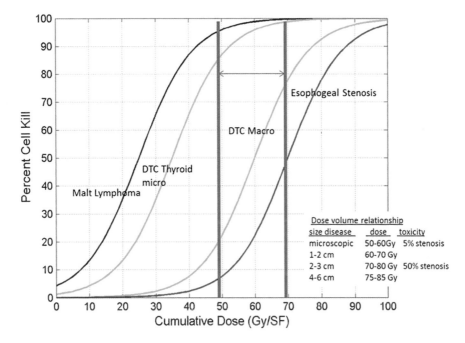

Fig. 14.1 Theoretical cell survival curves for a very radiosensitive MALT lymphoma, moderately radiosensitive microscopic and macroscopic aggregate of DTC thyroid cells, and the normal esophageal mucosa. Larger cumulative doses increase the likelihood of cell kill and sterilization of tumor, and also damage to normal tissues. The therapeutic ratio, the balance between the likelihood for cure and toxicity, is defined by the separation of the curves at two different dose points

60 Gy/SF, the challenge to eradicate large ATC tumors or bulky recurrent DTCs becomes obvious. Dose escalation, within acceptable constraints, may be facilitated by improvements in targeting, however, with a limitation specifically defined by the tumor's proximity to critical structures. Often, as in the case of most thyroid cancers, the cumulative dose of radiation (RT) is constrained by the tolerance of adjacent structures and such is often insufficient to effectively sterilize bulk measurable disease. As an exception, however, thyroid lymphomas are intrinsically more radiosensitive, requiring relatively much less dose (30–45 Gy/SF) for eradication even of bulk disease, with correspondingly minimal risk to surrounding structures.

In the treatment of any cancer, there must always be a balance as to the anticipated kill of tumor versus damage to the adjacent normal tissues, this defining the "therapeutic ratio." Importantly, different normal tissues have varying sensitivities to EBRT, not only on an absolute basis but also relative to the volume of normal tissue irradiated. Normal tissue effects are also dependent on cellular kinetics, environmental/oxygenation factors, as well has host factors (age and comorbidities). In radiobiology, the "normal tissue tolerance" is defined by doses that give a certain probability for a specific clinical complication at 5 years. Late tissue tolerance doses are cited as 5% (TD5/5) and 50% (TD5/50) probabilities defined at 5 years. Furthermore, "acceptable risks" of complications are relevant to the severity of the complication balanced by the intent and likelihood of success of EBRT. For the treatment of thyroid cancers, the critical structures of concern include the parotid glands (tolerance: mean dose <25 Gy at standard fractionation), the esophagus (TD5/5 55–60 Gy), the spinal cord (TD5/5 47–50 Gy), and brachial plexus (TD5/5 65–77 Gy) [14].

Side effects from EBRT are referred in the literature as both acute (0–6 months) and late (6–24 months+) toxicities. Both types of effects are accounted for by the tissues within the path of the radiation beam and the absorbed dose, the latter dictated both by physical parameters of the patient and by technical aspects of the beam. For the specific treatment of the thyroid and neck region, the anticipated acute and late effects are dependent on the inclusion, or exclusion, of the oral cavity, parotids, vocal cords, and lung. If the oral cavity is included in the field, at 2 weeks there will be an onset of change in taste and at 3–4 weeks the onset of skin erythema and loss of hair in the treatment fields. At about the same time, esophagitis will ensue. At 4–5 weeks, there will be hoarseness and difficulty swallowing roughage. Generalized fatigue will ensue and last for approximately 6 weeks. After completion of therapy, these acute effects typically subside within weeks, although return of taste may take months, and some return of salivary flow may take up to a year. Submental edema develops in a few months and lasts for approximately a year. Serious late effects, including esophageal stenosis, are cited at 5–10%, depending on total dose and length of esophagus irradiated. If the upper mediastinum and supraclavicular regions are included, asymptomatic fibrosis is anticipated. Carotid artery atherosclerosis is a very late effect, usually of concern in the treatment of young patients. Brachial plexopathy is rare if doses are constrained to less than 66 Gy. For those without thyroidectomy, and specifically noted in the treatment of thyroid lymphomas, there is a likelihood of iatrogenic hypothyroidism, which often does not become apparent for many months.

Radiation treatment planning is a critical process in defining outcome. Conformal radiation therapy, including 3D CT scan-based dosimetry and IMRT, has been instrumental in improving the targeting of tumors, while minimizing exposure of critical structures. IMRT utilizes inverse treatment planning whereby targeted structures are outlined on a planning CT scan and the limits of both constraints, as well as priorities, are defined by the treating physician (Figs. 14.2 and 14.3). This involves sophisticated, time-consuming treatment planning involving both highly trained physicist/dosimetrists and the radiation oncologist. Technically, dose delivery is accomplished by varying/modulating the intensity of the beam across multiple treatment fields, thereby conforming to irregular shapes and resulting in a preferable inhomogeneous dose distribution. Dose–volume histograms (DVHs), see Fig. 14.3, graphically illustrate the distribution of doses to both the tumor and critical structures over the entire course of therapy, often lasting 6–7 weeks. Recently, there are emerging reports attesting to the efficacy of IMRT in the treatment of thyroid cancers, allowing improved coverage with higher doses and reduced toxicity to normal tissues [5, 15–20].

External Beam Radiation Therapy for Differentiated Thyroid Cancer: An Overview

The literature supports that EBRT is an effective modality for the treatment of DTC. However, it is rarely indicated because of the availability of ^{131}I, the concern for late morbidity that has historically been associated with EBRT and the relatively indolent clinical course even those patients who demonstrate recurrences.

In the adjuvant setting, EBRT has a limited role. [131]I and TSH suppression (sTSH) therapies, with the inherent advantages of providing systemic coverage and facilitating long-term surveillance, have evolved to become a standard of care for patients deemed at risk for recurrence [1–4, 21–23]. A supplementary role for EBRT may be appropriate for only a small cohort of 10–15% of patients who meet two criteria: (1) are assessed to be at very high risk for locoregional recurrence based on tumor, patient, and prior treatment factors and (2) are unlikely to have recurrent tumor salvaged with additional surgery, ^{131}I, or other options [18, 24–26]. Rather than any single criterion, patients should likely have a constellation of risk factors justifying the addition of EBRT to frontline therapy.

In contrast to the controversial role of EBRT in the adjuvant treatment of small volume disease, the use of EBRT in the treatment of unresectable or measurable disease to achieve local control is more straightforward, yet technically more challenging. In the setting of gross disease, most authorities recommend a dose intensification strategy, employing

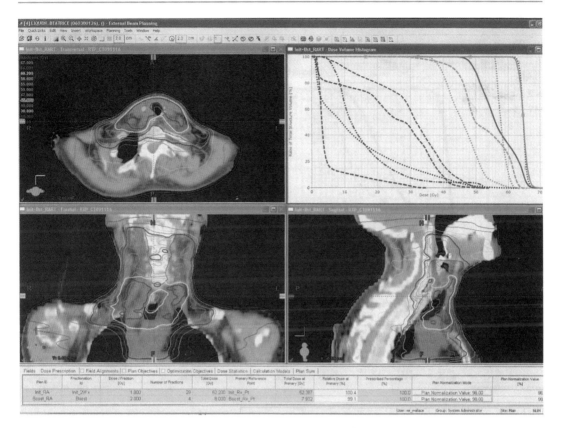

Fig. 14.2 An IMRT treatment plan, as depicted three-dimensionally by CT simulation, for a patient with residual thyroid disease in the surgical bed. Anatomical dose distributions are illustrated overlying physician defined colored normal tissue and tumor targets. The cumulative dose distributions over the entire treatment for both the defined critical structures and different (presumed microscopic, gross) dose targets are illustrated by respective curves on the dose–volume histogram

both primary EBRT and ^{131}I along with TSH suppression. Notably, recent innovations in the diagnostic realm (high-resolution ultrasonography, PET/CT scans, and MRI) coupled with advances in therapeutic radiology, including IMRT, may facilitate identifying and more effectively sterilizing relatively small-volume macroscopic disease, even for those with non-iodine-avid disease.

Role of EBRT in Preventing Locoregional Recurrence, Impact on Survival/Quality of Life

The rationale for the adjuvant use of EBRT is to prevent a locoregional recurrence that would otherwise significantly impact on survival and/or quality of life. The efficacy of EBRT must always be assessed in the context of competing alternatives and its long-term morbidity. Despite the current standard of care, overall recurrence rates for DTCs are reported in the 8–23% range [27–32]. Specifically with regard to locoregional recurrences, DTC demonstrates a relatively slow median time to local failure ranging from 2 to 9 years (range 0.3–25 years), mirroring generally slow growth and response kinetics [4, 27, 29, 32–34].

Most DTC recurrences are nodal and/or distant; a few (<10%) are in the thyroid surgical bed. Although outcomes are contingent on the demographics of the study populations, especially as to the percentage of tumors exhibiting extrathyroidal extension (ETE), the pattern of recurrences based on three separate large unselected populations (each composed of greater than a 1,000 patients) is remarkably consistent: nodal 9–13%, surgical bed 6–11%, and distant

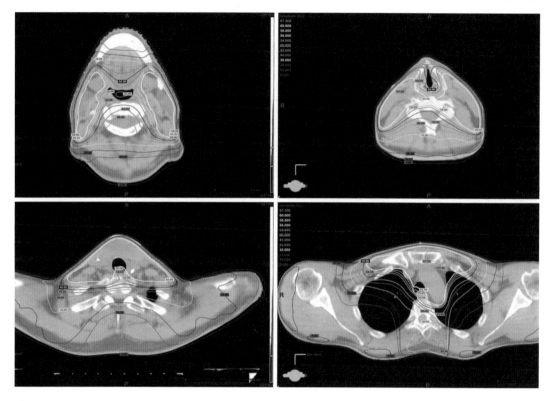

Fig. 14.3 IMRT rotational arc treatment plan, as illustrated on sequential cephalid to caudal axial CT projections, for a patient with small-volume postoperative residual disease in the surgical bed and upper mediastinum. Note the curvilinear distributions that minimize dose to the spinal cord, larynx, and lungs, while maintaining adequate coverage to the surgical bed and nodal regions

metastasis 4–9% [3, 35, 36]. Unfortunately, especially relevant to the indications for EBRT, most all of the historical radiotherapy literature did not discriminate between central versus regional recurrences and many did not specify as to the extent of ETE, or size of postoperative residuum, both important prognostic variables especially predictive for central recurrences.

Regional recurrences in the cervical neck nodes are the most common type of recurrence. At diagnosis, the incidence of subclinical nodal disease is on the order of 21–82% [36, 37]. The observation that only 3–15% of patients not completing an initial neck dissection develop a subsequent nodal relapse suggests that adjuvant ^{131}I/sTSH in high-risk patients successfully controls much of the subclinical residual disease [36]. Furthermore, recurrent nodal disease often retains iodine avidity and hence can often be salvaged with subsequent neck dissection and/or ^{131}I therapy [34, 36, 38].

Although controversial, some authorities recommend consideration for supplementary EBRT at the time of initial diagnosis for those presenting with large (>2 cm) nodal bulk disease or exhibiting any extracapsular extension (ECE) [29, 36, 39]. Others, however, recommend EBRT only if nodal disease persists or recurs despite a modified neck dissection and prior [131]I [6, 38].

Central recurrences are especially challenging for both surgery and EBRT and are the major impetus to consider supplementary EBRT. Of those who succumb from DTC, 20% of deaths occur within the first year after surgery; most are of older patients. Nearly half of all deaths from PTC are due to uncontrolled disease in the central compartment [36, 38]. Following standard therapy, the majority of surgical bed recurrences are associated with tumors initially diagnosed with ETE to nearby organs (oETE) and most are found not to concentrate iodine at the time of recurrence, having been previously treated with surgery plus ^{131}I/sTSH [19, 34, 36, 40]. Patients demonstrating central recurrences are much more likely to die from disease, with a reported mortality of 50–75% [19, 34, 36, 40–43]. Importantly, although current treatment standards have decreased the incidence of all locoregional recurrences, still less than 50% of central recurrences can be salvaged [36, 40]. This relatively poor salvage rate is often consequential to both the technical risks and challenges of reoperation into the prior surgical bed as well as the relative nonavidity of many recurrent tumors [5, 34, 44]. Accordingly, upfront initial adjuvant EBRT remains an important consideration specifically for patients deemed at "very high risk" specifically for central recurrences, i.e., older patients (often with comorbidities as deterrents for surgery), having infiltrative disease with questionable margins, that likely does not concentrate ^{131}I, and especially for those with higher-grade tumors.

An improvement in survival is the strongest testimony as to the efficacy of any adjuvant therapy. Conceptionally, those patients deemed at "very high risk", especially for central failures, have the most to gain from adjuvant EBRT, beyond that offered by the standard post-thyroidectomy ^{131}I/sTSH. There is literature attesting to this degree of benefit; however, interpretation can be challenged because of confounding or uncounted for prognostic variables, variation in the use of ^{131}I, and methods of data reporting. Statistically improved survival with adjuvant EBRT is reported in the older Canadian literature, specifically for patients having confirmed microscopic (R1) positive margins as compared to surgery alone [3] or on comparing groups treated "with" versus "without EBRT." [6, 45] Simpson noted a 10-year cause-specific-survival (CSS) advantage with 35–50 Gy (over 3–5 weeks) of postoperative EBRT, as compared to surgery alone (with or without sTSH): 95% 10-year CSS with surgery plus sTSH and EBRT versus 85% with surgery plus sTSH alone or versus 58% for surgery alone ($p = 0.04$) [3]. However, a similar advantage was also seen with adjuvant ^{131}I alone and there was no direct comparison made between the adjuvant therapies. Both Tsang and

Brierley sequentially reported a relatively small but statistically significant survival advantage for patients with PTCs having specifically microscopic (R1) positive margins and treated "with" versus "without" EBRT, 100% versus 95% 10-year CSS [6, 45] Additionally, Brierley (acknowledging problems with obtaining pathology reports adequately specifying margin status) defined a "presumed" surrogate for microscopic positive margins as tumors having intraoperative assessment of ETE but without gross residuum after resection. He also introduced age into the analysis and noted a significant difference in outcome between those 45–60 and especially over 60 years of age. For 70 patients over 60 years of age, having either PTC or FTC tumors with "presumed" microscopically positive margins, there was a significant survival advantage, 81% versus 65% 10-year CSS ($p = 0.04$) for those treated with versus without EBRT [45]. Notably, with the exception of Simpson's earlier data, most reports in the RT literature, including those of Tsang and Brierley, practiced the method of reporting outcomes by "bundling" results of the four different patient cohorts and submitted data only for two patient groups, those treated "with" versus "without" EBRT. Both the disproportional use of [131]I (type II bias) between the two groups (many "with" EBRT also received ^{131}I/sTSH) and the inclusion of high-risk patients treated with surgery alone (type III bias) included in the "without EBRT" group confound interpretation as to the true merits of EBRT over and above that of adjuvant ^{131}I alone. As later elucidated by Brierley, 54% of Tsang's "without EBRT" R1 subgroup included patients treated with surgery alone and 70% of R1 patients treated "with EBRT" also received ^{131}I, as compared to only 46% of R1 patients treated "without EBRT" [45].

With the exception of these three Canadian studies reported by Simpson, Tsang, and Brierley, most of the subsequent RT literature either did not adequately review or demonstrated only equivalent (importantly not inferior) overall or cause-specific survivals [29, 36, 39, 46, 47]. In contrast to the Canadian and European literature, a few U.S. reports, including from Mazzaferri and

Samaan, demonstrated inferior survivals; yet, on review, this is likely explained by patients treated with EBRT having significantly worse prognostic variables, as compared to those treated without EBRT [21, 31]. Importantly, with one questionable exception [39], adverse patient selection type I bias whereby EBRT patients were relatively older, had more extensive infiltrative disease and sometimes even more distant metastasis present as compared to those treated "without RT" in most all of the RT literature [3, 6, 29, 36, 45–47] Accordingly, results demonstrating equivalent survivals may actually imply a survival benefit conferred by EBRT for patients deemed at high risk for central recurrence.

In contrast to its controversial impact on survival, there is ample evidence that moderate-dose EBRT decreases the locoregional recurrence of those same very high-risk patients. However, for similar reasons, whether there is additional benefit over standard adjuvant therapy is unclear, given conflicting biases [6, 36, 47]. Noteworthy, Kim demonstrated similar survivals despite all three types of biases negatively impacting on outcomes with EBRT [46].

Prognostic Variables Predictive for Locoregional Recurrence

The early literature identified tumor, patient, and treatment-related variables predictive for locoregional recurrence. Although often inter-related and notably contingent on the demographics of the study population (and the selected variables for review), the list also includes prior treatment-related factors, as these are known to subsequently impact on the outcome of secondary treatments, such as EBRT. A review of the literature cites the following prognostic variables predictive for a locoregional recurrence: (1)patient age>45, especially >60 years [27, 39, 42, 45, 47]; (2) any ETE, especially oETE [29, 34, 36, 41, 45–47]; (3) advanced cervical nodal disease, especially >2 cm nodes or having ECE [29, 36, 39, 46]; (4) high-grade histologies, especially those shown to be PET positive [5, 19, 42, 48]; and (5) recurrent disease, especially centrally located

[18, 36, 44]. Treatment factors include the use of [131]I [3, 6, 36, 45], the extent of surgical resection (specifically the size of postoperative residuum) [3, 4, 6, 36, 42, 44, 45], and the selected use of EBRT, with several studies having confirmed the favorable impact of RT by multivariate analysis [39, 46, 47].

To elucidate both the rationale for postoperative EBRT and the anticipated outcome, it is worthwhile to review several of these prognostic factors, including (1) the size of postoperative residuum, (2) the extent of ETE, (3) high-grade histologies, and (4) recurrent disease status.

Significance of the Volume of Postoperative Residuum: Microscopic, Macroscopic, Gross Disease

Understandably, with rare exception, [19] the volume of residual disease, especially within the surgical bed, has been shown to be highly prognostic for locoregional control, [3, 5, 6, 18, 44, 45],often also for overall survival comparing treatment of microscopic versus gross residuum [5, 18, 44]. For patients having measurable recurrences specifically in the thyroid remnant or in regional nodes, for whom surgery and/or ^{131}I remain successful salvage measures, there is less likely a compromise in survival, as compared for those having true central recurrences [40, 43].

In accordance with the "dose volume tenet" of radiotherapy, the strongest predictors for disease control in the surgical bed with EBRT are the aggregate volume of disease and the cumulative dose delivered.

Four studies have evaluated the outcome after EBRT prescribed for study populations having locally advanced disease, defined by a high percentage (>50%) of ETE and/or postoperative residuum. Outcomes were analyzed according to the volume of residuum, comparing results of similar RT doses given for R1 microscopic (or after gross total resection, R0, R1) versus R2, R3 gross disease (compare results noted in Table 14.1 section III vs. Table 14.4 section I). Two of these study populations were comprised of exclusively well-DTCs [18, 44] and two had significant

Table 14.1 Literature adjuvant EBRT for DTC (PTC): microscopic (R1) or very small volume residuum

Author refs #	n	Constellation of risk factors** for EBRT			With EBRT (+/-)		Without EBRT (S+/-I)			cEBRT		sEBRT	
		sRS	Any ETE	+ Risks: Age or LN	Iodine C EBRT (%)	10-year LRC (%)	:0-year LC (%)	Surgery alone (%)	^{131}I (%)	10 year CSS (%)	p	10 year CSS(%)	p
I Canadian studies: 45–50 Gy/(2.25 Gy/Fx)				Tx scheme:									
Simpson [3]	s172	R1**		S alone		none	26% (cum)	100% S	none		ss	58%/85%	ss
				S+RT	0%I	90% (cum)				95%			
				S+/-I+/-R	100% I	86% (cum)	82% (cum)	none	100%I	92%	ss	92%	ss
Tsang [6]	s155	R1**			70%I	93%	78%	54% S	46%I	100%	ss	95%	ss
Brierley [45]	s154	R1**			na	94%	84%	na	na	100%	ss	95%	ss
	s70	GTR*(R1, R0) &	ETE** &	>60 year**	na	86%	66%	na	na	81%	ss	65%	ss
II Korean studies: 50–63 Gy/SF													
Keum [47]	s43	R1	& oETE**		4%Iov	93% (cum)	50% (cum)		4%I			na	na
	68	R0,R1,mR2	& oETE**		4%I	89%	38%	70%S ov	30%I	63% (os)	ss	79% (os)	ns
Kim [46]	91	R1,mR2	& ETE**	or cLN**	52%I	95% (5y)	67% (5y)	none	100%I	90%	ss	98%	ns
III US studies: 60 Gy (equivalent)–65 Gy/SF													
Meadows [18]	s22	R1,diffuse**			39%I	100% (5 year)				90% (5y)			
Azrif [44]	s29	R0, R1**	or ETE**	or ECE**	100%I	89% (5y)				91% (5y)			
IV Populations with high-grade histologies: 60–70 Gy/SF (higher doses)													
O'connell [42]	s74	R1PTC+FTC	47% ov	22%HGHov	65%Iov	81% (cum)				60% (10y)			
	s43	R1 (PTC)	''	''	''	84% (cum)							
Schwartz [5]	s37	R1	96% ov	26%HGHov	82%Iov	85% (5+10y)				50% (10y) (os)			
	s111	GTR(R0R1)	96% ov		''	86% (4y)				79% (4y) (os)/50% (10y) (os)			
Terezakis [19]	s24	R1	84% ov	56%HGHov	74%Iov	87% (4y)				68% (5y) (os)			

Anticipate 90–93% LRC (EBRT alone) and 93–94% (EBRT+I-131); for HGHs anticipate 84–87% control

S subpopulation, *SRS* surgical resection status, *R0* negative, *R1* microscopic, *mR2* macroscopic margins, *ETE* extrathyroidal extension, *LRC* locoregional control, *CSS* cause-specific survival, *os* overall survival, *Cum* cumulative, *ss* statistically significant, *ns* not significant, *na* not available, *I* iodine, *ov* for overall population, *HGH* high-grade histologies, *cLN* cervical lymph nodes, *ECE* extracapsular extension, **major indicator for inclusion EBRT. Indications for I-131=positive whole-body Iodine scan (WBIS) for same high risk (**) population, all comparative studies EBRT patients had worse prognostic variables (older age, more ETE) as compared to those treated without EBRT

proportions of high-grade histologies [5, 19]. For the treatment of well-differentiated but locally advanced thyroid cancers, both Meadows ($p=0.02$ and $p=0.03$) and Azrif ($p=0.03$ and $p=0.01$) confirmed significant differences in both locoregional control and cause-specific survival (respectively) between those treated having microscopic versus gross residuum [18, 44]. Both studies used similar doses, an equivalence of 60–65 Gy, prescribed to all patients irrespective of volume of disease. Despite a differential proportional use of ^{131}I (39% and 100%, respectively) both authors reported quite similar outcomes for patients securing a gross tumor resection (R0, R1), citing a 89%–100% 5-year locoregional control (Table 14.1; III). Furthermore, despite a differential inclusion of distant metastasis (21% versus none, respectively), survival was also quite similar between the studies, for R1 patients having well-differentiated tumors a 90–91% 5-year cause-specific survival. Both Schwartz and Terezakis also reported on the impact of the volume of residuum for populations having locally advanced tumors but, also having a high percentage of high-grade histologies. As compared to the well-differentiated patient studies, both prescribed somewhat higher doses of 60–70 Gy, often with IMRT technology [5, 19] (Table 14.4). Similar to results with well-differentiated tumors, Schwartz cited a significant difference in all outcomes, including locoregional recurrence ($p<0.0001$), cause-specific survival ($p<0.0001$), and overall survival ($p=0.0001$) between patients treated for microscopic (following gross tumor resection) versus gross disease. On multivariate analysis, both gross residual disease (hazard ratio, HR, 10.8) and high-grade histologies (HR 3.61) were the only variables predictive of locoregional recurrence, while high-grade histologies (HR 2.8), gross residuum (2.5), and distant metastasis (0.38 HR) were predictive for cause-specific survival [5]. In contrast to these three studies, Terezakis reported that the extent of surgical resection status did not significantly impact on any outcomes after EBRT: locoregional recurrence ($p=0.52$) or overall survival ($p=0.64$). Despite similar prescribed doses, the overall inclusion of somewhat more patients having distant metastasis (36% vs. 28%), and more

high-grade histologies (56% vs. 28%), patients treated specifically for microscopic disease fared similarly as compared to R1 patients treated by Schwartz, especially with regard to the 4–5-year locoregional controls, 87% vs. 85–86%, as well as 4–5-year overall survivals, 68% vs. 79%, respectively (Table 14.1, IV). However, the outcomes for those treated for gross disease were quite different between these two studies. As can be seen in Table 14.4 II, those treated by Terezakis having gross disease fared distinctively better, both with regard to 4–5-year locoregional recurrence (62% vs. 22%) and 4-year overall survival (46% vs. 32%), despite nearly twice as many high-grade histologies and more metastasis overall compare to Schwartz data. Accordingly, relatively better results for the treatment of gross disease may account for insignificant difference in the outcomes between those treated for microscopic versus gross disease, unique for Terezakis' population. Although the populations may have varied in other important prognostic variables, including 16% of Terezakis' overall population comprised of medullary thyroid cancers, such dramatic differences in outcomes may have also been influenced by the greater use of IMRT (63% vs. 44%) and the addition of radiation-sensitizing chemotherapy (30% vs. none). Terezakis noted that although local control was achieved for most, outcomes for all patients were overshadowed by other very high-risk features dictating survival outcomes, especially high-grade histologies and extensive ETE. Furthermore, while follow-up is limited, the local progression-free curves (local control) between those having no versus microscopic versus macroscopic residuum are noted to separate at 4 years; however, by 4 years overall survival already decreased to 68% [19]. In conclusion, these four studies give testimony to the importance, of the size of residuum and emphasize the importance of securing at least a gross total resection in the interest of both local control and survival.

Although aggregate volume of disease remains a critical variable predictive for outcome after any given dose of EBRT, only the early Canadian studies evaluated the endpoint of locoregional control for populations stratified according to the volume of postoperative residuum, specifically microscopic R1 residuum. Importantly, most other authors evaluating the impact of "positive margins" do not quantitate volume and the spectrum includes microscopic as well as measurable R2 disease [29, 36, 39, 47]. For the RT literature reviewing outcomes for patients having microscopic R1 disease on one extreme, and that reporting on bulky unresectable R3 disease at the other extreme, there remains a wide spectrum of generally poorly defined measurable R2 disease. As on review of the radiation literature, as reported in Table 14.1 I & III, DTC patients treated for microscopic disease with EBRT alone have a reported 10-year or cumulative locoregional control of 90–93% [3, 47] I-III, while those treated with EBRT with some variable amount of ^{131}I have shown a quite similar locoregional control of 93–94% [3, 6, 18, 45]. In comparison, as seen in Table 14.3, those few studies reporting on presumed small-volume measurable disease (speculated to be on the order of 0.5–2 cm) with well-differentiated tumors have reported locoregional recurrences of 80–88%, when treated with 50–63 Gy of EBRT and varying amounts of "supplementary" ^{131}I [4, 6, 29, 36, 47]. Notably, the definition of durable local control for these patients is best represented by a plateau in locoregional control curves spanning over greater than 10 years.

In contrast to the generally concordant outcomes for the treatment of microscopic or small-volume measurable disease, treatment of DTC patients having bulky measurable, palpable, or varying amounts of unresectable (R3) disease results (Table 14.4, I) in a wide range of reported locoregional controls of 22–63%, notably without plateau, for between 5 and 10 years, despite doses of 60–65 Gy [4, 18, 36, 44]. Generally in the literature, "control" of bulky measurable disease is defined by stabilization, with no evidence of radiographic progression. Importantly, the clinical response of measurable well-differentiated tumors disease to EBRT is slow, with a median time to maximum local response ranging from 6 months to 2 years [3, 5, 6].

Besides the aggregate volume of targeted disease, the cumulative dose of EBRT is the other important determinant of the dose–volume tenet of RT. There is suggestion in the literature that increasing dose improves outcome for any given volume of disease [4, 18, 49]. The early RT literature reported on doses often inadequate to control even microscopic disease. Improvements in targeting should enhance efficacy. Ford noted improved local control with increasing doses ranging from <50 Gy/SF to >54 Gy/SF [49]. Tubiana noted a 15% in-field locoregional recurrence with lower doses and inferior technology, as compared to 5% locoregional recurrence after 50 Gy/SF and megavoltage EBRT [4]. Meadows reported no failures, even with gross disease, with doses over 64 Gy/SF, although the median follow-up was only 4 years [18]. It should be emphasized that dose constraints imposed by adjacent critical structures, notably the esophagus, set a limit to the benefits of EBRT and a "ceiling" even with IMRT technology, especially when treating measurable bulk residual disease. However, as illustrated in Fig. 14.3, the use of IMRT technology can, to some extent, bend the high-dose profile around the esophagus, likely resulting in less late esophageal stenosis as was historically observed even with 3D conformal radiotherapy. IMRT may be especially relevant for those patients with relatively small-volume (0.5–2 cm) but measurable residual disease who require doses in excess of that required for sterilization of microscopic disease.

In conclusion, there is strong evidence to suggest that microscopic disease can be eradicated by either adjuvant ^{131}I or moderate doses of EBRT. Adjuvant ^{131}I/sTSH has become the preferred frontline therapy as it offers more comprehensive coverage. However, EBRT may be more efficacious for tumors that have lost their ability to concentrate iodine, especially for older patients and/or high-grade tumors. There is suggestion that high-grade tumors of microscopic proportion can be adequately controlled with EBRT, not fully benefiting from ^{131}I therapy alone. Measurable, but small-volume, well-differentiated disease may especially benefit from the combined use of ^{131}I/sTSH and EBRT (dose intensification), or, especially relevant for higher-grade tumors, also benefit from the use of IMRT (dose escalation). Large volumes of residuum remain a challenge and likely only "temporized" by currently attainable doses of EBRT.

Significance of Extrathyroidal Extension

The significance of ETE has been extensively reviewed as it impacts on both outcomes of locoregional recurrence and survival [5, 24, 30, 36, 39, 41, 50–58]. ETE has been further categorized into three degrees of extension: minimal extension into adjacent connective tissues (minETE), extension to adjacent organs (oETE), and extensive infiltration into unresectable structures (eETE). Such categorization is instrumental in directing the aggressiveness and combination of treatment options, especially the indications for EBRT. Understandably, with more extensive tumor infiltration, there is an associated higher likelihood for positive margins; this incidence increases substantially with disease extending to adjacent organs. On reporting on a large cohort of patients having an overall incidence of 40% ETE, Chow correlated the extent of ETE with the incidence of observed positive margins: with min ETE, 27%; with oETE, 86%; and with eETE, 96% [36]. For patients treated with surgery alone, the 10-year locoregional recurrence with minETE was 33%, while for oETE it was 59%. Tuttle notes that ETE, along with presence of distant metastasis are the only two risk factors predictive of death in all of the published risk group systems [50]. He cites that on multivariate analysis for patients having ETE, the use of EBRT was the only predictor for both improvement in cause-specific survival ($p = 0.02$) and overall survival ($p = 0.06$) [55].

There is observed a strong association between ETE and older patients and those with high grade histologies [50]. Additionally, the clinical impact of having ETE as well as any additional risk factor, including positive surgical margins [36], older age >45 or >60 years [24, 39, 45], and concomitant cervical nodal disease [29, 39], magnifies the deleterious impact on both survival and locoregional control. Farahati observed that when nodal status was introduced into the analysis,

EBRT impacted on locoregional control only for those having oETE as well as being >40 years of age and with cervical lymph nodes [39]. Chow recommended supplementary EBRT in addition to standard ^{131}I/sTSH only for patients having evidence for both oETE and confirmed (any) positive margins. Treatment with EBRT (plus ^{131}I/sTSH), as opposed to without EBRT, more than halved the LR from 58% to 23% ($p < 0.001$). [36] Anderson observed that older patients having tumors with ETE demonstrated poorer survival, as compared to those without ETE, regardless of whether the tumors were completely resected. In contrast, younger patients with ETE showed comparable survival as those patients not having ETE as long as the tumors could be completely resected [24]. Importantly, although tumors having had initial evidence for extensive ETE have been observed to be less iodine-avid at the time of recurrence, [34] they are not necessarily more resistant to or less effectively treated by EBRT, other than as dictated by the aggregate volume of the residuum. In summary, the specific use of EBRT, in addition to standard therapy, is often recommended when ETE is associated with at least one other known high-risk variable, including documented positive margins, [36, 46] extensive nodal disease [39, 46], advanced age, [24, 39, 48] or high-grade histologies [5, 19, 38, 52].

Significance of High-Grade Histology: Poorly Differentiated PTC, FTC, Hurthle Cell, Clear Cell, and Tall Cell Variants

The older radiation literature often did not analyze outcomes according to histological grade, acknowledging that such tumors were rare. In Simpson's large database, less than 10% of PTCs were poorly differentiated [3]. Chow comments that grade was not analyzed as it was not available on the pathology report [27]. Given their rarity, there is a paucity of literature analyzing the impact of either EBRT or ^{131}I, given alone or in combination, for high-grade histology thyroid cancers. Much of the literature is comprised only of observations as to their natural history or case reports [41, 59–62]. Invariably, most authorities acknowledge common features, including a high incidence of ETE, nodal disease, and distant metastasis [50] . Most also agree that high-grade histologies are typically less iodine-avid; the role of ^{131}I said by some to remain undefined [48, 52, 59]. These variants of DTC are especially at risk for locoregional recurrence, especially within the surgical bed [60, 62] Several authors have suggested that the threshold to add EBRT needs to be lowered; this in contrast to the more general recommendations for adopting a "watchful waiting" approach toward EBRT as an adjuvant therapy for most other DTCs [5, 34, 38].

Three authors have reported on outcomes of populations having relatively high percentages (22–56%) of high-grade histologies treated with EBRT and varying amounts ^{131}I [5, 19, 41]. Recent data with short follow-up have demonstrated a reasonable 4–10-year locoregional controls of 84–87% (see Table 14.1, IV), when specifically microscopic high-grade histologies are treated with moderately high doses of 60–70 Gy of postoperative adjuvant EBRT, with or without ^{131}I. This is approximately 10% less (Table 14.1, I–III) than the typical results observed for the adjuvant treatment of microscopic well-DTC. With the loss of avidity, especially at the time of recurrence, or as validated by PET positivity, relatively higher doses of EBRT may be warranted, as compared to well-differentiated tumors, even for the treatment of microscopic disease. Furthermore, some may retain partial capacity to concentrate iodine, thereby supporting the strategy to supplement EBRT with ^{131}I as a form of dose intensification. However, for the treatment of gross disease (Table 14.1, II) there are relatively poor and quite variable locoregional control rates of 22–62%, despite doses of 60–70 Gy/SF. Schwartz noted that on multivariate analysis the variable of high-grade histology (hazard ratio 10.8) was second only to volume of gross residuum (hazard ratio 3.6) as predictive for locoregional recurrence, while for survival hazard ratios were 2.8 and 2.5, respectively [5].

For high-grade variants, the reported survivals are also appreciably less than for those of more DTC. This is understandable given the inherently higher incidence of metastasis and more extensive ETE at diagnosis (correlating with risk for occult distant metastasis). The observed 4-year survivals for R1 (Table 14.1; IV) and for R2/R3 (Table 14.4; II) disease, and are 68–79% and 32–46%, respectively.

In conclusion, given more rapid kinetics, with mean time to local failure of 1.5 years [5, 19, 32] (as compared to 5 years for DTCs), the variable production of Tg as a surveillance tool, and less effective systemic options, it appears advantageous to intervene earlier with EBRT in the treatment of high-grade variants, as compared to a more conservative approach adopted for most other well-DTC [5, 19, 38, 52]. Both Sanders and Schwartz make recommendation for consideration of EBRT as de novo adjuvant therapy for high grade histology tumors if there is even minimal ETE or extensive cervical adenopathy with ECE [5, 38]. However, similar to the impact of improved surveillance tools for DTC, PET/CT scans may be useful surveillance tools for high-grade tumors and hence also instrumental in changing the treatment paradigm. Several authors have reported that PET positivity correlates with ^{131}I resistance and is predicative for survival. Relevant to the use of EBRT, PET/CT scans may lead to earlier detection of ^{131}I-resistant tumors, whether in the neck or systemically. Should a PET scan detect early distant metastasis, then the justification for "adjuvant" of EBRT to the neck should be assessed on a case-by-case basis, depending on the competing threats of uncontrolled central versus distant disease [19, 38]. On the other hand, should the PET/CT show only neck positivity, without distant disease, then the role of EBRT may be elevated, in an attempt both to control the primary and to better circumvent distant dissemination. As noted, small volume of high-grade histologies may be effectively sterilized with dose-escalated IMRT (Table 14.1, IV), while treatment of measurable disease is far less effective (Table 14.4, II).

Significance and the Treatment of Recurrent Disease

As noted, there is controversy as to the impact of a recurrence on overall survival. In general, the ability to successfully treat DTC recurrences is dependent on patient, tumor, and treatment variables, both at the time of the initial diagnosis and at the time of recurrence. Specific prognostic variables relevant to the outcome of the treatment of recurrent disease include: patient age, the ability of tumor to concentrate iodine, the site of recurrence, and the initial extent (ETE) and bulk of disease both at of initial diagnosis and at the time relapse [34, 38, 40, 41, 43]. Several authors have reported worse survivals [36, 44], while others have reported no significant difference in outcomes for patients treated for recurrent disease, as compared to survivals of patients not having recurrence [5, 18, 54]. As previously noted, in general, only 50% of central recurrences can be surgically salvaged and many do not concentrate iodine [40, 43]. For surgical bed failures, differences in reported outcomes can likely be accounted for by differences in the success of re-resection, correlated with the degree of ETE at the time of both the initial and salvage surgeries. Chow noted a 10-year cause-specific survival of only 58% for those who suffered a local surgical bed relapse after initial standard therapy, including EBRT for selected high-risk patients having gross residuum or extensive ETE and/or extensive nodal disease [36]. This was significantly worse as compared to the 97% cause-specific survival for those who did not relapse ($p < 0.0001$). He did not, however, specify prognostic variables accounting for such recurrences, specifically the success of initial surgery in accomplishing at least a gross total resection. Similarly, Azrif also reported on the outcome of 12 relapsed patients from a study population of DTC, 78% having ETE at diagnosis and none with distant metastasis treated with both EBRT (equivalent dose 60 Gy) and [131]I [44]. Of the recurrences, one-third were in the central compartment and two-thirds in the cervical nodes. The 5-year cause-specific survival was worse for those who relapsed, as compared to those who maintained control, 59% versus 91%. Although the p value was not cited, the differences in survival curves were impressive with a plateau in survival after 3 years for those without relapse and no plateau out 10 years for those who suffered a local relapse. For those

with local relapse, the 10-year cause-specific survival was only 20%. Furthermore, 66% of those who had a local failure died within 4 years of the initial diagnosis. Azrif noted that only 50% (three of six) patients could be surgically salvaged after EBRT and [131]I. Notably, however, many of these patients were likely initially ineffectively treated with EBRT having been left with gross residuum: 39% had gross residuum and 16% had inoperable disease at the time of RT; attempted salvage of progressive gross disease remained equally ineffective. Multivariate analysis demonstrated that the single most important factor predictive for a favorable outcome was the margin status at the time of initial therapy [44].

Although some authors have voiced a concern that EBRT may hamper future surgical salvage, this has been refuted by others [7, 39]. There may be some increased risk for surgery after EBRT, but the difference in outcome may reflect the inherent biological aggressiveness and the extent of the initial disease, as opposed to adverse effects of moderate doses of EBRT in a clinician good hands [3, 5, 19, 39, 46].

Several authors have emphasized that the survival outcome is best correlated with the attainment of gross tumor resection, followed by further adjuvant therapy. Palme noted that survival at first recurrence was similar to survival at diagnosis, with plateau; however, subsequent recurrences were more detrimental, without a plateau over years [54]. Three authors, Meadows [18], Terezakis [19], and Schwartz [5], have reported on the use of EBRT specifically in the management of recurrent disease; all reporting on populations consisting of approximately half (48–58%) treated specifically for recurrent disease. Only Meadows reported on a population comprised only of well-differentiated tumors (the percentage of ETE was not reported) who were treated with 65 Gy; 38% also received [131]I. He alone specifically compared outcomes of those treated for de novo disease versus recurrent disease and cited improved outcome for de novo patients, with cause-specific survivals of 86% versus 71% for those treated for recurrent disease. This, however, was not statistically significant, $p = 0.25$. Unfortunately, Meadow's analysis as to the significance of recurrent disease is limited by patients not having been stratified according to volume of residuum at the time of RT, although notation made that half of the overall population had not attained a gross tumor resection [18]. In contrast to Meadows, both Schwartz and Terezakis reported on populations having other significant risk variables, including high-grade histologies (28%–56%), which confound analysis as to impact of recurrence status. Both of these study populations also had greater than 80% ETE, were treated with 60–70 Gy EBRT, and 74–82% received supplementary ^{131}I. As reported by Terzakis, patients having locoregional recurrences fared poorly, commenting that half of those patients who died of disease had been treated for recurrent disease [19]. However, Terezakis did not analyze outcome according to the surgical resection status or by histology. Schwartz did not submit data, although he specifically commented that recurrent status did not impact on local control or overall survival, as long as a gross total resection was accomplished [5].

In summary, although a "watchful waiting" approach, assuming appropriate initial standard therapy and adequate surveillance, may be an appropriate initial strategy for many. EBRT should be an important consideration at the time of first recurrence, ideally after a gross tumor resection. Early detection, prior to progression to unresectable disease or distant metastasis is crucial in predicting outcome. This strategy for close surveillance is important given the narrow window of opportunity for effective salvage, especially with EBRT. Chow noted a median time to distant metastasis of 7 years, 2 years beyond that of the median time to locoregional recurrence [27]. On the other hand, high-grade histologies show both shorter time to local recurrence and likely faster time to distant metastasis.

Interpretation of the Radiation Literature: Confounding Variables

With regard to the choice of adjuvant therapy for patients thought to be at risk for locoregional recurrence, there are no prospective randomized trials; a European effort was aborted because of poor accrual [63, 64]. There are only retrospective reviews, with inherent limitations, for which to guide therapy.

Prior to the accepted standard of adjuvant ^{131}I/sTSH, the older literature compared outcomes between EBRT alone versus ^{131}I alone. Although outdated, these early studies remain important in validating the efficacy of EBRT for projecting outcomes in the treatment of iodine-non-avid disease, and identifying important prognostic variables predictive for locoregional recurrence. However, there are multiple problems with these studies, which are discussed in the following.

Selection Bias

Most of the older study populations were stratified according to status of the postoperative residuum and categorized by the different treatment options. Often, there is mention, though no reporting as to the distribution or influence, of other prognostic variables such as age, lymph node status, and the measurable volume of residuum. Invariably, there was often strong patient allocation type I bias with patients known to have worse prognostic variables (larger initial tumors, more extensive ETE, larger postoperative residuum, and older patients) preferentially treated with EBRT, hence, understandably expected to have worse survival [31], though often found to have equivalent survival [29, 46, 47]; and at times improved survival [3, 6]. Inclusion criteria were often ambiguous: many of the early studies noted that ^{131}I was given only with a positive post ablation scan, although the methodology of ^{131}I was likely often inadequate [3]. Additionally, in the larger studies, many patients were given radiotherapy that were unlikely to derive benefit [5, 6]. On the other hand, subgroup analysis or evaluations of smaller more homogeneous study populations were often underpowered and demographics of subpopulations not segregated for analysis.

Disproportional Allocation of Treatment Variables

A common inadequacy in the early studies evaluating the role of EBRT as an adjuvant modality was the tendency of bundling treatment regimens, when reporting outcome data. This often resulted in a disproportional use of ^{131}I between treatment regimens with EBRT, as opposed to those without EBRT. As noted in Tables 14.1: I,III and 14.2, such type II bias conferred an inherent [46, 47] disadvantage or advantage [6, 36] for the EBRT treatment regimen. On the other hand, some studies noted that high-risk patients who were treated with surgery alone were grouped in the without EBRT regimen, leading to an inherent advantage for the with EBRT regimen [6, 27, 36, 47]. Additionally, a type III bias is present when high risk patients are treated with surgery alone but the outcome is included in "without RT" group.

Strong Institutional Bias

This also confounds a comparative review between reported series. Noteworthy is the brevity of US reports specifically analyzing the impact of EBRT, seemingly favoring the use of [131]I. Most of the EBRT literature has been generated from the Royal Marsden Hospital in the UK, Princess Margaret Hospital in Canada, or Asian institutions [3, 6, 27, 36, 45, 65]. Importantly, these large cohorts of study patients from Canada and Asia demonstrated a relatively high incidence of any ETE (30–60%), as compared to the US incidence of 10% [24, 55, 58, 66]. This facilitated review as to the impact of EBRT in such high-risk patients. Nevertheless, between institutions there was often variation as to treatment technique and radiotherapy fractionation schedule and doses. Most use the standard fractionation schedule (SF) of 1.8–2.0 Gy/fxn; the Canadian [3, 6, 45] schedule was 45–50 Gy with 2.25 Gy/fxn. Azrif, from the UK, prescribed a hypofractionated course of 45 Gy at 2.75 Gy/fxn, said to be biologically equivalent to 60 Gy/SF [44].

Time Bias

The long indolent natural history of DTC requires a long study period to validate outcomes of tumor control, survival, and late RT toxicities. Innovations in diagnostic tools (MRI, PET/CT, ultrasonography, and Tg), refinements in treat-

ment methodology (EBRT technology and ^{131}I preparation/doses), as well as surgical philosophy and expertise impacted on outcomes even within a reported study period [3, 4, 45, 67]. These transitions, as well as the change in 2002 staging as to the importance of minimal ETE, all account for unstable and confounding variables during a given protracted study time.

Omissions and Ambiguities

Finally, much of the literature has ill-defined or important omissions with regard to data analysis. The early American literature often invariably omitted important EBRT treatment factors, including dose, fractionation schedule, and fields [31, 68]. Many studies showed wide variation in doses delivered, often reporting only median dose [3, 24]. The extent of "positive margin" and "any" ETE was also often poorly defined. Definition of local control and survival varies between reports, as does the stratification of known prognostic variable for subgroup populations. Local control is often represented by absolute cumulative control over duration of study versus local progression-free survival. For some, survival was not reviewed [36, 39]; others reported cause-specific survival [3, 6, 45, 47], although occasionally overall survival [5, 19, 29]. Finally, there is an obvious deficiency as to the description, success, and morbidities associated with salvage therapies.

Review of RT Literature: Adjuvant, Macroscopic, Gross Disease

Evolutionary refinements in the use of ^{131}I and suppressed TSH, as well as the introduction of Tg as a powerful surveillance tool, eventually supported the preferential use of ^{131}I as frontline adjuvant treatment for the approximately 80% of patients having iodine-avid tumors at diagnosis. [1, 22, 23] In comparison with EBRT, ^{131}I/sTSH therapy also offered a more comprehensive systemic coverage option for ongoing close surveillance and repeat salvage attempts. With the acceptance of ^{131}I/sTSH therapy as standard of care, the appropriate question became what added benefit, and for whom, does EBRT give an important advantage over [131]I? To date, only three authors have investigated the role of EBRT as a supplement to standard adjuvant therapy of ^{131}I/sTSH after subtotal/total thyroidectomy in the treatment of DTCs [27, 29, 36, 39]. While all validated a favorable impact of treatment with as compared to without EBRT on locoregional control, only one [29] reviewed the impact on survival. All reported that EBRT, in the range of 50–60 Gy/SF, is well tolerated and reported toxicities are acceptable.

Adjuvant EBRT

The early pivotal trials reviewing the role of EBRT as an adjuvant modality of DTC, prior to current standard guidelines, are listed in (Table 14.1; I,II). Table 14.2 cites the three trials that reported results on the use of EBRT in accord with current guidelines. As an overview, the treatment of DTC (mostly PTC) with adjuvant EBRT, in the range of 50–63 Gy/SF prescribed for confirmed or presumed microscopic residuum in the surgical bed, significantly increased the 10-year locoregional control from 26% when treated with surgery alone [3] to 90–93% with the addition of postoperative EBRT alone [3, 47], or to 93–94% with EBRT, with varying percentages of sequential [131]I [6, 18, 43, 45–47].

A literature review notes increased survival (and locoregional control) for treatment with EBRT for patients: (1) With confirmed microscopic (R_1) positive surgical margins, as compared with surgery alone [3] and as compared to treatment without EBRT [6, 45], OR (2) With extensive ETE (oETE) (with gross total resection) and age > 60 years [45].

Improvement in locoregional control "with" EBRT, as compared to "without" was observed for patients with: (1) Microscopic residum [6, 45], OR (2) Positive surgical and ETE [36, 46, 47], OR (3) Positive cervical lymph nodes and

positive surgical margin [46], OR (4) ETE and >40 years [39].

As noted in Table 14.2, after the adoption of ^{131}I/sTSH as standard therapy (given to all patients), three authors reported on the benefit of EBRT added to ^{131}I/sTSH for patients with confirmed positive margins or suspected microscopic residuum with ETE into the surrounding organs [27, 29, 36, 39]. Both Farahati et al. and Philips and colleagues reported on small populations having relatively short follow-up of 5–8 years [29, 39]. Phlips et al. did not report statistical analysis for local control although the addition of 55 Gy/SF of EBRT to ^{131}I improved the overall local control (79% vs. 97%) for 94 patients left with positive surgical margins (R1 or R2) or cervical adenopathy, especially having extranodal extension of tumor [29]. Farahati et al. noted a significant benefit in 10-year local control (free from locoregional and distant failure) favoring the addition of 50–60 Gy/SF of EBRT: 45% versus 90% ($p=0.0009$) for patients having a constellation of PTC histology and ETE and age >40 years [39]. Notably, when Farahati introduced the cervical LN status into his analysis, the results were then only significant for those 31 patients also having confirmed positive cervical LNs with reported freedom from locoregional or distant failure of 20% versus 90%; $p=0.01$[39].

Also, as noted in Table 14.2, a more recent and much larger-scale analysis as to the potential selective benefit of EBRT in the adjuvant treatment of DTC, specifically PTC, was reported by Chow in 2002 and a more detailed analysis in 2006 [27, 36]. He reported on a large Chinese population of 1,297 patients with PTC, treated between 1960 and 2000, with 10-year follow-up. In his 2006 report, he evaluated the treatment with EBRT, as compared to without EBRT, according to multiple prognostic variables, including (a) margin status; (b) extent of disease: minETE, oETE, and eETE; and (c) cervical LN or repeated Survival outcomes. There was no analysis as to the impact of age on reported survival outcomes in the 2006 analysis. As did others, Chow reported outcomes with results bundled "with" versus "without" EBRT; however, he gave more detailed results of all four treatment options for those with

Table 14.2 Literature adjuvant EBRT for DTC (PTC): EBRT with 131I versus 131I alone (Standard recommendation)

| Author refs# | n | Constellation of risk factors** for EBRT | | | With EBRT (+ I) | | | Without EBRT (S+I131) | | | | cRT | sRT | |
		sRs	Any ETE	Age or LN / OR cLN/ECE**	Dose	^{131}I cRT (%)	LRC 10-year	LRC 10-year	Salone (%)	^{131}I (%)	p	OS 5 year	OS 5 year	p
Philips [29]	94	R1mR2 (+sm)**		OR cLN/ECE**	55 Gy	100%I	97% (5y)	79% (5y)	none	100%*	na	84	94	na
Farahati [39]	s137	na	ETE**	& >40 year	50–60 Gy	100%I	90% (5y)	45% (5y)	None	100%	ss	na		
	s31	na	ETE**	& >40 year+cLN	"	100%	90% (5y)	20% (5y)	None	100%	ss	na		
				Tx scheme:										
Chow [36]	s51	R1,mR2 (+sm)		s Alone	-	-	-	32%	100%	None	ss	na		
		"		S+I	-	-	-	80%	None	100%				
		"		S+RT	60 Gy	None	57%	-	-	-				
		"		S+RT +I	"	100%I	90%	-	-	-				
	s131	RoR1,R2(71%)	oETE	S Alone	-	-	-	41%	100%	None	ss	na		
			"	S+I	"	-	-	72%	None	100%				
			"	S+RT	"	60 Gy	None	60%	-	-	-			
			"	S+RT +I	"	"	100%I	88%	-	-	-			
	s142	R1,mR2(+sm)	& oETE	S+RT +I/–I	60 Gy	Most	77%	42%	na	Most	ss	na		
	s222			cLN	60 Gy	Most	80%	58%	na	Most	ss	na		
	s114			LN>2 cm	60 Gy	Most	81%	56%	na	Most	ss	na		
Chow [36]	s51	R1,mR2 (+sm)		-	-	-	-	32%	100%	None	ss	na		
		"		-	-	-	-	80%	None	100%				

**Major indicator for inclusion EBRT, except for Chow (see text); indicators for ^{131}I: +whole-body ^{131}I scan for Philips
+sm = positive surgical margins; other abbreviations see Table 14.1, text.

positive surgical margins, minETE, and oETE. Importantly, this was a prospective protocol with inclusion criteria for adjuvant ^{131}I in accordance with current standards. EBRT was to be given after ^{131}I/sTSH therapy only if there was gross residuum, extensive ETE, and/or extensive LNs. In contrast to all prior literature, the indication for the use of ^{131}I included tumor >1 cm, older than 40 years, any ETE, and/or the presence of distant metastasis. Notably, there were protocol deviations, including many high-risk patients, some with confirmed positive surgical margins or oETE (9%) treated with surgery alone and bundled along with ^{131}I-treated patients. Also, despite guidelines, some patients received EBRT, without [131]I. For those patients with tumors having any positive surgical margins, treatment with EBRT alone improved the locoregional control, as compared to surgery alone (57% vs. 32%; $p < 0.0001$); however, so did the use of [131]I (80% vs. 32%; $p < 0.009$), as did the combined use of ^{131}I and EBRT (90% vs. 32%). Furthermore, the difference in outcome between ^{131}I alone and the combined use of ^{131}I and EBRT did not differ appreciably (80% vs. 90%). Similarly, for those with oETE, the use of only adjuvant EBRT, as compared to surgery alone, showed improvement in locoregional control (60% vs. 41%); however, so did the use of [131]I (72% vs. 41%), as did the combined use of EBRT and [131]I (88% vs. 41%). Similar to the analysis with positive margins, the combined use did not differ appreciably for ^{131}I alone (72% vs. 88%). Chow recommended the use of ^{131}I alone for patients having oETE or positive margins. However, he emphasized that for those patients whose tumors demonstrated both oETE and confirmed positive margins, treatment with EBRT, as compared to without EBRT, more than halved the locoregional recurrence from 58% to 23%, $p < 0.001$ (local control improved from 42% to 77%). Chow qualified that the added morbidity of EBRT is justified for those with a constellation of risk factors: PTC histology, oETE, and confirmed positive margins [36].

Four authors have specifically evaluated the role of EBRT in the treatment of patients having cervical nodal disease [29, 36, 39, 46]. Three reported locoregional control outcomes with EBRT versus without EBRT, while using current standard treatment of ^{131}I/sTSH. As noted, Farahati found improvement with EBRT only for those PTC patients having cervical LNs and oETE and age >40 years [39]. Philips noted improvement for those 12 patients having cervical LNs demonstrating ECE (extranodal extension): locoregional control 34% vs. 84% [29]. Chow reported a significant advantage with EBRT for those PTC patients having cervical LNs (58% vs. 80%; $p < 0.02$) or for LNs >2 cm (56% vs. 81%; $p = 0.008$) [36]. Chow further commented that those who were treated for a nodal recurrence, after standard therapy, demonstrated worse survivals, as compared to those who did not (10-year cause-specific survival of 79% vs. 96%, $p < 0.0001$).

In summary, there is a strong suggestion, although only from retrospective studies, that adjuvant EBRT improves on the locoregional recurrence for patients having PTC histology and the following constellation of variables: (1) confirmed microscopic positive margins [3, 6, 45] or (2) extensive ETE (oETE and eETE), without gross residuum, especially if combined with additional variables of (a) positive margins [36, 46, 47], or (b) advanced age [24, 39, 45], or (c) also having advanced cervical adenopathy [39]. It should also be considered for patients presenting with extensive cervical lymph nodes, likely in addition to some other risk factor such as primary tumor with oETE or nodes >2 cm or nodes with extranodal extension or advanced age [29, 36, 39, 46]. EBRT has an advantage over radioactive iodine treatment in patients whose tumors have lost the ability to concentrate iodine. Patients having deeply infiltrating tumors or older in age, or having larger volumes of residuum or recurrent central disease are those most likely to have lost iodine avidity [34, 42].

Treatment of Macroscopic or Small-Volume Disease (Table 14.3)

Although more straightforward with regard to indications for EBRT, the treatment of gross disease is technically more challenging than that of small-volume likely microscopic disease. As

Table 14.3 EBRT OF macroscopic (small volume), but gross disease (mR2)

Author; refs #	n	sRs	With EBRT		Locoregional Control%				Without EBRT				
			EBRT dose (median)	131I with EBRT**(%)	5 year	10 year	15 year	20 year	Locoregional Control%				131I with surgery(%)
									5 year	10 year	15 year	20 year	
Tubiana [4]	s97	mR2	50 Gy/SF	none		85% (cum*)			na	68% (cum*)			S+23%I
Tsang [6]	s33	mR2	45 Gy(2.25/fxn)	60% I	62%	62%	62%	62%					S
Keum [47]	s13	mR2	50-63 Gy/SF	4% I		87% (cum*)				0 (cum*)			S+30%I
	68	R0R1, mR2(19%)	"	"	89%	89%			60%	38%			"
Phlips [29]	s15	mR2	55 Gy/SF	100%I	100% (cum*)				33% (cum*)				S+100%I
Chow [36]	s137	Nonpalpable R2	60 Gy/SF	Most I	92%	80%	80%	80%	52%	39%	35%	30%	Most I

Anticipate with 50–63 Gy. (+/–I) 80–88% LRC (10 y), with plateau

Ref# reference number, *s* subpopulation, rt=sRS surgical resection status, *R0* negative margins, *R1* microscopic, *mR2* macroscopic, *mR2* macroscopic gross residuum, *n* # patients, *SF* standard fractionation (1.8–2.0 Gy/fraction),I 131I; *S* surgery, *y* years*cum* cumulative, Tubiana had minimum follow-up of 8 years for 97 patients treated with EBRT and 57 patients treated with S+/–131I, Keum had average follow-up of 8.5 years, Phlips median of 5.5 years**%I for overall population

previously noted, outcome is understandably correlated with volume of residuum.

Only a few studies discuss the outcome of postoperative small-volume macroscopic disease. (Table 14.3) Importantly, these are the tumors that may likely derive the maximum benefit from dose intensification strategies, including the concomitant use of both ^{131}I and dose-escalated IMRT. Successful treatment should be defined by a plateau of the rates of locoregional control noted on long-term follow-up. As noted in Table 14.3, recent data cite an approximate 10-year locoregional control rate of approximately 80–88% with 50–63 Gy of EBRT [4, 6, 36, 47]. Tsang et al. reported on 33 patients having macroscopic residual disease and treated with EBRT, with 60% also receiving [131]I [6]. After treatment with 45 Gy (2.25 Gy/fxn) of EBRT, the 5/10/15- and 20-year local relapse-free survivals were sustained, all at 62%. The 5-year cause-specific survival was 65%. Speculatively, most patients had small-volume macroscopic disease. Keum et al. noted that for high-risk patients all having tracheal involvement and left with "macroscopic residuum," there was a significant difference in local control (87% vs. 0%; $p=0.005$) for those treated with 50–63 Gy/SF, as compared to those treated "without EBRT", although 60% of these patients were treated with surgery alone [47]. As noted, for the population as a whole, those treated with EBRT (with only 4% with ^{131}I) showed a plateau in local control (progression-free survival rate) after 1 year with the 5/10-year progression-free survival rate of 89%/89% versus 60%/38% and no plateau for those treated with surgery (30% with ^{131}I) [47]. There is a paucity of data comparing the results of treatment of macroscopic disease with EBRT vs. [131]I. Wilson cites that ^{131}I can likely eradicate disease less than 2 cm [41]. Larger tumor volumes require more intensive measures, especially if it does not concentrate iodine. Chow subdivided gross residuum into palpable and nonpalpable disease [36]. For the 137 patients with gross, but nonpalpable (macroscopic), disease, the use of 60 Gy EBRT (most with ^{131}I), as compared to ^{131}I alone, doubled the 10-year locoregional control from 39% to 80% ($p<0.001$). [36]Tubiana also reported on

97 patients having macroscopic residuum who showed 85% 10-year locoregional control with EBRT alone; EBRT halved locoregional progression from 32% to 15% [4].

Treatment of Locally Advanced Gross or Unresectable Disease (Table 14.1)

The use of EBRT in the treatment of locally advanced, gross residual disease is straightforward, often technically challenging, but typically disappointing. (Table 14.4) Radioactive iodine treatment alone is generally inadequate to eliminate or control gross residual disease [27, 29]. In the treatment of bulk DTC disease in the neck, the literature qualifies a wide range of 23–70% 5-year tumor control with EBRT, effectively delaying progression of disease, often for a lifetime [3, 6, 42, 69, 70]. More recent data, with dose escalation, cite a 70% 5-year local control [18, 44]. However, more typically, there is still a relentless drop in local control and overall survival over time without a plateau for either outcome. Variations in local control and survival are accounted for by both the study population (including R3 versus gR2 disease) and the inclusion of high-grade histologies.

In consideration of the long indolent clinical course of DTC, control of the primary site remains a priority, as distant metastases are often delayed. Chow notes a 2-year difference between development of time to locoregional failure (5 years) and time to distant metastasis (7 years) [27]. For unresectable or bulk residual disease, most advocate a dual approach with both the use of ^{131}I and EBRT [3, 27, 36, 71]. EBRT doses in excess of 60 Gy/SF, using conformal CT-based planning systems, are recommended so as to maintain durable control, with acceptable morbidity [5, 18, 19, 42]. Tubiana reported on 17 patients, all having bulk (R3), unresectable disease. Relapse-free survival and overall survival at 5 and 10 years were 55%/60% and 60%/27%, respectively, without a plateau. Only two patients (12%) showed long-term control [4].

Table 14.4 EBRT for measurable, bulk (gR2)OR unresectable (R3) disease

Author	n	sRs	With EBRT (±% I-131)						Without EBRT (S±/-I-131)				
			EBRT dose	%I-131 C EBRT	% LRC		% OS Survival		% LRC		%S alone	%CS Survival	
					5year	10y	5y	10y	5y	10y		5y	10y
I WDTC/PTC													
Chowref [27]	s124	gR2+R3(noDM)	60 Gy	most	70%	56%			40%	24%	na		58% ns
Chow [36]	s217	gR2+R3 (all)	60 Gy	88%I	na	63%		74% (css)	na	24%	43%		50% (ss)
Chow [36]	s51	gR2,R3palpable	"	most	23% (2y)		na		6% (2y)				
Tubiana [4]	s17	R3 (100%)	50–60 Gy	Few	55% (rfs*)	22%	60%	27%	na				
Azif #[44]	s19	gR2+R3(42%)	60 Gy(eq)	100%I	69%	35%	58% css	30% css	na				
Meadows [18]	s20	gR2+R3(30%)	65 Gy	36%ov	70%	na	69%	na	na				
II High-grade histologies													
O'Connell [42]	s49	gR2+R3(49%) 22% HGH	60 Gy	65%ov	na	na	27%	13%	na				
Schwartz [5]	s15	gR2+R3 (na) 26% HGH	60–70 Gy 44%IMRT	82%ov	22% (4y)	na	32% (4y)	≤10%	na				
Terezakis [19]	s41	gR2+R3(20%) 56%HGH	60–70 Gy 63% IMRT 30% CTX	74%ov	62% (4y)	na	46% (4y)	na	na				

Anticipate 35–63% 10 year LRC with 60–70 Gy/SF (no plateau) # reference number, *s* subpopulation, *sRs* surgical resection status, *gR2* gross residuum, R3 unresectable disease, *ov* for overall study population, *n* number, *os* overall survival, *css* cause-specific survival, *HGH* high-grade histologies (poorly differentiated PTC or FTC, Hurthle cell, Tall Cell, Clear cell), *na* not available, *S* surgery, *LRC* locoregional control, *eq* equivalent dose, I ^{131}I, *IMRT* Intensity-Modulated Radiation Therapy, *CTX* chemotherapy

Sheline found that for patients with unresectable disease (R3), the 5/10/15-year local control rates were 55%, 22%, and 7%, without plateau [69]. In 1994, O'Connell reported on 49 patients having gross disease, 46% (22 patients) had R3 disease [42]. He noted that after 60 Gy/SF the overall objective response rate was 62%, 37% demonstrated a complete clinical response, 25% a partial response, and 37% were nonresponders. Local control was not evaluated, but the 5- and 10-year overall survival rates were 27 and 12%. For the overall population, 44% of the patients who died had a component of local failure.

Chow and colleagues also reported on the role of EBRT in the treatment of gross residual disease [27, 36]. On multivariate analysis, the presence of postoperative gross residual disease (gR2) was the strongest variable impacting on outcomes, overriding all other prognostic variables. The use of EBRT significantly decreased the 10-year local recurrence for patients with gross disease, as compared to those treated without EBRT. For the 124 patients having gR2 disease, the use of EBRT (with or without ^{131}I) resulted in half the local recurrence, with local control improving from 24% to 56% ($p=0.0019$), as compared to no EBRT (surgery alone or postoperative ^{131}I) [27]. With additional patients, Chow reported in 2006 that on multivariate analysis, the use of EBRT (with or without ^{131}I) notably improved not only the local control but the 10-year cause-specific survival as well [36]. For the 217 patients with gR2 residuum, the use of EBRT doubled the local control from 24% to 63% ($p<0.001$) and significantly improved the 10-year cause-specific survival from 50% to 74% ($p=0.01$) as compared to "without EBRT". The majority (88%) had received both ^{131}I and EBRT. The results can be criticized given that those without EBRT included 38 patients (43% of the "without EBRT" group) who were treated with surgery alone. As previously noted, Chow subdivided gross disease into those with nonpalpable (likely small-volume macroscopic residuum) and palpable disease. For the 51 patients with gross, palpable disease the outcomes were poor; nonetheless, treatment with EBRT (mostly in addition to ^{131}I/sTSH) still improved the 2-year local con-

trol as compared to those who did not receive EBRT (6% vs. 23%; $p=0.03$).

Azif and colleagues reported on 19 patients having gross residum (gR$_2$) from well differentiated thyroid carcinoma, including 42% with unresectable R$_3$ disease [44]. Contrary to most schedules, ^{131}I was given 3 weeks after completion of a hypofractionated course of EBRT, said to be equivalent to 60 Gy/SF. The observed 5- and 10-year local recurrence-free rates were 69% and 35%, and the 5- and 10-year cause-specific survival rates were 58 and 30%, respectively. On multivariate analysis, the bulk of disease was the most important factor predictive for both locoregional recurrence and cause-specific survival. Meadows reported similar outcomes for 20 patients treated for gross well differentiated thyroid carcinoma, including 6/20 (30%) with R3 treated to somewhat higher doses of EBRT (65 Gy/SF), some with IMRT [18]. Outcomes were similar to those of Azif et al. with 5-year local control of 70% and 5-year cause-specific survival of 69%. Half of the six patients with unresectable disease were treated with EBRT alone and remained controlled for more than 3 years, all dying of intercurrent disease. Two of the six died from local disease. Notably, no patient who received >64 Gy developed a locoregional recurrence during follow-up ranging from 0.2 to 32 years, with a median of 4 years.

Use of IMRT, Treatment Fields, Doses

The radiation literature is currently evolving with regard to the use of IMRT in the treatment of thyroid cancers. Emerging reports out of the United States, notably from MD Anderson Cancer Center [5, 20], Memorial Sloan Kettering Cancer Center [19, 72], University of California San Francisco [73], and University of Florida [18], as well as the United Kingdom [15–17], have validated its usefulness in circumventing dose constraints imposed especially by the spinal cord, and parotid glands (Table 14.5). Currently, IMRT rotational arc therapy may facilitate avoidance of the esophagus in the very-high dose region, while adequately treating subclinical or microscopic disease near the

Table 14.5 Significant EBRT toxicities

author	Refs #	*n*	Acute (0–6 months)	Late (6 months–2 years±)
Simpson	[3]	201	Common esophagitis	
Tubiana	[4]	95		1% carotid stenosis
				2% brachial plexopathy
				1% tracheal constriction
Phlips	[29]	38	2% Grade 3 dysphagia	2% severe neck fibrosis
Farahati	[39]	99	33% Erythema, esophagitis	None; RT did not compromise subsequent surgeries
Tsang	[6]	185	7% acute esophagitis	3% neck fibrosis
Kim	[46]	23	Common mild esophagitis	None; RT did not compromise subsequent surgeries
MSDS	[63, 64]	22	8% grade 3 esophagitis	Not evaluable
Schwartz	[5]	131		12% esophageal stenosis with 3D-conformal EBRT
				vs 2% esophageal stenosis with IMRT
Terezakis	[19]	76	14% treatment break	7% grade 3 xerostomia
			11% tracheostomy tube	4% tracheostomy, 3% laryngeal edema
			29% short term PEG	5% permanent PEG (2 years)
				9% overall late-grade 3/4 toxicity (30% with CTX)
Rosenbluth	[72]	20	Most grade 3 mucositis	None (9 months)

Ref reference number, *n* number of study population, grade ¾ toxicities typically defined by need for medical intervention, *PEG* percutaneous endoscopic gastrostomy tube, *MSDS* Multicenter Trial Differentiated Thyroid Carcinoma

tracheal–esophageal groove (Fig. 14.3). Besides offering better avoidance of critical structures, the expectation is that dose escalation will also improve tumor control, especially for those who harbor small macroscopic disease on the order of 0.5–2 cm disease residuum.

In the treatment of thyroid cancers, including for DTCs and high-grade histologies, standards have evolved to prescribe doses to second echelon lymph node stations on the order of 45–54 Gy, to first echelon stations (high suspicion for microscopic residuum) of 54–60 Gy, and to gross residual disease of 66–70 Gy, with a standard fractionation schedule of 1.8–2.0 Gy per day. This can be accomplished by a technique of multiple sequential "shrinking fields," these combined into a composite plan with an illustrative dose–volume histogram (DVH), and using either IMRT (inverse treatment planning) or 3D conformal (forward treatment) planning. IMRT offers the possibility for one initial treatment plan incorporating a "dose painting" technique whereby different targets are given different radiobiologically equivalent doses in the same number of overall treatment fractions.

On reviewing the specific role of IMRT, it is challenging to be able to conclusively validate improvements in local control or survival; this is likely confounded by a disease typically having slow kinetics with a protracted overall clinical course and literature devoid of any prospective randomized trials. Of interest, prior to even 3D conformal technology, doses were often limited by the varying position of the spinal cord. Nutting demonstrated the superiority of IMRT over 3D conformal RT in increasing the dose to the thyroid bed, while limiting the dose to the spinal cord within the tolerance of 45–50 Gy/SF [16]. Early toxicity has been reported, awaiting longer follow-up as IMRT technology has largely been available only since 2000. Terezakis notes that for his overall population of 76 patients developed significant short-term toxicities including 11% tracheotomy, 29% required percutaneous feedings, and 14% required a treatment break [19]. Late-grade ¾ toxicities included 9% (seven patients, with overall 4% requiring long-term) tracheotomy and 5% long-term percutaneous feedings. Overall, there was no notable difference in toxicity between IMRT and 3D conformal RT. However, it can be speculated that, given the methodology of dose prescription, patients prescribed IMRT likely received relatively higher targeted tumor doses. Furthermore, Schwartz reported that the use of IMRT decreased toxicity as compared to 3D conformal EBRT (2% vs. 12%), although p value was not reported for this small population [5]. Esophageal stenosis requiring dilatation was the most common late effect, most occurring within the first year, all within 2 years. There were eight patients who required dilation, two tracheotomy, and one percutaneous required gastrostomy; nine out of ten of these were after 3D conformal EBRT, although those patients said to have longer follow-up.

In conclusion, IMRT offers both dose intensification and normal tissue avoidance (Figs.14.2 and 14.3). There are suggestions for improvements in tumor control, especially relevant for patients who are deemed at very high risk for central recurrence, harboring tumors likely resistant to [131]I. Despite its theoretical advantage in being able to increase tumor dose, while maintaining constraints for normal tissues, its efficacy likely still remains limited to the treatment of relatively small-volume disease. Although the spinal cord (dose constraint 45–50 Gy/SF) no longer limits dose delivery, the tolerance of the esophagus is notably on the order of 60 Gy/SF, with this being a marginally adequate dose alone for eradication of visible small-volume disease. Sequential ^{131}I hopefully may serve a supplementary role for some tumors. Furthermore, diagnostic advances, including PET/CT scan, ultrasensitive ultrasonography, and MRI technology may offer a window of opportunity so as to diagnosis recurrences earlier, either facilitating gross tumor resection or detecting small-volume disease amenable to IMRT. PET identifies patients who have likely non-iodine-avid disease, hence more likely to respond to EBRT. Robbins reported a median survival of 4.5 years after detection of FDG positivity [74]. The same authors reported that FDG-avid metastatic lesions are relatively resistant to ^{131}I therapy [75].

Adequate treatment of thyroid tumors can be one of the most challenging of clinical setups for a radiation oncologist. The typical radiation fields include the thyroid bed at the nape of the neck and thoracic inlet. The most cephalad portion of the central target reaches superiorly to just lateral to the true vocal cords. The full length of the upper cervical esophagus is typically included in the low to moderate RT dose region (50–60 Gy), but there should be attempts to spare long segments of the entire upper esophagus from the high-dose (>60–66 Gy) regions. Tumors that involve the esophagus need include that segment in the high-dose region, but this may then limit the maximum permissible cumulative dose. The design of the bilateral neck fields is contingent on the extent of central and lateral cervical nodal disease. Clinically involved lateral cervical nodal chains prompt that the fields need be higher than the level of the hyoid, at least on the involved side. Having the chin tilted upward may decrease exposure to the oral cavity, thus minimizing effects on taste for higher neck fields. IMRT has been shown to minimize the dose to the parotid glands, especially if high neck regions need to be included. The lower extent of most fields should include the upper superior mediastinum (manubrium to brachiocephalic vein) as a next echelon nodal region. For tumors that extend inferiorly to clinically involve the upper mediastinum, there should be consideration for treatment to the carina [44]; however, that will increase the length of esophageal treatment and also lung exposure. Azrif commented that the rarity of mediastinal recurrences as isolated events does not support prophylactic elective irradiation of the region of the mediastinal extending from the brachiocephalic vein to the carina. He notes that restricting dose to this area may also facilitate dose escalation (using only 3D conformal RT) so as to improve locoregional control and avoid mediastinal radiation toxicity [44]. Treatment of the mediastinum to doses above 45–50 Gy is further challenged by having the arms typically positioned to the side (with head and neck immobilized by a face mask), which limits the angle of arcs required to restrict dose to the spinal cord and may compromise lung parenchyma within the angled beams.

A recent publication by Kim et al. compared control outcome between a limited field of radiotherapy, including only the surgical bed and clinically involved nodal chain, versus an extended field which included regional cervical nodes and upper mediastinum in addition to the surgical bed [76]. Both cohorts received the same cumulative dose of 62.5 Gy (range 60–69 Gy); those with extended field also received a median dose of 50 Gy to regional cervical nodes and upper mediastinum. There was a significant difference in locoregional recurrence at 5 years favoring the extended field (40% vs. 89%, $p=0.041$). There was a nonsignificant trend toward improved overall survival (88% vs. 67%, $p=0.475$). The acute or late toxicities were similar.

Treatment of Metastatic Disease

The overall incidence of distant metastasis is reported in 7–23% of patients with DTC, and is present at the time of diagnosis in only 1–4% of patients. Distant metastases are typically in lung and bones. In general, when the size of tumor is considered, location is less prognostic. It is thought that the poor responsiveness of bone metastasis to radioactive iodine is likely linked to the size of the disease [67, 77, 78]. Although significant portions of the lung cannot tolerate even moderate doses of EBRT, limited thoracic treatment is applicable for those who present with the superior vena cava syndrome, or localized tumor deposits, not amenable to resection. Surgery is preferable for bone metastasis at risk for fracture and some solitary bone metastasis. However, if the patient is not a surgical candidate, EBRT can provide sustained long-term palliation. With an abbreviated hypofractionated course of EBRT, Falkmer et al. noted that significant relief was obtained in >80% of patients and for >6 months in 50% [77]. Schlumberger and colleagues suggest higher doses (40–50 Gy), along with ^{131}I, for patients having longer projected survivals [78]. Importantly, acknowledging the risk of a flare with ^{131}I in the treatment of spinal cord or brain metastasis, EBRT may be the preferred modality

[79–81]. Limited brain metastases, observed in 5% of patients, may be treated with stereotactic radiosurgery [82, 83].

Summary: Current Guidelines

According to the 2009 guidelines of the American Thyroid Association: "The use of EBRT to treat the primary tumor should be considered inpatients over age 45 with grossly visible ETE at the time of surgery and a high likelihood of microscopic residual disease, and for those patients with gross residual tumor in whom further surgery or ^{131}I would likely be ineffective. The sequence of EBRT and ^{131}I therapy depends on the volume of gross residual disease and the likelihood of the tumor being ^{131}I responsive." [1]

References

1. Cooper D, Doherty G, Haugen B, et al. Revised American Thyroid Association Management Guidelines for patients with thyroid nodules and differentiated thyroid cancer. Thyroid. 2009;19(11):1167–214.
2. Powell C, Newbold K, Harrington K, Bhide S, Nutting C. External beam radiotherapy for differentiated thyroid cancer. ClinOncol (R CollRadiol). 2010; 22(6):456–63. Epub 2010 Apr 27.
3. Simpson W, Panzarella T, Carruthers J, Gospodarowicz M, Sutcliffe S. Papillary and follicular thyroid cancer: impact of treatment in 1578 patients. Int J Radiat Oncol Biol Phys. 1988;14(6):1063–75.
4. Tubiana M, Haddad E, Schlumberger M, Hill C, Rougier P, Sarrazin D. External radiotherapy in thyroid cancers. Cancer. 1985;55(9 Suppl):2062–71.
5. Schwartz D, Lobo M, Ang K, et al. Postoperative external beam radiotherapy for differentiated thyroid cancer: outcomes and morbidity with conformal treatment. Int J Radiat Oncol Biol Phys. 2009;74(4): 1083–91.
6. Tsang R, Brierley J, Simpson W, Panzarella T, Gospodarowicz M, Sutcliffe S. The effects of surgery, radioiodine, and external radiation therapy on the clinical outcome of patients with differentiated thyroid carcinoma. Cancer. 1998;82(2):375–88.
7. Kim J, Leeper R. Treatment of anaplastic giant and spindle cell carcinoma of the thyroid gland with combination Adriamycin and radiation therapy. A new approach. Cancer. 1983;52(6):954–7.
8. Tallroth E, Wallin G, Lundell G, Löwhagen T, Einhorn J. Multimodality treatment in anaplastic giant cell thyroid carcinoma. Cancer. 1987;60(7):1428–31.

9. Thames HD, Peters LJ, Withers HR, Fletcher GH. Accelerated fractionation vs hyperfractionation: rationales for several treatments per day. Int J Radiat Oncol Biol Phys. 1983;9(2):127–38.

10. Bonner JA, Harari PM, Giralt J, et al. Radiotherapy plus cetuximab for locoregionally advanced head and neck cancer: 5-year survival data from a phase 3 randomised trial, and relation between cetuximab-induced rash and survival. Lancet Oncol. 2010;11(1):21–8.

11. Bonner JA, Harari PM, Giralt J, et al. Radiotherapy plus cetuximab for squamous-cell carcinoma of the head and neck. N Engl J Med. 2006;354(6):567–78.

12. Kim S, Prichard C, Younes M, et al. Cetuximab and irinotecan interact synergistically to inhibit the growth of orthotopic anaplastic thyroid carcinoma xenografts in nude mice. Clin Cancer Res. 2006;12(2):600–7.

13. Shukovsky L, Fletcher G. Time-dose and tumor volume relationships in the irradiation of squamous cell carcinoma of the tonsillar fossa. Radiology. 1973; 107(3):621–6.

14. Emami B, Lyman J, Brown A, et al. Tolerance of normal tissue to therapeutic irradiation. Int J Radiat Oncol Biol Phys. 1991;21(1):109–22.

15. Harmer C, Bidmead M, Shepherd S, Sharpe A, Vini L. Radiotherapy planning techniques for thyroid cancer. Br J Radiol. 1998;71(850):1069–75.

16. Nutting C, Convery D, Cosgrove V, et al. Improvements in target coverage and reduced spinal cord irradiation using intensity-modulated radiotherapy (IMRT) in patients with carcinoma of the thyroid gland. Radiother Oncol. 2001;60(2):173–80.

17. Urbano T, Clark C, Hansen V, et al. Intensity Modulated Radiotherapy (IMRT) in locally advanced thyroid cancer: acute toxicity results of a phase I study. Radiother Oncol. 2007;85(1):58–63.

18. Meadows K, Amdur R, Morris C, Villaret D, Mazzaferri E, Mendenhall W. External beam radiotherapy for differentiated thyroid cancer. Am J Otolaryngol. 2006;27(1):24–8.

19. Terezakis S, Lee K, Ghossein R, et al. Role of external beam radiotherapy in patients with advanced or recurrent nonanaplastic thyroid cancer: Memorial Sloan-Kettering Cancer Center experience. Int J Radiat Oncol Biol Phys. 2009;73(3):795–801.

20. Bhatia A, Rao A, Ang K, et al. Anaplastic thyroid cancer: clinical outcomes with conformal radiotherapy. Head Neck. 2010;32(7):829–36.

21. Mazzaferri E, Young R. Papillary thyroid carcinoma: a 10 year follow-up report of the impact of therapy in 576 patients. Am J Med. 1981;97:418–28.

22. Mazzaferri E. Thyroid remnant ^{131}I ablation for papillary and follicular thyroid carcinoma. Thyroid. 1997;7(2):265–71.

23. McGriff N, Csako G, Gourgiotis L, Lori CG, Pucino F, Sarlis N. Effects of thyroid hormone suppression therapy on adverse clinical outcomes in thyroid cancer. Ann Med. 2002;34(7–8):554–64.

24. Andersen P, Kinsella J, Loree T, Shaha A, Shah J. Differentiated carcinoma of the thyroid with extrathyroidal extension. Am J Surg. 1995;170(5):467–70.

25. Patel K, Shaha A. Locally advanced thyroid cancer. Curr Opin Otolaryngol Head Neck Surg. 2005;13(2): 112–6.

26. Carcangiu M, Zampi G, Pupi A, Castagnoli A, Rosai J. Papillary carcinoma of the thyroid. A clinicopathologic study of 241 cases treated at the University of Florence, Italy. Cancer. 1985;55(4):805–28.

27. Chow S, Law S, Mendenhall W, et al. Papillary thyroid carcinoma: prognostic factors and the role of radioiodine and external radiotherapy. Int J Radiat Oncol Biol Phys. 2002;52(3):784–95.

28. Benbassat C, Mechlis-Frish S, Hirsch D. Clinicopathological characteristics and long-term outcome in patients with distant metastases from differentiated thyroid cancer. World J Surg. 2006;30(6): 1088–95.

29. Phlips P, Hanzen C, Andry G, Van Houtte P, Früuling J. Postoperative irradiation for thyroid cancer. Eur J Surg Oncol. 1993;19(5):399–404.

30. Mazzaferri E, Jhiang S. Long-term impact of initial surgical and medical therapy on papillary and follicular thyroid cancer. Am J Med. 1994;97(5):418–28.

31. Samaan N, Schultz P, Hickey R, et al. The results of various modalities of treatment of well differentiated thyroid carcinomas: a retrospective review of 1599 patients. J Clin Endocrinol Metab. 1992;75(3):714–20.

32. Palme C, Waseem Z, Raza S, Eski S, Walfish P, Freeman J. Management and outcome of recurrent well-differentiated thyroid carcinoma. Arch Otolaryngol Head Neck Surg. 2004;130(7):819–24.

33. Stojadinovic A, Shoup M, Ghossein R, et al. The role of operations for distantly metastatic well-differentiated thyroid carcinoma. Surgery. 2002;131(6):636–43.

34. Vassilopoulou-Sellin R, Schultz P, Haynie T. Clinical outcome of patients with papillary thyroid carcinoma who have recurrence after initial radioactive iodine therapy. Cancer. 1996;78(3):493–501.

35. Hay ID. Papillary thyroid carcinoma. Endocrinol Metab Clin N Amer. 1990;19:545–76.

36. Chow S, Yau S, Kwan C, Poon P, Law S. Local and regional control in patients with papillary thyroid carcinoma: specific indications of external radiotherapy and radioactive iodine according to T and N categories in AJCC 6th edition. Endocr Relat Cancer. 2006; 13(4):1159–72.

37. Noguchi S, Noguchi A, Murakami N, et al. Papillary carcinoma of the thyroid I. Developing pattern of metastasis cancer. 1970;26:1053–60.

38. Sanders EJ, LiVolsi V, Brierley J, Shin J, Randolph G. An evidence-based review of poorly differentiated thyroid cancer. World J Surg. 2007;31(5):934–45.

39. Farahati J, Reiners C, Stuschke M, et al. Differentiated thyroid cancer. Impact of adjuvant external radiotherapy in patients with perithyroidal tumor infiltration (stage pT4). Cancer. 1996;77(1):172–80.

40. Stojadinovic A, Shoup M, Nissan A, et al. Recurrent differentiated thyroid carcinoma: biological implications of age, method of detection, and site and extent of recurrence. Ann Surg Oncol. 2002;9(8): 789–98.

41. Wilson P, Millar B, Brierley J. The management of advanced thyroid cancer. Clin Oncol (R Coll Radiol). 2004;16(8):561–8.

42. O'Connell M, A'Hern R, Harmer C. Results of external beam radiotherapy in differentiated thyroid carcinoma: a retrospective study from the Royal Marsden Hospital. Eur J Cancer. 1994;30A(6):733–9.

43. Grant C, Hay I, Gough I, Bergstralh E, Goellner J, McConahey W. Local recurrence in papillary thyroid carcinoma: is extent of surgical resection important? Surgery. 1988;104(6):954–62.

44. Azrif M, Slevin N, Sykes A, Swindell R, Yap B. Patterns of relapse following radiotherapy for differentiated thyroid cancer: implication for target volume delineation. Radiother Oncol. 2008;89(1):105–13.

45. Brierley J, Tsang R, Panzarella T, Bana N. Prognostic factors and the effect of treatment with radioactive iodine and external beam radiation on patients with differentiated thyroid cancer seen at a single institution over 40 years. Clin Endocrinol (Oxf). 2005; 63(4):418–27.

46. Kim T, Yang D, Jung K, Kim C, Choi M. Value of external irradiation for locally advanced papillary thyroid cancer. Int J Radiat Oncol Biol Phys. 2003;55(4): 1006–12.

47. Keum K, Suh Y, Koom W, et al. The role of postoperative external-beam radiotherapy in the management of patients with papillary thyroid cancer invading the trachea. Int J Radiat Oncol Biol Phys. 2006; 65(2):474–80.

48. Foote R, Brown P, Garces Y, McIver B, Kasperbauer J. Is there a role for radiation therapy in the management of Hürthle cell carcinoma? Int J Radiat Oncol Biol Phys. 2003;56(4):1067–72.

49. Ford D, Giridharan S, McConkey C, et al. External beam radiotherapy in the management of differentiated thyroid cancer. Clin Oncol (R Coll Radiol). 2003;15(6):337–41.

50. Tuttle R, Leboeuf R, Martorella A. Papillary thyroid cancer: monitoring and therapy. Endocrinol Metab Clin North Am. 2007;36(3):753–78. vii.

51. Shah J. Exploiting biology in selecting treatment for differentiated cancer of the thyroid gland. Eur Arch Otorhinolaryngol. 2008;265(10):1155–60.

52. Shaha A. Treatment of thyroid cancer based on risk groups. J Surg Oncol. 2006;94(8):683–91.

53. Nishida T, Nakaok A, Hashimoto T. Local control in differentiated thyroid carcinoma with extrathyroidal extension. Am J Surg. 2000;179(2):86–91.

54. Palme C, Freeman J. Surgical strategy for thyroid bed recurrence in patients with well-differentiated thyroid carcinoma. J Otolaryngol. 2005;34(1):7–12.

55. Hu A, Clark J, Payne R, Eski S, Walfish P, Freeman J. Extrathyroidal extension in well-differentiated thyroid cancer: macroscopic vs microscopic as a predictor of outcome. Arch Otolaryngol Head Neck Surg. 2007; 133(7):644–9.

56. Cady B. Seminars in surgical oncology on thyroid cancer. J Surg Oncol. 2006;94(8):646–8.

57. Shaha A. Thyroid carcinoma: implications of prognostic factors. Cancer. 1998;83(3):401–2. discussion 403–404.

58. Shah J, Loree T, Dharker D, Strong E, Begg C, Vlamis V. Prognostic factors in differentiated carcinoma of the thyroid gland. Am J Surg. 1992;164(6):658–61.

59. Mills S, Haq M, Smellie W, Harmer C. Hürthle cell carcinoma of the thyroid: Retrospective review of 62 patients treated at the Royal Marsden Hospital between 1946 and 2003. Eur J Surg Oncol. 2009;35(3):230–4.

60. Carling T, Ocal I, Udelsman R. Special variants of differentiated thyroid cancer: does it alter the extent of surgery versus well-differentiated thyroid cancer? World J Surg. 2007;31(5):916–23.

61. Falvo L, Catania A, Grilli P, Di Matteo F, De Antoni E. Treatment of "locally advanced" well-differentiated thyroid carcinomas. Ann Ital Chir. 2004;75(1):17–21.

62. Falvo L, Catania A, D'Andrea V, Grilli P, D'Ercole C, De Antoni E. Prognostic factors of insular versus papillary/follicular thyroid carcinoma. Am Surg. 2004;70(5):461–6.

63. Biermann M, Pixberg M, Schuck A, et al. Multicenter study differentiated thyroid carcinoma (MSDS). Diminished acceptance of adjuvant external beam radiotherapy. Nuklearmedizin. 2003;42(6):244–50.

64. Biermann M, Pixberg M, Riemann B, et al. Clinical outcomes of adjuvant external-beam radiotherapy for differentiated thyroid cancer - results after 874 patient-years of follow-up in the MSDS-trial. Nuklearmedizin. 2009;48(3):89–98. quiz N15.

65. Chow S, Law S, Au S, et al. Changes in clinical presentation, management and outcome in 1348 patients with differentiated thyroid carcinoma: experience in a single institute in Hong Kong, 1960–2000. Clin Oncol (R Coll Radiol). 2003;15(6):329–36.

66. Mazzaferri E, Kloos R. Clinical review 128: Current approaches to primary therapy for papillary and follicular thyroid cancer. J Clin Endocrinol Metab. 2001; 86(4):1447–63.

67. Haq M, Harmer C. Differentiated thyroid carcinoma with distant metastases at presentation: prognostic factors and outcome. Clin Endocrinol (Oxf). 2005; 63(1):87–93.

68. Kebebew E, Clark O. Differentiated thyroid cancer: "complete" rational approach. World J Surg. 2000; 24(8):942–51.

69. Sheline G, Galante M, Lindsay S. Radiation therapy in the control of persistent thyroid cancer. Am J Roentgenol Radium Ther Nucl Med. 1966;97(4): 923–30.

70. Glanzmann C, Lütolf U. Papillary and follicular thyroid carcinoma: long-term course in 339 patients of the Zurich University Hospital 1960 to 1988 and review. Schweiz Rundsch Med Prax. 1992;81(15):457–67.

71. Tuttle M, Robbins R, Larson S, Strauss H. Challenging cases in thyroid cancer: a multidisciplinary approach. Eur J Nucl Med Mol Imaging. 2004;31(4):605–12.

72. Rosenbluth B, Serrano V, Happersett L, Shaha A, Tuttle M, et al. Intensity-modulated radiation therapy

for the treatment of nonanaplastic thyroid cancer. Int J Radiat Oncol Biol Phys. 2005;63(5):1419–26.

73. Posner M, Quivey J, Akazawa P, et al. Dose optimization for the treatment of anaplastic thyroid carcinoma: a comparison of treatment planning techniques. Int J Radiat Oncol Biol Phys. 2000;48(2):475–83.

74. Robbins R, Wan Q, Grewal R, et al. Real-time prognosis for metastatic thyroid carcinoma based on 2-[18 F]fluoro-2-deoxy-D-glucose-positron emission tomography scanning. J Clin Endocrinol Metab. 2006;91(2):498–505.

75. Wang W, Larson S, Tuttle R, et al. Resistance of [18 F]-fluorodeoxyglucose-avid metastatic thyroid cancer lesions to treatment with high-dose radioactive iodine. Thyroid. 2001;11(12):1169–75.

76. Kim T, Chung K, Lee Y, et al. The effect of external beam radiotherapy volume on locoregional control in patients with locoregionally advanced or recurrent nonanaplastic thyroid cancer. Radiat Oncol. 2010; 5:69.

77. Falkmer U, Järhult J, Wersäll P, Cavallin-Ståhl E. A systematic overview of radiation therapy effects in skeletal metastases. Acta Oncol. 2003;42(5–6): 620–33.

78. Schlumberger M, Challeton C, De Vathaire F, et al. Radioactive iodine treatment and external radiotherapy for lung and bone metastases from thyroid carcinoma. J Nucl Med. 1996;37(4):598–605.

79. Greenblatt D, Chen H. Palliation of advanced thyroid malignancies. Surg Oncol. 2007;16(4):237–47.

80. Datz F. Cerebral edema following iodine-131 therapy for thyroid carcinoma metastatic to the brain. J Nucl Med. 1986;27(5):637–40.

81. Holmquest D, Lake P. Sudden hemorrhage in metastatic thyroid carcinoma of the brain during treatment with iodine-131. J Nucl Med. 1976;17(4):307–9.

82. Kim I, Kondziolka D, Niranjan A, Flickinger J, Lunsford L. Gamma knife radiosurgery for metastatic brain tumors from thyroid cancer. J Neurooncol. 2009;93(3):355–9.

83. McWilliams R, Giannini C, Hay I, Atkinson J, Stafford S, Buckner J. Management of brain metastases from thyroid carcinoma: a study of 16 pathologically confirmed cases over 25 years. Cancer. 2003;98(2):356–62.

Targeted Therapy of Thyroid Cancer

Stephen W. Lim

Introduction

The primary therapy of thyroid cancer is surgical resection. For locally advanced or metastatic well-differentiated thyroid cancer (DTC), radioactive iodine is often curative. The adverse prognostic characteristics for DTC are well known, including age, positive lymph nodes, increased tumor size, and distant metastasis [1]. Positron emission tomography positive disease is also a negative prognostic marker [2]. These patients have a higher risk for the development of metastatic disease and have a shorter survival. Once the disease has become radioiodine refractory, the systemic therapeutic options are limited due to poor response rates and high toxicity.

When to treat patients with advanced or metastatic well-differentiated thyroid carcinoma poses a clinical dilemma. Locally advanced or metastatic disease is often asymptomatic and slowly progressive. Because of this, the survival of patients with advanced disease is commonly measured in years, or even decades. One must also balance the marginal benefit of conventional systemic chemotherapy with the associated significant toxicity. For the more aggressive thyroid cancers, medullary thyroid cancer, poorly differentiated thyroid cancer, and anaplastic thyroid cancer, there are no standard systemic chemotherapy regimens due to the lack of significant response.

Recently, there has been research that has provided greater insight into the molecular pathology of thyroid cancers. It is hoped that, with this improved understanding, new targeted therapies directed against unique cellular abnormalities can be developed into therapeutic options for patients with advanced or aggressive thyroid cancers. Newly developed multi-tyrosine kinase inhibitors, developed for other solid tumors, hold promise in thyroid carcinomas. Greater insight into the molecular pathophysiology of thyroid cancer has also provided hope for redifferentiation of dedifferentiated tumors. Agents of clinical interest include retinoic acid, PPAR-gamma antagonists, demethylating agents, and histone deacytelase inhibitors.

Conventional Systemic Cytotoxic Chemotherapy

Clinical trials define response rate according to the Response Evaluation Criteria in Solid Tumors (RECIST). By RECIST, complete response is the disappearance of all target lesions, while a partial response is at least a 30% decrease in the sum of the longest dimensions. Stable disease is reduction of less than 30% and progression not more than 20% of the sum of the longest dimension.

S.W. Lim (✉)
Department of Medicine and Samuel Oschin
Comprehensive Cancer Center, Cedars-Sinai Medical
Center, 8700 Beverly Boulevard, Room AC-1072,
Los Angeles, CA 90048, USA
e-mail: limsw@cshs.org

G.D. Braunstein (ed.), *Thyroid Cancer*, Endocrine Updates 30,
DOI 10.1007/978-1-4614-0875-8_15, © Springer Science+Business Media, LLC 2012

Progressive disease is an increase of at least 20% of the sum of the longest dimensions [3]. The response rate for systemic chemotherapy in thyroid cancer is relatively low. In a randomized clinical trial of patients with advanced differentiated, medullary, and anaplastic thyroid cancer, single-agent doxorubicin at 60 mg/m^2 given intravenously every 3 weeks had a partial response rate of 17% [4]. Doxorubicin at the same dose combined with cisplatin at 40 mg/m^2 given intravenously every 3 weeks had a complete plus partial response rate of 26%. Of the 43 patients in the combination group, there were six partial responses and five complete responses. Four of the five complete responders survived more than 2 years. The difference in overall response between the two arms was not statistically significant. Side effects included severe hematologic toxicity, nausea, and vomiting, though none were fatal.

Another study of patients with all types of advanced thyroid cancer using doxorubicin at 60 mg/m^2 with cisplatin at 60 mg/m^2 reported only two brief partial responses, for a response rate of 9.1%. There was significant toxicity and one drug-related death [5]. In a single institution's report of their experience over 10 years with various regimens, including single-agent doxorubicin, cisplatin, elliptinium acetate, combination doxorubicin and cisplatin, and combination doxorubicin, etoposide, 5-fluorouracil, and cyclophosphamide, resulted in two objective responses, for a response rate of only 3% [6].

In medullary thyroid cancer, the use of single-agent doxorubicin has been described [7]. In this report of three patients, there was a decrease in the serum calcitonin in one patient while on therapy, but there were no objective radiographic responses. In 20 patients with advanced medullary thyroid cancer treated with alternating doses of 5-fluorouracil with streptozocin and 5-fluorouracil with dacarbazine, there were three partial responses and 11 patients with disease stabilization. Toxicity with this regimen was low [8]. Another small trial, also with 20 patients, substituted the 5-fluorouracil in combination with streptozocin with doxorubicin. The results were nearly identical with three partial responses and

ten patients with stable disease. Toxicity was low and there were no treatment-related deaths [9].

More recently, single-agent oral capecitabine has been described in five patients, three with metastatic medullary thyroid cancer and two with radioiodine-resistant follicular thyroid carcinoma [10]. Two of the three patients with medullary thyroid carcinoma had disease stabilization or regression and both patients with follicular thyroid carcinoma had stable disease.

Poorly differentiated and anaplastic thyroid carcinomas are clinically aggressive cancers with short median survival. When diagnosed at an early stage, management usually involves multimodality therapy including surgery, radiation therapy, and chemotherapy [11–13]. These thyroid carcinomas have very low response rates to systemic chemotherapy. Combination chemotherapy with cisplatin, doxorubicin, etoposide, and peplobycin in ten patients with anaplastic thyroid carcinoma yielded only two partial responses lasting 2 and 3 months, respectively [14]. In patients with anaplastic thyroid carcinoma, continuous infusion paclitaxel over 96 h has been reported to give a 53% total response rate with one complete response rate and nine partial responders out of 19 subjects [15]. In 13 patients with anaplastic thyroid carcinoma, Higashiyama reported an overall response rate of 33% with one complete response and three partial responses [16]. More recently, Kawada et al. described an overall response rate of 14% in seven patients with anaplastic thyroid cancer and a median time to progression of only 6 weeks [17].

Low-dose doxorubicin administered intravenously weekly has been used with concurrent external radiation therapy as a radiosensitizer for locally advanced thyroid carcinoma [18]. There was no increased toxicity compared to radiation therapy alone.

Despite modest response rates in patients with advanced well-differentiated thyroid cancer and in patients with poorly differentiated thyroid cancers, conventional cytotoxic chemotherapy has not shown any improvement in the overall survival in these patients. Another type of systemic therapy is needed for these types of patients.

Targeted Therapy in Oncology

Cytotoxic chemotherapy in the treatment of human malignancy is a nonspecific process. It relies on causing lethal cellular damage in malignant cells that may not have robust repair mechanisms and are more sensitive to apoptosis. Conventional cytotoxic chemotherapy in treating cancer has a narrow therapeutic window. Suboptimal doses have a reduced efficacy, while higher doses have significant toxicity, and may be lethal.

Targeted therapy, delivering an effective drug directly to the malignant cell, has been the goal in order to both improve efficacy and reduce toxicity. An early example of targeted therapy includes radioactive iodine in well-differentiated thyroid cancer. This relies on the unique metabolism of thyroid carcinoma and the uptake of iodine. Other targeted strategies rely on unique proteins on the cancer cells. These include rituximab targeting CD20 on malignant B-cell lymphomas [19] and trastuzumab targeting the epidermal growth factor receptor (EGFR) in women with her2/neu-positive breast cancers [20].

Molecularly Targeted Therapy

Another attractive strategy is to target abnormalities within the cancer that are unique to the malignant cells. Many of these targets are related to cell signaling and cellular proliferation and structural proteins.

The first highly successful use of a small molecule in cancer was imatinib therapy in chronic myelogenous leukemia [21]. Imatinib blocks the ATP-binding site of a constitutively activated tyrosine kinase formed by the translocation of the bcr gene with the abl proto-oncogene. Imatinib is an oral agent and in CML has a response rate of 90% at 5 years and mild manageable side effects. The multikinase inhibitors sorafenib and sunitinib are approved for renal cell carcinoma; sorafenib also is approved in hepatocellular carcinoma. Other molecular targets include vascular endothelial growth factor receptor (VEGFR) and endothelial growth factor receptor (EGFR) in lung and colon cancers.

Molecular Abnormalities in Thyroid Cancer

Differentiated Thyroid Cancers

Papillary Thyroid Cancer

Papillary thyroid cancer comprises 80% of thyroid cancers. Several molecular abnormalities in papillary thyroid cancer have been described. Most mutations found in papillary thyroid carcinoma involve the common signaling pathway involving RET/PTC-RAS-BRAF (see Fig. 15.1). The biological effects of this pathway include changes in the cytoskeleton, cell proliferation, and differentiation [22].

The most common molecular abnormalities in papillary thyroid cancer are in BRAF, occurring in approximately 45% of PTC [23]. BRAF is one of three serine–threonine kinases including ARAF and CRAF/RAF1. Most BRAF mutations are a valine to glutamine substitution at residue 600. These mutations result in the continuous phosphorylation of the downstream mitogen-activated/ERK kinase, MEK [24]; BRAF mutations have a high association with the tall cell variant of papillary thyroid cancer [25]. Mutation in BRAF portends a worse prognosis [26–29].

The second most common molecular abnormality in papillary thyroid cancer are mutations of RET, occurring from 20 to 30% of cases [30]. RET encodes for a transmembrane receptor tyrosine kinase [31]. Mutations of RET are described in multiple endocrine neoplasia type 2 and Hirshprung's disease [32–35]. RET mutations are common in patients with papillary thyroid cancer who have had prior radiation exposure [36–39]. Most of the mutations in RET are chromosomal rearrangement linking the promoter of an unrelated gene to RET resulting in a constitutively activated product.

Abnormalities of RAS are described in 10–20% of cases of papillary thyroid cancer [40, 41]. RAS is a GTPase that functions as a cell signaling protein [42]. It is downstream of many receptor tyrosine kinases, such as RET, and upstream of many cell signaling pathways. RAS mutations are found in both benign and malignant thyroid

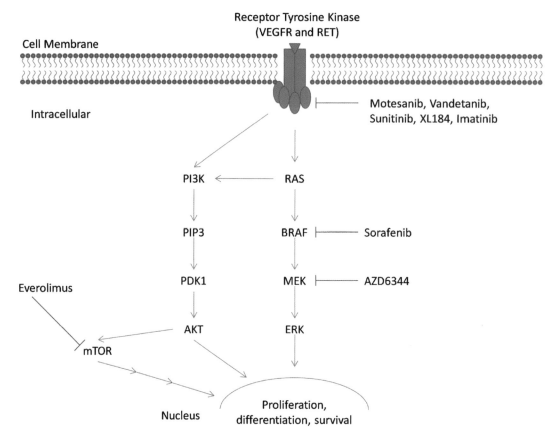

Fig. 15.1 Molecular abnormalities in thyroid carcinoma. Thyroid carcinomas commonly overexpress the receptor tyrosine kinase (RTK) vascular endothelial growth factor (VEGFR). The RTK RET is mutated in nearly all hereditary medullary thyroid carcinomas and in approximately 50% of sporadic medullary thyroid carcinomas. Other common mutations in well-differentiated thyroid carcinoma involve BRAF. Several drugs that are in clinical trials and their mechanism of inhibition are listed

neoplasms [43]. Mutations of RAS are associated with a more aggressive clinical course [44].

These mutations in the RET/PTC-RAS-BRAF pathway appear to mainly be nonoverlapping and mutually exclusive. Therefore, each probably occurs early in oncogenesis.

Follicular Thyroid Cancer

RAS abnormalities are described in 20–50% of follicular thyroid cancer [40, 41, 45–47]. The rate of RAS mutation in follicular thyroid carcinomas has been described as being higher in iodine-deficient areas (50%) versus iodine-sufficient areas (10%) [48]. It is also probably an early occurrence. The RAS mutation is described in high aneuploidy cells. Another abnormality in

follicular thyroid cancer is PAX8-PPARγ (35%) and is associated with t(2;3)(a13;p25) that fuses the promoter of paired box 8 (PAX8) with peroxisome proliferator-activated receptor γ (PPARγ) [46]. These two mutations in follicular thyroid cancer appear to be nonoverlapping.

Medullary Thyroid Cancer

Approximately 25% of medullary thyroid cancers (MTC) are hereditary, associated with the multiple endocrine neoplasias MEN2A and MEN2B 70–80% of the time [49]. The germline mutations predominantly affect RET, located on chromosome 10q11.2. RET encodes a membrane tyrosine kinase receptor. RET affects the downstream pathways RAS/MEK/ERK, PI3K/AKT/

NFkB, p38, MAPK, Jak/STAT, and protein C kinase. RET is mutated in almost 100% of the hereditary MTC and in 50% of the sporadic MTC [50]. The genotypes, grouped into three risk categories based on codon mutation, correlate with clinical aggressiveness [51–53].

Poorly Differentiated and Anaplastic Thyroid Carcinomas

Mutations in BRAF have also been described in poorly differentiated and anaplastic thyroid carcinomas (ATC) [25]. BRAF mutations were found in two (13%) poorly differentiated carcinomas and three (10%) anaplastic thyroid carcinomas. Utilizing microdissection techniques, thyroid cancer specimens containing both well-differentiated papillary areas in one sample of poorly differentiated and one sample of anaplastic thyroid carcinoma were analyzed for BRAF mutations. Both samples were found to contain mutations in the well-differentiated areas and the poorly differentiated and anaplastic components. This suggests that the BRAF mutation was an early clonal event that arose from well-differentiated thyroid cancer before dedifferentiating into a more aggressive subtype.

PIK3CA gene mutations have been described in 23% of ATC [54]. PIK3A encodes the catalytic subunit phosphatidylinositol 3′-kinase (PI3K). When a well-differentiated component is found in association with ATC that is found to have a mutation of PIK3Ca, the well-differentiated tissues do not harbor the mutation. This suggests that this mutation is involved in the dedifferentiation and progression to a more clinically aggressive cancer. Hou et al. described PIK3CA gene alterations, resulting in a gain of copy number, in 20% of differentiated thyroid cancers (28% of follicular thyroid carcinoma and 12% of papillary thyroid carcinoma), 42% of anaplastic thyroid carcinoma, and 17% of benign thyroid adenomas. BRAF mutation was found in 29% of ATC, and 43% of ATC that had a BRAF mutation also had a PI3K/AKT genetic alteration [55]. This suggests a pathogenic role of the PI3K/AKT pathway in the transformation of PTC to ATC.

Mutations in p53 tumor suppressor gene result in loss of function and are implicated in a large number of human cancers. However, mutations in p53 have been described in only approximately 10% thyroid cancer [56, 57]. They are thought to be rare in well-differentiated thyroid carcinomas [58, 59]. P53 mutations may be more prevalent in a subset of anaplastic thyroid carcinomas that are derived from papillary carcinomas with a BRAF mutation [60].

Clinical Trials of Targeted Therapy in Thyroid Cancer

Sorafenib

Sorafenib is an oral multi-kinase inhibitor with multiple targets including BRAF, VEGFR1, and VEGFR2. Sorafenib is currently FDA approved for the treatment of renal cell carcinoma and hepatocellular carcinoma (Table 15.1).

A phase II trial was performed in patients with advanced, iodine-refractory thyroid carcinoma [61]. Thirty patients were enrolled. Papillary and follicular/Hurthle cell were the main subtypes. There were two patients with poorly differentiated/anaplastic and one patient with medullary thyroid carcinoma. Patients received sorafenib 400 mg orally twice a day. Responses were measured radiographically every 2–3 months. The study endpoints included response rate, progression-free survival, and best response by response evaluation criteria in solid tumors. The partial response rate was 23%. The stable disease rate was 53%. The median overall progression-free survival was 79 weeks. There was no significant difference in progression-free survival between follicular and papillary subtypes. Of the 19 patients who had thyroglobulin levels available, 17 (95%) had a marked reduction in their levels. The mean decrease was 70% within 4 months of starting treatment.

Six patients, 20%, withdrew from the study due to adverse events. Dose reductions were required in 47% of the patients and a drug holiday was required in 63% of patients. Side effects were mostly mild and included palmar and plantar erythema, rash, fatigue, stomatitis/mucositis, weight loss, and musculoskeletal pain. More serious

Table 15.1 Results of targeted therapies in clinical trials for thyroid carcinoma

Drug	Target	Phase	Subtype of thyroid cancer	N	Results	References
Sorafenib	BRAF, VEGFR, PDGFR, FLT3, KIT, RET	II	Papillary, follicular, medullary, poorly differentiated	30	PR 23%, SD 53% PD 3%	[61]
		II	Papillary, follicular, medullary, poorly differentiated	56	Of 41 pts with PTC-PR 15%, SD 56%	[62]
		II	Medullary, hereditary and sporadic	21	Sporadic (16 pts)-PR 6.3%, SD 87.5%	[63]
		III	Papillary, follicular		Open to enrollment	
Motesanib	VEGFR, PDGFR, KIT	II	Papillary, Hurthle cell, follicular	93	PR 14%, SD 67%, PD 8%	[64]
		II	Medullary	91	PR 2%, SD 81%, PD 8%	[65]
Axitinib	VEGFR, PDGFR, KIT	II	Papillary, follicular, Hurthle cell, medullary, anaplastic	60	PR 30%, SD 38%, PD 7%	[66]
Vandetanib	RET, VEGFR, EGFR	II	Medullary	30	PR 20%, SD 73%, PD 3%	[67]
Imatinib	Bcr-Abl, PDGFR, KIT, RET	II	Medullary	15	No PR, 4 pts with SD for greater than 24 months	[68]
Sunitinib	PDGFR, VEGFR, FLT3, KIT	Case report	Papillary, follicular	2	Partial metabolic response (1 pt), SD (1 pt)	[70]
Gefitinib	EGFR	II	Papillary, follicular, anaplastic, medullary, Hurthle cell	27	No PR, SD 48%	[72]

VEGFR vascular endothelial growth factor receptor; *PDGFR* platelet derived growth factor receptor; *EGFR* endothelial growth factor receptor; *PR* partial response; *SD* stable disease; *PD* Progressive disease

toxicities included hypertension, rash, weight loss, diarrhea, palmer and plantar erythema, fatigue, pruritus, anorexia, anxiety, and elevated lipase and amylase. The idiosyncratic symptom of palmer–plantar erythema was treated with anti-inflammatory agents, drug interruptions, and dose reductions. Ten patients, 33%, were found to have an increase in the serum TSH level. Overall, sorafenib was effective and well tolerated. It had a clinical benefit rate of 77% in patients with iodine-refractory, metastatic thyroid cancer.

A second trial utilizing sorafenib in 56 patients with metastatic thyroid cancer has been reported [62]. Sorafenib was administered at an initial dose of 400 mg orally twice a day. Of the 41 patients with papillary thyroid cancer, the partial response rate was six of 33 patients, 15%. Clinical benefit, partial responses or stable disease for greater than 6 months was noted in 23 (56%) patients. Sixty-four percent of chemotherapy-naive PTC patients had a thyroglobulin response. The thyroglobulin response did not correlate with the objective response in the 14 patients assessed by PET imaging.

Side effects in this trial were also mild, although 52% of patients required dose reduction. Side effects included hand–foot skin reactions, diarrhea and weight loss, hypertension, fatigue, arthralgia, musculoskeletal chest pain, and mouth pain. Sorafenib is now undergoing a randomized phase III trial in well-differentiated metastatic thyroid cancer.

In a phase II trial, sorafenib has also been studied in patients with metastatic medullary thyroid cancer [63]. In 15 evaluable subjects with spo-radic MTC, there was one (6.3%) partial response and 14 (87.5%) with stable disease. The median progression-free survival was 17.9 months. Toxicities were similar to other trials of sorafenib with thyroid carcinoma, but there was one reported death due to a sepsis-like syndrome and wide-spread *Clostridium* infection of the bowel.

Motesanib

Motesanib is an oral multi-kinase inhibitor that targets the VEGFR1, 2, and 3, platelet-derived growth factor (PDGF), and KIT. It has been stud-ied in phase I trials in patients with advanced solid tumors.

Motesanib was studied in a single-armed, phase II trial of 93 patients, who had progres-sive, locally advanced or metastatic, radioiodine-resistant differentiated thyroid cancer [64]. The major subtype was papillary thyroid cancer. Other subtypes included in the study were follicular and Hurthle cell. The dose of motesanib was 125 mg orally once a day.

Objective response was seen in 13 patients (14%), all who had a partial response. The median time to the response was 15 weeks. Stable disease was seen in 62 patients (67%). Seventy-four per-cent of patients had a decrease in tumor measure-ments from baseline, while 8% of patients had disease progression. There was no obvious differ-ence in response between the histologic subtypes. In 33 patients, tumors were screened for various mutations. There was no association between the presence or absence of the BRAF V600E muta-tion and clinical outcome.

Of the patients who had thyroglobulin mea-sured, 81% had a decrease from baseline during the study. A correlation was observed between a decrease from baseline of 50% or more in thyro-globulin concentration and a tumor response of the target lesions.

Thirteen percent of the patients discontinued the study due to adverse events. The most com-mon side effects were diarrhea, hypertension, and weight loss. Moderate to severe side effects occurred in 55% of the patients. These included

hypocalcemia, hyperuricemia, hypokalemia, cerebral hemorrhage, confusion, agitation, and oliguria. In 22% of the patients an increase in thyrotrophin concentration, hypothyroidism, or both were seen.

Motesanib was also studied in a phase II trial in patients with advanced or metastatic medul-lary thyroid cancer [65]. Motesanib was adminis-tered at 125 mg orally daily. Of the 91 patients, there were two (2%) objective responses and 81% stable disease rate. The median progression-free survival was 48 weeks. The most common side effects were diarrhea, fatigue, hypothyroidism, hyperthyroidism, and anorexia.

Axitinib

Axitinib is an oral inhibitor of VEGFR1, 2, and 3, PDGF, and KIT. A phase I trial of axitinib determined the dose to be 5 mg twice daily. A study of advanced thyroid cancer, of any histology, was conducted in 60 patients [66]. If patients toler-ated the 5 mg twice daily dose, they could be escalated to 7 mg PO twice daily and then to 10 mg twice daily. Half of the patients had papil-lary histology. Follicular and Hurthle cell variant comprised another 25%. There were 18% of patients with medullary thyroid cancer and 3% had anaplastic thyroid cancer. A majority of patients had prior therapy, primarily radiotherapy and radioactive iodine. Fifteen percent had prior chemotherapy and 8% had prior investigational therapy. A partial response was seen in 30% of the patients. Stable disease was seen in another 38%, while 7% had progressive disease. There was no association between the response and the histologic type. Of the responders, 72% had not had progression at the time of the publication of the report. The median progression-free survival was 18.1 months. Seventeen percent of patients discontinued treatment because of lack of effi-cacy and 13% of patients discontinued treatment because of adverse events. The most common side effects included fatigue, diarrhea, nausea, anorexia, hypertension, stomatitis, weight loss, and headache. Of the patients who had med-ullary thyroid carcinoma and had calcitonin measurements, those with a partial response had a marked decrease in calcitonin, patients with stable disease had a slight reduction, and those who had progressive disease had no change in calcitonin concentration. The authors of the study concluded that axitinib was active in all histologic subtypes of metastatic thyroid cancer with the overall response rate of 30%. An additional 38% of patients had stable disease for 16 weeks or more by standard RECIST criteria.

Vandetanib

Vandetanib is an oral inhibitor of the RET kinase. An open-label, phase II, multicenter trial was conducted in 30 patients with locally advanced or metastatic medullary thyroid cancer with a confirmed clinical diagnosis of MEN2A, MEN2B, or familial medullary thyroid cancer and a germline RET mutation [67]. Subjects were given vandetanib 300 mg orally daily. A partial response was seen in six (20%) of the patients. The median duration of response was 10.2 months. Durable, stable disease was seen in 53% of the patients. Disease control, defined as partial response and stable disease, was observed in 73%. There was no association between RET germline mutation and response to vandetanib treatment. A decrease from baseline in serum calcitonin levels was seen in 80% of patients. All six patients who had a partial response by RECIST criteria had a decrease in serum calcitonin ranging from 73 to 99%. Diarrhea was the most commonly reported side effect, and 24 patients required either a dose reduction or an interruption. Adverse affects were usually mild and included diarrhea, fatigue, rash, and nausea. Grade 3 adverse events included QTc prolongation diarrhea, nausea, and hypertension.

Imatinib

Imatinib is a multikinase inhibitor affecting bcr-abl, PDGFRa, PDGFRb, c-FMS, KIT, and RET. It is FDA approved for the treatment of chronic myelogenous leukemia, Philadelphia chromosome–positive acute lymphoblastic leukemia, and gastrointestinal stromal tumors. Imatinib was administered in a phase II trial to 15 patients with metastatic medullary thyroid carcinoma [68]. There were no objective responses, but four patients had stable disease over 24 months. Side effects included fatigue, nausea, rash, and malaise. The dose of thyroid hormone supplementation needed to be escalated due to hypothyroidism in nine patients.

Sunitinib

Sunitinib is a selective oral tyrosine kinase inhibitor of PDGFR, VGFR, fms-like tyrosine kinase (flt3), and KIT. It is currently FDA approved for the treatment of advanced renal cell carcinoma. Sunitinib has shown in vitro inhibitory activity against RET/papillary thyroid cancer kinases [69]. In a phase I trial, two patients, one with papillary thyroid carcinoma and the other with follicular thyroid carcinoma, had sustained clinical response to sunitinib [70]. In a case report, a patient with metastatic medullary thyroid carcinoma who received sunitinib had resolution of diarrhea, reduction in size and number of pulmonary metastasis, and reduction in serum calcitonin and carcinoembryonic antigen levels [71].

Gefitinib

Gefitinib is an oral inhibitor of the tyrosine kinase domain of VEGFR. Gefitinib is indicated for patients with locally advanced or metastatic non-small-cell lung cancer. Twenty-seven patients were studied in an open-label phase II trial [72]. Histologic subtypes included papillary, follicular, anaplastic, medullary, and Hurthle cell carcinomas. No objective responses were seen. Stable disease was reported in 48%, 24%, and 12% of subjects at 3, 6, and 12 months, respectively. The median progression-free survival was 3.7 months and the overall survival was 17.5 months. Five patients with stable disease had a reduction of greater than 90% from baseline for at least 3 months.

XL184

XL184 is a tyrosine kinase inhibitor that targets primarily MET, VEGFR2, and RET, and also has activity against KIT and flt3. It is currently in early clinical trials in patients with advanced solid tumors including glioblastoma multiforme [73]. A phase I trial with XL184 in 55 patients, 13 with medullary thyroid carcinoma, reported reductions in serum calcitonin and some objective responses along with stabilization of disease [74]. Toxicity included palmar/plantar erythema, abnormalities of liver function, mucositis, and diarrhea. Sixty percent of patients had no drug-related toxicity greater than grade 1. XL184 is currently in phase III trials in patients with medullary thyroid carcinoma [75].

AZD6244

AZD6244 is a specific inhibitor of the MAPK kinases, MEK1 and MEK2, which are immediately downstream of BRAF. AZD6244 causes growth inhibition of thyroid carcinoma cell lines, with greater inhibition of lines with BRAF mutations compared to wild type [76]. AZD6244 was studied in a phase I trial with 57 patients having advanced cancers [77]. Nine patients were reported to have stable disease for greater than 5 months, including one patient with thyroid carcinoma who had stable disease for 19 months. Rash was the most common dose-limiting toxicity.

Everolimus

Everolimus (RAD001) is an inhibitor of mammalian target of rapamycin (mTOR), a kinase that is downstream of PI3K. Everolimus is approved for use in advanced renal cell carcinoma and is being studied in other solid tumors. Dose-dependent growth inhibition has been described in anaplastic thyroid carcinoma cell lines [78]. Clinical trials of everolimus in thyroid carcinoma are ongoing.

Other Targeted Therapies in Early Clinical Trials

Redifferentiation Therapy

Retinoic Acid

A case of the spontaneous reappearance of ^{131}iodine uptake in a patient who previously had low ^{131}iodine uptake was described by Oyen in 1995 [79]. Retinoids have been used in re-differentiation therapy in acute promyelocytic leukemia and in solid tumors. Retinoic acid has been shown to re-differentiate thyroid carcinoma cell lines [80]. This phenomenon appears to be mediated by the upregulation of the sodium/iodide symporter by retinoic acid [81, 82].

Clinically, Simon et al. described the administration of 13-cis retinoic acid to ten subjects with advanced thyroid carcinoma [83]. Four of the ten had renewed uptake of radioiodine that allowed for further radioiodine therapy. Since that first clinical report, others have described mixed response to retinoic acid re-differentiation therapy and an uncertain impact on overall outcome [84–92].

Rosiglitazone

Peroxisome proliferator-activated receptors (PPAR) are nuclear receptor proteins that function as transcription factors. The thiazolidinediones have shown antiproliferative activity in human follicular and anaplastic thyroid carcinoma cell lines [93, 94]. The thiazolidinedione, rosiglitazone, is a PPAR agonist and is approved for use as a hypoglycemic agent in patients with diabetes mellitus. Patients with high expression of PPARγ may undergo redifferentiation of their thyroid carcinoma by the administration of rosiglitazone [95]. Kebebrew described 5 of 20 patients who failed to take up iodine having positive radioiodine scans following rosiglitazone treatment [96]. Clinical trials with rosiglitazone in differentiated thyroid carcinoma are ongoing.

Azacitidine

Epigenetics describes the silencing of genes through methylation of cytosine in cytosine–guanine pairs comprising CpG islands. Thyroid transcription factor-1 (TTF-1) is expressed in both normal thyroid tissue and well-differentiated thyroid carcinomas. TTF-1 expression is lost in undifferentiated thyroid carcinomas. The decreased production of TTF-1 is correlated with increased methylation in the CpG of the TTF-1 promoter [97]. The DNA demethylating agent 5-aza-deoxycitidine was able to restore TTF-1 expression in thyroid carcinoma cell lines. Restoration of radioactive iodine uptake in human thyroid cancer cell lines has been demonstrated by the activation of sodium–iodine symporter gene transcription by a combination of 5-azacitidine and sodium butyrate [98]. Azacitidine (5-azacitidine) is active in the therapy of myelodysplastic syndromes [99]. Azacitidine has been studied in a phase I trial of patients with advanced cancers, including thyroid carcinoma, in conjunction with valproic acid [100].

Histone Deacetylase Inhibitors

Histone deacetylase (HDAC) plays a role in regulating gene expression by tightly coiling chromatin. HDAC inhibitor may reverse the silencing of tumor suppressor genes and allow transcription of antigrowth and proapoptotic genes. HDAC inhibitors, such as suberoylanilide hydroxamic acid (SAHA), have been found to have in vitro and in vivo activity against thyroid cancer cell lines [101–104]. In a phase II trial, 19 patients with differentiated and medullary thyroid carcinoma received oral vorinostat [105]. No patient had a partial or complete response. Adverse events included fatigue, dehydration, ataxia, deep vein thrombosis, and severe thrombocytopenia. Other trials with HDAC inhibitors in thyroid cancer are ongoing.

Antiangiogenic Agents

Several antiangiogenic agents have been studied in thyroid carcinoma. Thalidomide is an immunomodulatory agent with antiangiogenic properties and is very active in patients with multiple myeloma. Thalidomide's activity in patients with thyroid carcinoma has been reported [106]. In 28

of 36 evaluable subjects, there were five (18%) patients with a partial response and nine (32%) with stable disease. The median PR duration was 4 months and the SD duration was 6 months. The most common side effect was fatigue. Other side effects included infection, one pericardial effusion, and one pulmonary embolus.

Combretastastin A4 phosphate (fosbretabulin) is a novel antiangiogenic agent that preferentially inhibits blood flow through the blood vessels of malignant tumors. It has shown activity against anaplastic and medullary thyroid cancer when used in combination with chemotherapy in vitro [107] and in vivo in a mouse model [108, 109]. A phase II trial of single-agent fosbretabulin in 26 patients with advanced anaplastic thyroid carcinoma reported stable disease in seven patients with a median duration of response of 12.3 months [110]. There were no objective responses seen. Toxicity included QTc prolongation causing delay and discontinuation of therapy. Other trials with fosbretabulin are ongoing.

Other Issues in Targeted Therapy

Limitations of RECIST in Thyroid Cancer

As noted, the efficacy of chemotherapy in the treatment of solid tumors has been standardized by using the RECIST criteria. This defines the measurement criteria for a given response such as complete response, partial response, stable disease, and progression, but these criteria may be too stringent for thyroid cancer.

Prior studies with the tyrosine kinase inhibitors in thyroid cancer have shown only very few partial responses and very rare complete responses by RECIST. The majority of these patients appear to have stable disease by RECIST. In studies with hepatocellular carcinoma, a majority of patients also had stable disease that correlated with improvement in overall survival. Some of the radiographic studies utilizing CT were able to show central necrosis despite no obvious reduction by bi-dimensional measurements.

The dilemma for the future of clinical trials using TKIs in thyroid cancer is finding an appropriate endpoint besides the classical reduction in tumor size by RECIST [111]. Ideally, overall survival would be the gold-standard measurement for the efficacy of an antineoplastic agent. Given the long and variable natural course of untreated metastatic radioiodine-refractory thyroid cancer trials utilizing overall survival would need to occur over many years, even possibly decades. For thyroid cancer studies utilizing TKIs, one may need to use less desirable outcome measures including partial response, stable disease, and progression-free survival.

One must also balance efficacy against side effects. Many patients, if not most, are relatively asymptomatic from their metastatic disease. Only those with a large tumor burden, particularly metastatic bone or lung disease, are truly symptomatic. Although the TKIs has a much lower side-effect profile compared to chemotherapy, in an otherwise asymptomatic population, even this degree of adverse events may not be acceptable.

Thyroidal Effects of TKIs

The administration of TKIs may induce hypothyroidism [112]. De Groot described a series of patients who had had thyroidectomy and were on levothyroxine who then received imatinib and subsequently developed hypothyroidism [68]. In several of the clinical trials described above hypothyroidism was reported. If further clinical trials show that targeted therapy with the tyrosine kinase inhibitors is active in various histologies for thyroid cancer, clinicians will need to be aware of this effect. In a recent review of TKI-related hypothyroidism, the authors recommended monitoring TFTs before and during TKI therapy, including during the first few weeks of therapy and then monthly [113].

Summary

The therapeutic options for patients with advanced thyroid carcinoma have been limited due to poor efficacy and relatively high toxicity. Recently, great strides have been made to elucidate the molecular abnormalities in the various histologies of thyroid carcinomas. This greater under-

standing into thyroid carcinoma pathophysiology has provided the ability to rationally select new agents for clinical trials utilizing drugs that target these known cellular abnormalities. Several early-phase clinical trials across all subtypes of thyroid carcinoma have shown clinical response, specifically stabilization of disease. Unfortunately, response by conventional RECIST criteria has been low. Long-term improvements in outcomes, such as overall survival, have not yet been proven. The new agents studied in these clinical trials, primarily orally administered kinase inhibitors, have had mild, predictable, and reversible toxicities. Phase III trials with some of these agents are currently underway. Results of clinical trials utilizing other approaches, including antiangiogenesis agents and redifferentiating agents, are pending completion and publication.

References

1. Passler C, Scheuba C, Prager G, et al. Prognostic factors of papillary and follicular thyroid cancer: differences in an iodine-replete endemic goiter region. Endocr Relat Cancer. 2004;11(1):131–9.
2. Wang W, Larson SM, Fazzari M, et al. Prognostic value of [18F]fluorodeoxyglucose positron emission tomographic scanning in patients with thyroid cancer. J Clin Endocrinol Metab. 2000;85(3):1107–13.
3. Eisenhauer EA, Therasse P, Bogaerts J, et al. New response evaluation criteria in solid tumours: revised RECIST guideline (version 1.1). Eur J Cancer. 2009; 45(2):228–47.
4. Shimaoka K, Schoenfeld DA, DeWys WD, Creech RH, DeConti R. A randomized trial of doxorubicin versus doxorubicin plus cisplatin in patients with advanced thyroid carcinoma. Cancer. 1985;56(9): 2155–60.
5. Williams SD, Birch R, Einhorn LH. Phase II evaluation of doxorubicin plus cisplatin in advanced thyroid cancer: a Southeastern Cancer Study Group Trial. Cancer Treat Rep. 1986;70(3):405–7.
6. Droz JP, Schlumberger M, Rougier P, Ghosn M, Gardet P, Parmentier C. Chemotherapy in metastatic nonanaplastic thyroid cancer: experience at the Institut Gustave-Roussy. Tumori. 1990;76(5):480–3.
7. Husain M, Alsever RN, Lock JP, George WF, Katz FH. Failure of medullary carcinoma of the thyroid to respond to doxorubicin therapy. Horm Res. 1978;9(1):22–5.
8. Schlumberger M, Abdelmoumene N, Delisle MJ, Couette JE. Treatment of advanced medullary thyroid cancer with an alternating combination of 5 FU-streptozocin and 5 FU-dacarbazine. The Groupe d'Etude des Tumeurs a Calcitonine (GETC). Br J Cancer. 1995;71(2):363–5.

9. Nocera M, Baudin E, Pellegriti G, Cailleux AF, Mechelany-Corone C, Schlumberger M. Treatment of advanced medullary thyroid cancer with an alternating combination of doxorubicin-streptozocin and 5 FU-dacarbazine. Groupe d'Etude des Tumeurs a Calcitonine (GETC). Br J Cancer. 2000;83(6): 715–8.

10. Gilliam LK, Kohn AD, Lalani T, et al. Capecitabine therapy for refractory metastatic thyroid carcinoma: a case series. Thyroid. 2006;16(8):801–10.

11. Haigh PI, Ituarte PH, Wu HS, et al. Completely resected anaplastic thyroid carcinoma combined with adjuvant chemotherapy and irradiation is associated with prolonged survival. Cancer. 2001;91(12):2335–42.

12. Busnardo B, Daniele O, Pelizzo MR, et al. A multimodality therapeutic approach in anaplastic thyroid carcinoma: study on 39 patients. J Endocrinol Invest. 2000;23(11):755–61.

13. De Crevoisier R, Baudin E, Bachelot A, et al. Combined treatment of anaplastic thyroid carcinoma with surgery, chemotherapy, and hyperfractionated accelerated external radiotherapy. Int J Radiat Oncol Biol Phys. 2004;60(4):1137–43.

14. Chemotherapy Committee, The Japanese Society of Thyroid Surgery. Intensive chemotherapy for anaplastic thyroid carcinoma: combination of cisplatin, doxorubicin, etoposide and peplomycin with granulocyte granulocyte colony-stimulating factor support. Jpn J Clin Oncol. 1995;25(5):203–7.

15. Ain KB, Egorin MJ, DeSimone PA. Treatment of anaplastic thyroid carcinoma with paclitaxel: phase 2 trial using ninety-six-hour infusion. Collaborative Anaplastic Thyroid Cancer Health Intervention Trials (CATCHIT) Group. Thyroid. 2000;10(7):587–94.

16. Higashiyama T, Ito Y, Hirokawa M, et al. Induction chemotherapy with weekly paclitaxel administration for anaplastic thyroid carcinoma. Thyroid. 2010;20(1): 7–14.

17. Kawada K, Kitagawa K, Kamei S, et al. The feasibility study of docetaxel in patients with anaplastic thyroid cancer. Jpn J Clin Oncol. 2010;40(6):596–9.

18. Kim JH, Leeper RD. Treatment of locally advanced thyroid carcinoma with combination doxorubicin and radiation therapy. Cancer. 1987;60(10):2372–5.

19. Schulz H, Bohlius J, Skoetz N, et al. Chemotherapy plus Rituximab versus chemotherapy alone for B-cell non-Hodgkin's lymphoma. Cochrane Database Syst Rev. 2007;(4):Cd003805.

20. Cobleigh MA, Vogel CL, Tripathy D, et al. Multinational study of the efficacy and safety of humanized anti-HER2 monoclonal antibody in women who have HER2-overexpressing metastatic breast cancer that has progressed after chemotherapy for metastatic disease. J Clin Oncol. 1999;17(9):2639–48.

21. Druker BJ, Guilhot F, O'Brien SG, et al. Five-year follow-up of patients receiving imatinib for chronic myeloid leukemia. N Engl J Med. 2006;355(23): 2408–17.

22. van Weering DH, Bos JL. Signal transduction by the receptor tyrosine kinase Ret. Recent Results Cancer Res. 1998;154:271–81.

23. Kimura ET, Nikiforova MN, Zhu Z, Knauf JA, Nikiforov YE, Fagin JA. High prevalence of BRAF mutations in thyroid cancer: genetic evidence for constitutive activation of the RET/PTC-RAS-BRAF signaling pathway in papillary thyroid carcinoma. Cancer Res. 2003;63(7):1454–7.

24. Giordano TJ, Kuick R, Thomas DG, et al. Molecular classification of papillary thyroid carcinoma: distinct BRAF, RAS, and RET/PTC mutation-specific gene expression profiles discovered by DNA microarray analysis. Oncogene. 2005;24(44):6646–56.

25. Nikiforova MN, Kimura ET, Gandhi M, et al. BRAF mutations in thyroid tumors are restricted to papillary carcinomas and anaplastic or poorly differentiated carcinomas arising from papillary carcinomas. J Clin Endocrinol Metab. 2003;88(11):5399–404.

26. Elisei R, Ugolini C, Viola D, et al. BRAF(V600E) mutation and outcome of patients with papillary thyroid carcinoma: a 15-year median follow-up study. J Clin Endocrinol Metab. 2008;93(10):3943–9.

27. Xing M, Westra WH, Tufano RP, et al. BRAF mutation predicts a poorer clinical prognosis for papillary thyroid cancer. J Clin Endocrinol Metab. 2005;90(12): 6373–9.

28. Lupi C, Giannini R, Ugolini C, et al. Association of BRAF V600E mutation with poor clinicopathological outcomes in 500 consecutive cases of papillary thyroid carcinoma. J Clin Endocrinol Metab. 2007;92(11): 4085–90.

29. Kebebew E, Weng J, Bauer J, et al. The prevalence and prognostic value of BRAF mutation in thyroid cancer. Ann Surg. 2007;246(3):466–70. discussion 470–471.

30. Nikiforov YE. RET/PTC rearrangement in thyroid tumors. Endocr Pathol. 2002;13(1):3–16.

31. Jhiang SM. The RET proto-oncogene in human cancers. Oncogene. 2000;19(49):5590–7.

32. Miya A, Yamamoto M, Morimoto H, et al. Expression of the ret proto-oncogene in human medullary thyroid carcinomas and pheochromocytomas of MEN 2A. Henry Ford Hosp Med J. 1992;40(3–4):215–9.

33. Donis-Keller H, Dou S, Chi D, et al. Mutations in the RET proto-oncogene are associated with MEN 2A and FMTC. Hum Mol Genet. 1993;2(7):851–6.

34. Edery P, Lyonnet S, Mulligan LM, et al. Mutations of the RET proto-oncogene in Hirschsprung's disease. Nature. 1994;367(6461):378–80.

35. Romeo G, Ronchetto P, Luo Y, et al. Point mutations affecting the tyrosine kinase domain of the RET proto-oncogene in Hirschsprung's disease. Nature. 1994;367(6461):377–8.

36. Klugbauer S, Lengfelder E, Demidchik EP, Rabes HM. High prevalence of RET rearrangement in thyroid tumors of children from Belarus after the Chernobyl reactor accident. Oncogene. 1995;11(12):2459–67.

37. Fugazzola L, Pilotti S, Pinchera A, et al. Oncogenic rearrangements of the RET proto-oncogene in papillary thyroid carcinomas from children exposed to the Chernobyl nuclear accident. Cancer Res. 1995;55(23): 5617–20.

38. Bounacer A, Wicker R, Caillou B, et al. High prevalence of activating ret proto-oncogene rearrange-

ments, in thyroid tumors from patients who had received external radiation. Oncogene. 1997;15(11): 1263–73.

39. Rabes HM, Klugbauer S. Molecular genetics of childhood papillary thyroid carcinomas after irradiation: high prevalence of RET rearrangement. Recent Results Cancer Res. 1998;154:248–64.

40. Lemoine NR, Mayall ES, Wyllie FS, et al. Activated Ras oncogenes in human thyroid cancers. Cancer Res. 1988;48(16):4459–63.

41. Wright PA, Lemoine NR, Mayall ES, et al. Papillary and follicular thyroid carcinomas show a different pattern of Ras oncogene mutation. Br J Cancer. 1989; 60(4):576–7.

42. Stites EC, Ravichandran KS. A systems perspective of Ras signaling in cancer. Clin Cancer Res. 2009;15(5): 1510–3.

43. Namba H, Rubin SA, Fagin JA. Point mutations of Ras oncogenes are an early event in thyroid tumorigenesis. Mol Endocrinol. 1990;4(10):1474–9.

44. Zhu Z, Gandhi M, Nikiforova MN, Fischer AH, Nikiforov YE. Molecular profile and clinical-pathologic features of the follicular variant of papillary thyroid carcinoma. An unusually high prevalence of Ras mutations. Am J Clin Pathol. 2003;120(1):71–7.

45. Vasko V, Ferrand M, Di Cristofaro J, Carayon P, Henry JF, de Micco C. Specific pattern of RAS oncogene mutations in follicular thyroid tumors. J Clin Endocrinol Metab. 2003;88(6):2745–52.

46. Nikiforova MN, Lynch RA, Biddinger PW, et al. RAS point mutations and PAX8-PPAR gamma rearrangement in thyroid tumors: evidence for distinct molecular pathways in thyroid follicular carcinoma. J Clin Endocrinol Metab. 2003;88(5):2318–26.

47. Liu R-T, Hou C-Y, You H-L, et al. Selective occurrence of Ras mutations in benign and malignant thyroid follicular neoplasms in Taiwan. Thyroid. 2004; 14(8):616–21.

48. Shi YF, Zou MJ, Schmidt H, et al. High rates of Ras codon 61 mutation in thyroid tumors in an iodide-deficient area. Cancer Res. 1991;51(10):2690–3.

49. Lodish MB, Stratakis CA. RET oncogene in MEN2, MEN2B, MTC and other forms of thyroid cancer. Expert Rev Anticancer Ther. 2008;8(4):625–32.

50. Cerrato A, De Falco V, Santoro M. Molecular genetics of medullary thyroid carcinoma: the quest for novel therapeutic targets. J Mol Endocrinol. 2009;43(4): 143–55.

51. Szinnai G, Meier C, Komminoth P, Zumsteg UW. Review of multiple endocrine neoplasia type 2A in children: therapeutic results of early thyroidectomy and prognostic value of codon analysis. Pediatrics. 2003;111(2):E132–9.

52. Frank-Raue K, Buhr H, Dralle H, et al. Long-term outcome in 46 gene carriers of hereditary medullary thyroid carcinoma after prophylactic thyroidectomy: impact of individual RET genotype. Eur J Endocrinol. 2006;155(2):229–36.

53. Machens A, Dralle H. Genotype-phenotype based surgical concept of hereditary medullary thyroid carcinoma. World J Surg. 2007;31(5):957–68.

54. Garcia-Rostan G, Costa AM, Pereira-Castro I, et al. Mutation of the PIK3CA gene in anaplastic thyroid cancer. Cancer Res. 2005;65(22):10199–207.

55. Hou P, Liu D, Shan Y, et al. Genetic alterations and their relationship in the phosphatidylinositol 3-kinase/ Akt pathway in thyroid cancer. Clin Cancer Res. 2007;13(4):1161–70.

56. Olivier M, Eeles R, Hollstein M, Khan MA, Harris CC, Hainaut P. The IARC TP53 database: new online mutation analysis and recommendations to users. Hum Mutat. 2002;19(6):607–14.

57. Malaguarnera R, Vella V, Vigneri R, Frasca F. p53 family proteins in thyroid cancer. Endocr Relat Cancer. 2007;14(1):43–60.

58. Salvatore D, Celetti A, Fabien N, et al. Low frequency of p53 mutations in human thyroid tumours; p53 and Ras mutation in two out of fifty-six thyroid tumours. Eur J Endocrinol. 1996;134(2):177–83.

59. Wyllie FS, Haughton MF, Rowson JM, Wynford-Thomas D. Human thyroid cancer cells as a source of iso-genic, iso-phenotypic cell lines with or without functional p53. Br J Cancer. 1999;79(7–8):1111–20.

60. Quiros RM, Ding HG, Gattuso P, Prinz RA, Xu X. Evidence that one subset of anaplastic thyroid carcinomas are derived from papillary carcinomas due to BRAF and p53 mutations. Cancer. 2005;103(11): 2261–8.

61. Gupta-Abramson V, Troxel AB, Nellore A, et al. Phase II trial of sorafenib in advanced thyroid cancer. J Clin Oncol. 2008;26(29):4714–9.

62. Kloos RT, Ringel MD, Knopp MV, et al. Phase II trial of sorafenib in metastatic thyroid cancer. J Clin Oncol. 2009;27(10):1675–84.

63. Lam ET, Ringel MD, Kloos RT, et al. Phase II clinical trial of sorafenib in metastatic medullary thyroid cancer. J Clin Oncol. 2010;28(14):2323–30.

64. Sherman SI, Wirth LJ, Droz J-P, et al. Motesanib diphosphate in progressive differentiated thyroid cancer. N Engl J Med. 2008;359(1):31–42.

65. Schlumberger MJ, Elisei R, Bastholt L, et al. Phase II study of safety and efficacy of motesanib in patients with progressive or symptomatic, advanced or metastatic medullary thyroid cancer. J Clin Oncol. 2009;27(23):3794–801.

66. Cohen EEW, Rosen LS, Vokes EE, et al. Axitinib is an active treatment for all histologic subtypes of advanced thyroid cancer: results from a phase II study. J Clin Oncol. 2008;26(29):4708–13.

67. Wells SAJ, Gosnell JE, Gagel RF, et al. Vandetanib for the treatment of patients with locally advanced or metastatic hereditary medullary thyroid cancer. J Clin Oncol. 2010;28(5):767–72.

68. de Groot JWB, Zonnenberg BA, van Ufford-Mannesse PQ, et al. A phase II trial of imatinib therapy for metastatic medullary thyroid carcinoma. J Clin Endocrinol Metab. 2007;92(9):3466–9.

69. Kim DW, Jo YS, Jung HS, et al. An orally administered multitarget tyrosine kinase inhibitor, SU11248, is a novel potent inhibitor of thyroid oncogenic RET/ papillary thyroid cancer kinases. J Clin Endocrinol Metab. 2006;91(10):4070–6.

70. Dawson S-J, Conus NM, Toner GC, et al. Sustained clinical responses to tyrosine kinase inhibitor sunitinib in thyroid carcinoma. Anticancer Drugs. 2008; 19(5):547–52.

71. Kelleher FC, McDermott R. Response to sunitinib in medullary thyroid cancer. Ann Intern Med. 2008; 148(7):567.

72. Pennell NA, Daniels GH, Haddad RI, et al. A phase II study of gefitinib in patients with advanced thyroid cancer. Thyroid. 2008;18(3):317–23.

73. De Groot JF, Prados M, Urquhart T, Robertson S, Yaron Y, Sorensen AG, et al. A phase II study of XL184 in patients (pts) with progressive glioblastoma multiforme (GBM) in first or second relapse. J Clin Oncol. 2009;27:15s; abstr 2047.

74. Salgia R, Sherman S, Hong DS, Ng CS, Frye J, Janisch L, et al. A phase I study of XL184, a RET, VEGFR2, and MET kinase inhibitor, in patients (pts) with advanced malignancies, including pts with medullary thyroid cancer (MTC). J Clin Oncol. 2008;26:15S; abstr 3522.

75. Zhang Y, Guessous F, Kofman A, Schiff D, Abounader R. XL-184, a MET, VEGFR-2 and RET kinase inhibitor for the treatment of thyroid cancer, glioblastoma multiforme and NSCLC. IDrugs. 2010;13(2):112–21.

76. Ball DW, Jin N, Rosen DM, et al. Selective growth inhibition in BRAF mutant thyroid cancer by the mitogen-activated protein kinase kinase 1/2 inhibitor AZD6244. J Clin Endocrinol Metab. 2007;92(12): 4712–8.

77. Adjei AA, Cohen RB, Franklin W, et al. Phase I pharmacokinetic and pharmacodynamic study of the oral, small-molecule mitogen-activated protein kinase kinase 1/2 inhibitor AZD6244 (ARRY-142886) in patients with advanced cancers. J Clin Oncol. 2008;26(13):2139–46.

78. Papewalis C, Wuttke M, Schinner S, et al. Role of the novel mTOR inhibitor RAD001 (everolimus) in anaplastic thyroid cancer. Horm Metab Res. 2009;41(10): 752–6.

79. Oyen WJ, Mudde AH, van den Broek WJ, Corstens FH. Metastatic follicular carcinoma of the thyroid: reappearance of radioiodine uptake. J Nucl Med. 1995;36(4):613–5.

80. Schmutzler C, Brtko J, Bienert K, Kohrle J. Effects of retinoids and role of retinoic acid receptors in human thyroid carcinomas and cell lines derived therefrom. Exp Clin Endocrinol Diabetes. 1996;104 Suppl 4:16–9.

81. Schmutzler C, Winzer R, Meissner-Weigl J, Kohrle J. Retinoic acid increases sodium/iodide symporter mRNA levels in human thyroid cancer cell lines and suppresses expression of functional symporter in non-transformed FRTL-5 rat thyroid cells. Biochem Biophys Res Commun. 1997;240(3):832–8.

82. Jeong H, Kim Y-R, Kim K-N, Choe J-G, Chung J-K, Kim M-K. Effect of all-trans retinoic acid on sodium/iodide symporter expression, radioiodine uptake and gene expression profiles in a human anaplastic thyroid carcinoma cell line. Nucl Med Biol. 2006;33(7): 875–82.

83. Simon D, Kohrle J, Schmutzler C, Mainz K, Reiners C, Roher HD. Redifferentiation therapy of differentiated thyroid carcinoma with retinoic acid: basics and first clinical results. Exp Clin Endocrinol Diabetes. 1996;104 Suppl 4:13–5.

84. Grunwald F, Menzel C, Bender H, et al. Redifferentiation therapy-induced radioiodine uptake in thyroid cancer. J Nucl Med. 1998;39(11):1903–6.

85. Grunwald F, Pakos E, Bender H, et al. Redifferentiation therapy with retinoic acid in follicular thyroid cancer. J Nucl Med. 1998;39(9):1555–8.

86. Simon D, Korber C, Krausch M, et al. Clinical impact of retinoids in redifferentiation therapy of advanced thyroid cancer: final results of a pilot study. Eur J Nucl Med Mol Imaging. 2002;29(6):775–82.

87. Gruning T, Tiepolt C, Zophel K, Bredow J, Kropp J, Franke W-G. Retinoic acid for redifferentiation of thyroid cancer – does it hold its promise? Eur J Endocrinol. 2003;148(4):395–402.

88. Coelho SM, Corbo R, Buescu A, Carvalho DP, Vaisman M. Retinoic acid in patients with radioiodine non-responsive thyroid carcinoma. J Endocrinol Invest. 2004;27(4):334–9.

89. Coelho SM, Vaisman M, Carvalho DP. Tumour redifferentiation effect of retinoic acid: a novel therapeutic approach for advanced thyroid cancer. Curr Pharm Des. 2005;11(19):2525–31.

90. Courbon F, Zerdoud S, Bastie D, et al. Defective efficacy of retinoic acid treatment in patients with metastatic thyroid carcinoma. Thyroid. 2006;16(10):1025–31.

91. Fernandez CA, Puig-Domingo M, Lomena F, et al. Effectiveness of retinoic acid treatment for redifferentiation of thyroid cancer in relation to recovery of radioiodine uptake. J Endocrinol Invest. 2009;32(3):228–33.

92. Handkiewicz-Junak D, Roskosz J, Hasse-Lazar K, et al. 13-cis-retinoic acid re-differentiation therapy and recombinant human thyrotropin-aided radioiodine treatment of non-functional metastatic thyroid cancer: a single-center, 53-patient phase 2 study. Thyroid Res. 2009;2(1):8.

93. Bonofiglio D, Qi H, Gabriele S, et al. Peroxisome proliferator-activated receptor gamma inhibits follicular and anaplastic thyroid carcinoma cells growth by upregulating p21Cip1/WAF1 gene in a Sp1-dependent manner. Endocr Relat Cancer. 2008;15(2):545–57.

94. Antonelli A, Ferrari SM, Fallahi P, et al. Thiazolidinediones and antiblastics in primary human anaplastic thyroid cancer cells. Clin Endocrinol (Oxf). 2009;70(6):946–53.

95. Tepmongkol S, Keelawat S, Honsawek S, Ruangvejvorachai P. Rosiglitazone effect on radioiodine uptake in thyroid carcinoma patients with high thyroglobulin but negative total body scan: a correlation with the expression of peroxisome proliferator-activated receptor-gamma. Thyroid. 2008;18(7):697–704.

96. Kebebew E, Lindsay S, Clark OH, Woeber KA, Hawkins R, Greenspan FS. Results of rosiglitazone therapy in patients with thyroglobulin-positive and radioiodine-negative advanced differentiated thyroid cancer. Thyroid. 2009;19(9):953–6.

97. Kondo T, Nakazawa T, Ma D, et al. Epigenetic silencing of TTF-1/NKX2-1 through DNA hypermethylation and histone H3 modulation in thyroid carcinomas. Lab Invest. 2009;89(7):791–9.

98. Li W, Venkataraman GM, Ain KB. Protein synthesis inhibitors, in synergy with 5-azacytidine, restore sodium/iodide symporter gene expression in human thyroid adenoma cell line, KAK-1, suggesting transactive transcriptional repressor. J Clin Endocrinol Metab. 2007;92(3):1080–7.

99. Silverman LR, Demakos EP, Peterson BL, et al. Randomized controlled trial of azacitidine in patients with the myelodysplastic syndrome: a study of the cancer and leukemia group B. J Clin Oncol. 2002; 20(10):2429–40.

100. Braiteh F, Soriano AO, Garcia-Manero G, et al. Phase I study of epigenetic modulation with 5-azacytidine and valproic acid in patients with advanced cancers. Clin Cancer Res. 2008;14(19):6296–301.

101. Mitsiades CS, Poulaki V, McMullan C, et al. Novel histone deacetylase inhibitors in the treatment of thyroid cancer. Clin Cancer Res. 2005;11(10):3958–65.

102. Luong QT, O'Kelly J, Braunstein GD, Hershman JM, Koeffler HP. Antitumor activity of suberoylanilide hydroxamic acid against thyroid cancer cell lines in vitro and in vivo. Clin Cancer Res. 2006;12(18):5570–7.

103. Ning L, Jaskula-Sztul R, Kunnimalaiyaan M, Chen H. Suberoyl bishydroxamic acid activates notch1 signaling and suppresses tumor progression in an animal model of medullary thyroid carcinoma. Ann Surg Oncol. 2008;15(9):2600–5.

104. Borbone E, Berlingieri MT, De Bellis F, et al. Histone deacetylase inhibitors induce thyroid cancer-specific apoptosis through proteasome-dependent inhibition of TRAIL degradation. Oncogene. 2010;29(1):105–16.

105. Woyach JA, Kloos RT, Ringel MD, et al. Lack of therapeutic effect of the histone deacetylase inhibitor vorinostat in patients with metastatic radioiodine-refractory thyroid carcinoma. J Clin Endocrinol Metab. 2009;94(1):164–70.

106. Ain KB, Lee C, Williams KD. Phase II trial of thalidomide for therapy of radioiodine-unresponsive and rapidly progressive thyroid carcinomas. Thyroid. 2007;17(7):663–70.

107. Dziba JM, Marcinek R, Venkataraman G, Robinson JA, Ain KB. Combretastatin A4 phosphate has primary antineoplastic activity against human anaplastic thyroid carcinoma cell lines and xenograft tumors. Thyroid. 2002;12(12):1063–70.

108. Nelkin BD, Ball DW. Combretastatin A-4 and doxorubicin combination treatment is effective in a preclinical model of human medullary thyroid carcinoma. Oncol Rep. 2001;8(1):157–60.

109. Yeung S-CJ, She M, Yang H, Pan J, Sun L, Chaplin D. Combination chemotherapy including combretastatin A4 phosphate and paclitaxel is effective against anaplastic thyroid cancer in a nude mouse xenograft model. J Clin Endocrinol Metab. 2007; 92(8):2902–9.

110. Mooney CJ, Nagaiah G, Fu P, et al. A phase II trial of fosbretabulin in advanced anaplastic thyroid carcinoma and correlation of baseline serum-soluble intracellular adhesion molecule-1 with outcome. Thyroid. 2009;19(3):233–40.

111. Pacini F. Where do we stand with targeted therapy of refractory thyroid cancer? – Utility of RECIST criteria. Thyroid. 2008;18(3):279–80.

112. Torino F, Corsello SM, Longo R, Barnabei A, Gasparini G. Hypothyroidism related to tyrosine kinase inhibitors: an emerging toxic effect of targeted therapy. Nat Rev Clin Oncol. 2009;6(4):219–28.

113. Illouz F, Laboureau-Soares S, Dubois S, Rohmer V, Rodien P. Tyrosine kinase inhibitors and modifications of thyroid function tests: a review. Eur J Endocrinol. 2009;160(3):331–6.

Index

G.D. Braunstein (ed.), *Thyroid Cancer*, Endocrine Updates 30,
DOI 10.1007/978-1-4614-0875-8, © Springer Science+Business Media, LLC 2012